AF564798

Livestock
Health and Management

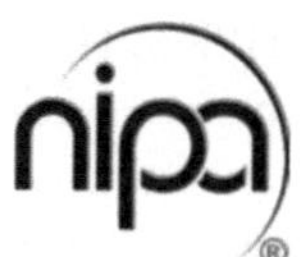

NIPA GENX ELECTRONIC RESOURCES & SOLUTIONS P. LTD.
New Delhi-110 034

About the Editors

Dr. Sudesh Radotra (born in 1963) joined Agricultural Research Services in 1991 the examination conducted by Agricultural Scientists Recruitment Board, New Delhi. After completion of training at the Academy of Agricultural Research Management Hyderabad, he joined ICAR- at Indian Grassland & Fodder Research Institute, Jhansi as Scientist Livestock Production & Management in 1992. He got posted at the Regional Research Centre of Indian Grassland & Fodder Research Institute (IGFRI) at Palampur (Himachal Pradesh) in 1996 where he served as Scientist In-charge from 2008- 2019. He did his Ph.D. in Animal Nutrition from CSK HPKV, Palampur. Presently, he is working as Principal Scientist at ICAR-Indian Veterinary Research Institute (IVRI) Regional Station, Palampur. He has a research experience of 25 years in fodder production, grassland management, pasture productivity, conservation, animal productivity, and rehabilitation of degraded grasslands in Western Himalaya. He has completed a number of institutes and externally funded projects and has published many research papers in peer reviewed National and International Journals. He has organised conferences and has presented research papers at National and International Conferences. He had served as Chairman/Co-chairman in many national and international conferences/ symposia. He has been awarded with seven best research paper/poster awards, fellow Range Management Society of India (RMSI) award, and fellow Indian Society of Agricultural Biochemistry (ISAB) award. He had been a National consultant for "Regional study on the adequacy of National Policies and Institutions for Rangeland Management in the Hindu Kush Himalaya at Kathmandu, Nepal. He provided Consultancy services as grassland/ pasture management expert in Himachal Pradesh Forest Ecosystem Climate Proofing Project. He served as an executive member of Animal Nutrition Association, ICAR-IVRI, Izatnagar, Bareilly (UP) and the Indian Society for Sheep and Goat Production and Utilization, ICAR- Central Sheep & Wool Research Institute, Avikanagar (Rajasthan). He was a Member/Expert for a project for nomads on fodder and nutrient management for Pashmina goats in Ladakh (UT) Department of Animal Husbandry, Dairying & Fisheries. Govt. of India, New Delhi. He was a member Scientific Advisory Committee of KVK, Kangra CSKHPKV, HP and KVK Samba SKUAST, Jammu J&K (UT). He is a life member of five National Profession Societies like The Indian Society of Animal Production and Management, Indian Society of Sheep and Goat Production and Management, Animal Nutrition Association, Indian Society of Agricultural Biochemists and Indian Academy of Veterinary Nutrition and Animal welfare.

Dr. Vijay Kumar Sharma, (born in 1957), joined Rajasthan Co-operative Dairy Federation Ltd. Jaipur as Animal Nutrition Officer in the year 1983 after completing his Ph.D., Dairying (Animal Nutrition) from National Dairy Research Institute, Karnal. Thereafter he joined CSKHP Agriculture University, College of Veterinary & Animal Sciences, Palampur in the year 1992 as a Sr. Scientist and attained the post of Head of Division in 2006 and served there till his retirement in 2017. He has about 44 research publications in his credit in the national and international journals besides having published 23 books and monographs and 21 book chapters. He has handled 14 internal and external funded research projects of National and International levels. He has been awarded 8 best paper awards besides Sr. Scientist Award by International Seabuckthorn Society, China for pursuit of research and teaching works. He has organised 10 conferences and has presented 58 research papers in National and 19 papers in International Conferences. He has been bestowed with number of times the responsibilities as Secretary, Rapporteur, Co-Chairman and Chairman in the Technical sessions of the conferences. He is a member of about 18 scientific societies besides an Editorial Member of 2 Research Journals. Editorial boards. He has delivered many radio and TV talks. He has visited Germany, Russia, China and Thailand for the pursuit of scientific knowledge. He has provided number of times the consultancy services to Dairy Farmers and Entrepreneurs in the field of Dairy development and animal nutrition.

Dr. Arun Kumar Sharma (Born in 1973) did his BVSc & AH, MVSc (Animal Nutrition) and Ph.D. (Animal Nutrition) from CSK Himachal Pradesh Krishi Vishvavidyalaya (CSKHPKV), Palampur (HP). He worked as a Junior Research fellow in Angora Rabbit Project at Veterinary College, CSKHPKV Palampur. He also worked as Veterinary Officer in state Animal Husbandry Department Himachal Pradesh. He joined in Animal Nutrition Department, CSKHPKV, Palampur in the year 2004 as Assistant Professor on deputation and was assigned duty of metabolic stall and feed unit apart from teaching, research and extension work. During his tenure as Incharge feed unit about forty different types of feeds were formulated for various livestock species and sold to Govt. agencies as well as to farmers of state and the turnover of feed plant increased to about nine crores per annum during this period. Thereafter, he joined as Senior Veterinary Officer at Animal Husbandry department HP. He was again deputed in Animal Nutrition Department in Veterinary College CSKHPKV Palampur and was assigned duties of teaching, research and extension apart from being given duties as Incharge of feed unit. Dr. Arun Sharma has attended number of national and international trainings and has also worked as visiting faculty at Kansas State Agriculture University, Kansas, USA. He worked on an extrusion programme and formulated feed for number of animal species through an extrusion process. He has also gone training of satellite remote sensing at National remote sensing institute in Hyderabad. He has authored and co-authored a number of research and review articles of national and international journals. He has written number of articles for farmers apart from writing books for farmers of state on Animal Husbandry related articles. He is also chief associate editor of international e- magazine. He has attended and presented his research in many national and an international conferences. He is consultant to number of NGOs and private as well as governmental agencies. He is a also deputed in Vice-Chancellor Technical cell office as a technical member in VC Secretariat. He is operating a revolving fund project in which not only production of feed is going but a number of research projects of PG as well as UG students are being undertaken. He is life member of many societies.

Dr. Daisy Wadhwa (born in 1964) joined as Assistant Professor in CSK Himachal Pradesh Agricultural University, Palampur in 2000. She did her Ph.D. in Animal Nutrition from University of Wales, Abrystwyth, U.K. Presently, she is working as Professor, in the Department of Animal Nutrition with an additional charge of Head, Department of Fisheries. She has a research experience of 28 years in the field of Animal Nutrition, with a special interest in feed formulation, alternate feed resources, fruit and vegetable industry byproducts, phytoadditives and treats for dogs. She has completed a number of externally funded research projects on the use of phytoadditives and fruit pomaces in animal feeding and has published many research papers and review articles in peer-reviewed National and International Journals, chapters in books, practical manuals of Animal Nutrition, besides presenting a large number of research articles and invited lectures in national and international societies. She has guided nine M.V.Sc. and one Ph.D. students and presently, three P.G. students are working with her. She had served as Chairman/ Co-chairman in many National and International Conferences/Symposia. She has been awarded with seven best research paper presentations, and one best review article. She provided consultancy services especially on feed formulation for dairy cattle and breeding bulls of Department of Animal Husbandry, Himachal Pradesh, consultancies to dog squads of BSF as well as various dog owners. She has also provided consultancies especially on clinical nutrition of dogs, presented in veterinary clinics. She is a life member of Professional Societies like Animal Nutrition Association, Indian Academy of Veterinary Nutrition and Animal welfare and the Himachal Veterinary council. Her Work on muzzle gland secretion, under a four-year ICAR research project found a place in the 4th edition (2010) of the book 'Mineral Nutrition of Livestock' by N.F. Suttle, Published by CAB INTERNATIONAL, Oxford Shire. Under this project, a diagnostic test was developed to detect sodium deficiency in large ruminants which was published in American Journal of Veterinary Research vol. 60:1074-1081, 1999.

Dr. Devi Gopinath (born in 1986) BVSc &AH, MVSc (Veterinary Medicine), Ph.D. (Veterinary Medicine) is posted as a Scientist at ICAR-Indian Veterinary Research Institute, Regional Station, Palampur (H.P.). After completing her BVSc & AH from Kerala Agricultural University, she was awarded prestigious ICAR-JRF for pursuing the masters from Indian Veterinary Research Institute, Bareilly. After that she completed Ph.D. from IVRI, Bareilly itself with ICAR-SRF fellowship. At the same time she was awarded DST-INSPIRE fellowship for her Doctoral studies. During Ph.D. program, she cleared ICAR-NET two times and got selected in ARS-2015. She is an expert in deficiency diseases of ruminants, canine diabetes and their amelioration through herbal extracts and small ruminant ectoparasitism. She has authored and co-authored a number of research and review articles of national and international high-impact journals. She has attended and presented her research in many national and international conferences. She is life member of Indian Society of Veterinary Medicine from 2012 onwards. She has reviewed manuscripts of many national and international journals and Naunyn-Schmiedeberg's Archives of Pharmacology (NAAS: 8.05) is one among them. She is member of health advisory committee of Dhauladhar Nature Park, Himachal Pradesh. Currently, her area of research is region specific animal diseases of North Western Himalayan Region with special emphasis on ectoparasitism and vector transmitted haemoprotozoan and rickettsial diseases of ruminants.

Dr. Gauri Jairath (born in 1987) B.V.Sc. & A.H. (Gold medallist), M.V.Sc. and Ph.D. in Livestock Products Technology is posted as a scientist at ICAR-Indian Veterinary Research Institute, Regional Station, Palampur (H.P.). She joined ICAR in 2016 and during training at NARM, Hyderabad, was awarded with Best Trainee Award. She has expertise in meat science and nutritional interventions for enhancing meat quality and has authored many research papers, review articles, popular articles, hindi booklet and book chapters in national and international journals and reputed magazines. She was awarded with DST INSPIRE fellowship for pursuing Ph.D. She has been awarded two times with Young Scientist Award by The Indian Society for Sheep and Goat Production and Utilization and Indian Association of Women Veterinarian in 2017. She is an editorial board member of Journal of Veterinary and Marine Sciences. She is a an Executive member of the Indian Meat Science Association. She is a reviewer of many national and international high impacted journals. She has presented research papers in five international and more than 10 national conferences and has been awarded with oral and poster awards and has also delivered a TV talk in Door Dharshan, Hisar in Kisan Programme. She is a life member of Indian Meat Science Association, Indian Association of Women Veterinarian, Indian Association of Veterinary Public Health Specialists and The Indian Society for Sheep and Goat Production.

Livestock Health and Management

Sudesh Radotra
Principal Scientist
ICAR-Indian Veterinary Research Institute
Regional Station, Palampur-176 061, Himachal Pradesh

VK Sharma
Retired Professor Animal Nutrition
Village Aima, Bhardwaj Colony, Palampur-176061, Himachal Pradesh

Arun Sharma
Assistant Professor
College of Veterinary and Animal Sciences
CSK Himachal Pradesh Agricultural University
Palampur-176062, Himachal Pradesh

Daisy Wadhwa
Professor
College of Veterinary and Animal Sciences
CSK Himachal Pradesh Agricultural University
Palampur-176062, Himachal Pradesh

Devi Gopinath
Scientist
ICAR-Indian Veterinary Research Institute
Regional Station, Palampur-176 061, Himachal Pradesh

Gauri Jairath
Scientist
ICAR-Indian Veterinary Research Institute
Regional Station, Palampur-176 061, Himachal Pradesh

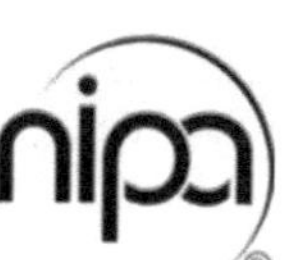

NIPA GENX ELECTRONIC RESOURCES & SOLUTIONS P. LTD.
New Delhi-110 034

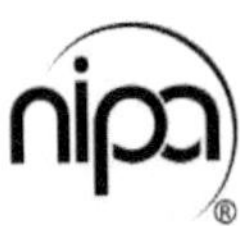

NIPA GENX ELECTRONIC RESOURCES & SOLUTIONS P. LTD.

101,103, Vikas Surya Plaza, CU Block
L.S.C.Market, Pitam Pura, New Delhi-110 034
Ph : +91 11 27341616, 27341717, 27341718
E-mail:newindiapublishingagency@gmail.com
www: www.nipabooks.com

For customer assistance, please contact
Phone: + 91-11-27 34 17 17 Fax: + 91-11- 27 34 16 16
E-Mail: feedbacks@nipabooks.com

ISBN: 978-93-90591-23-7

Composed and Designed by NIPA.

Dedicated to

All those who work for the cause of Animal Welfare and Nutritional Security

Preface

Animals and animal products have been a part of the human environment and heritage since prehistoric times. Animals provide a unique source of foods that have a high nutrient density and palatability. Animals are produced and utilized (for companionship, power, food) in all societies and geographic locations. The contribution of agriculture sector in the Indian economy is steadily declining, the livestock sector contributes significantly to the overall economy of the people in rural India. With the increase in human population, growing income and awareness of the importance of animal food as an integral component of a balanced diet, the demand for milk, meat, egg and fish is speculated to grow continuously at higher pace. Livestock production faces challenges in the form of optimum productivity and animal health vulnerability which adversely impact economics of animal production, public health and animal health welfare as well. The livestock sector is also a main source of family income and more than proportionally controlled by the poor. This book considers the present and future role of farm animals in sustainable agriculture or planet husbandry. It considers animal production, health and welfare, food safety the science of sustainable development climate change and economics of rearing farm animals to provide us food and other benefits.

The authors were encouraged to limit the prose to the extent necessary to facilitate use of the tabular information. The editors express their gratitude to several scientists, teachers especially to the organizations to they belong to.

Present publication is a compilation of the chapters contributed by different authors and invited papers presented as a part of the 3rd National Conference of Indian Academy of Veterinary Nutrition and welfare at CSK Himachal Pradesh Krishi Vishawvidyalaya of Himachal Pradesh.

We hope that present publication will serve its purpose as a reference book for teachers, scientists, students and industry personnel working in the area of animal production and in general animal health management and crop mixed farming for nutritional security.

Editors

Acknowledgements

The editors are greatly indebted to the scientists, authors and the institutions working on livestock crop mixed farming whose knowledge and work have been referred to and incorporated in the text of this book.

The editors also would like to acknowledge the contribution made by Indian Council of Agricultural Research, New Delhi and National Bank for Agriculture and Rural Development, Mumbai for funding to organize the 3rd National Conference of Indian Academy of Veterinary Nutrition and welfare at CSK Himachal Pradesh Krishi Vishvavidyalaya of Himachal Pradesh.

We sincerely thank Dr. Rinku Sharma and other colleagues who have assisted in preparing and improving the quality of the manuscript.

The editors would like to sincerely thank M/S NIPA Genx Electronic Resources & Solutions P. Ltd. for handling the manuscript expeditiously and giving the manuscript the present outlook.

Contents

List of Colour Plates

List of Colour Plates

Chapter 12: Freshwater Fish Transgenics: Implications and Issues

Chapter 21: Toxicological Study of Important Plants of North-Western Himalayan Region of India

1

Role of Livestock in Ensuring Food and Nutritional Security in India

A. K. Verma

Centre of Advanced Faculty Training in Animal Nutrition, Animal Nutrition Division ICAR-Indian Veterinary Research Institute, Izatnagar-243122

R. K. Mohanta

Subject Matter Specialist (Animal Science), Agriculture Science Centre National Rice Research Institute, Cuttack-753006, Odisha

Introduction

Food security is defined as "*a situation that exists when all people, at all times, have physical, social and economic access to sufficient, safe and nutritious food that meets their dietary needs and food preferences for an active and healthy life*" (The State of Food Insecurity, 2001) (see http://www.who.int/trade/glossary/story028/en/). As of 2015, the concept of food security has mostly focused on food calories rather than the quality and nutrition of food. Thus, food security usually emphasizes food quantity and therefore "nutrition security" is used for the quality dimension. The concept of food security has four dimensions: availability, accessibility, utilization and vulnerability. The interactions among them determine how food secure a country is or how adequate, steady and risk-free food consumption is at the household and individual levels (Kumar and Ayyappan, 2014). Though substantial progress has been achieved in reducing food insecurity, maintaining food security at the national and household level is a major challenge for India (Singh, 2014). The present article briefs about global and Indian scenarios on food security aspects, and the key role of livestock in achieving zero hunger by means of livestock-derived foods such as milk, egg and meat products.

The Global Challenge

Hunger and malnutrition pose more risk to global health; killing more people than AIDS, malaria, and tuberculosis combined. The increased population trend will further put pressure on food productivity, more particularly in the developing and underdeveloped countries and 50–70% increment will be needed by 2050 to feed the additional two billion people (Ingram *et al.*, 2010; Singh, 2014). About a billion of the world's population regularly goes to bed hungry and around two billion suffer from "hidden hunger," surviving on diets that fail to me*et al*l their nutritional needs, whereas 1.5 billion people suffer the effects of overconsumption (McMichael *et al.*, 2007).

Although the number and proportions of people living in the developing world who are undernourished are declining, it appears unlikely that this will be sufficient to meet the Millennium Development Goal of reducing by one-half the percentage of people suffering from chronic hunger by 2015 (FAO, 2012). Shockingly, therefore, at the start of the 21st century, most of the earth's inhabitants have suboptimal diets and more shockingly in India (Singh, 2014). Although poverty, food, and nutrition insecurity are intrinsically linked, these problems are not confined to poor countries; today 14% of U.S. citizens are classified as food insecure (Coleman-Jensen *et al.*, 2015). In a food secure nation, South Africa, is, 14.8% of the people in the sample were food secure, 5.8% were mildly food insecure, 26.4% were moderately food insecure and 53.1% were severely food insecure (De Cock *et al.*, 2013) and depended upon human capital (education, household size and dependency ratio), household income and location, while food production and access to land do not appear to be determinants of food security.

Indian Scenario

Farm families constitute the majority of India's population. A majority of small and marginal farm families as well as landless labourers suffer from undernutrition, because of inadequate income. Thus, we have to deal with three kinds of hunger if we are to achieve food and nutrition security for all. First, we have to help farm families overcome undernutrition as a result of deficiency in calories. Second, protein hunger is becoming serious due to the inadequate consumption of pulses and milk (in the case of vegetarians) and eggs, fish and meat (in the case of non-vegetarians). Third, there is widespread hidden hunger caused by the deficiency of micronutrients like iron, iodine, zinc, vitamin A, vitamin B_{12}, *etc.* in the diet (Das *et al.*, 2014). India is home to one-third of the world's undernourished children, one-third of its women are underweight, almost half of the children are stunted and 40% are underweight (Joshi *et al.*, 2011). This explains the severity of food and nutritional insecurity, which forced the Government of India to enact the National Food Security Act (NFSA), in September 2013 to ensure food security in India. Though India has achieved self sufficiency in food grains production, the production varies across regions and food insecurity arises due to the insufficient storage capacities and inefficient distribution and delivery systems to reach the people in need. However, the per capita production of food grains and availability of cereals hovered around 200 kg per annum and varied from 181–188 kg per annum (1983–2012), respectively. The increase in production and per capita availability has been much higher for horticulture, fish and livestock products compared to food grains. However, the consumption pattern of calories and proteins in rural and urban populations depicts a puzzling trend (Kumar and Ayyappan, 2014). Based on the data from NSSO, they reported that the per capita calorie intake and protein consumption for rural population declined from 2,240 kcal per day and 63.5 g per day in 1983 to 2,165 kcal per day and 58.5 g per day in 2011–2012. In urban areas, the per capita calorie intake increased slightly from 2,070 kcal in 1983 to 2,140 in 2011–2012 whereas the intake of proteins marginally declined from 58.1 to 57.4 g per day (Kumar and Ayyappan, 2014). They further reported that the level of calorie, protein and fat consumption for poor households is much below the norm and that too considerably lower in poor households than that in the rich households. One-fourth of the rural population and one-eighth of the urban population were undernourished in 2011–2012. Poverty and under-nutrition are highly correlated. The nutrition deficiency is mostly concentrated in poor households. 54% of the poor households were deficient in energy and 61.3% in protein intake in 2011–2012(Kumar and Ayyappan, 2014). This indicates only the gross indicators, the realistic values in terms of quantity and quality of nutrients are alarming. In the present days, there is a shift in demand for animal protein, particularly for their rich nutrient status.

Livestock for food security

The contributions made to the diets of the world's seven billion people by cattle, sheep, goats, pigs, chickens, and a dozen or so lesser-known, but locally important species (such as guinea fowl, yaks, and camels) are complex and multidimensional. They include direct and indirect impacts, which can be either beneficial or harmful to the overall food supply and food and nutrition security. Livestock plays a significant role in ensuring livelihood to millions of people in India. It contributed 537535 crores to Indian economy (4.11% of total GDP) out of 1828905 crores that come from agriculture and allied sectors (27.25%) in 2012-13 (Basic Animal Husbandry and Fisheries Statistics, 2014). Milk, meat (poultry, mutton, beef, pork) and eggs constitute the lions share, thereby indicating their role in national economy and food security. They also provide income and employment for producers and other working families; thereby proving as a crucial asset and safety net for the poor, especially for women and pastoralist groups. Further, they provide an important source of nourishment for billions of people irrespective of their food choice (Boogaard and Moyo, 2015). Livestock contributes to food supply by converting low-value materials, inedible or unpalatable for people, into milk, meat, and eggs (Devendra and Leng, 2011; Ertl *et al.*, 2015). Livestock directly contributes to nutrition security. Milk, meat, and eggs, the "animal-source foods," though expensive sources of energy, are one of the best sources of high quality protein and micronutrients that are essential for normal development and good health (FAO, 2012; Herrero *et al.*, 2013). But poor people tend to sell rather than consume the animal-source foods that they produce. The contribution of livestock to food, distinguished from nutrition security among the poor, is mostly indirect: sales of animals or produce, demand for which is rapidly growing, can provide cash for the purchase of staple foods, and provision of manure, draft power, and income for purchase of farm inputs can boost sustainable crop production in mixed crop-livestock systems (FAO, 2011a). Livestock has the potential to be transformative: by enhancing food and nutrition security, and providing income to pay for education and other needs, livestock can enable poor children to develop into healthy, well-educated, productive adults. The challenge is how to manage complex trade-offs to enable livestock's positive impacts to be realized while minimizing and mitigating negative ones, including threats to the health of people and the environment (FAO, 2011a, 2012).

Impact on Food Supply

Milk, meat, and eggs currently provide around 13% of the energy and 28% of the protein consumed globally; in developed countries, this rises to 20 and 48% for energy and protein, respectively (FAO, 2009). The livestock occurs in three main types of production systems: confined intensive, mixed crop–livestock, and open grazing systems (Herrero *et al.*, 2009, 2013). Estimates, based on data for 2001 to 2003, suggest that grazing systems supply 9% of the world's meat and 12% of milk; mixed crop–livestock systems contribute 46% of meat, 88% of milk, and 50% of cereals; while intensive systems provide 45% of meat (Steinfeld *et al.*, 2006). By consuming feedstuffs that people could consume directly, such as grains and legumes, animals reduce the total amount of food available. Today, about half the world's production of grain is fed to animals, especially monogastrics (IAASTD, 2009), and 77 million tonnes of plant protein are fed to livestock to produce 58 million tonnes of animal protein (Steinfeld *et al.*, 2006), contributing 13% of the energy to the world's diet. Feed crops occupy an estimated one-half a billion hectares of land (Steinfeld *et al.*, 2010). In 2011, almost 70% of the 900 million metric tons of global compounded feed went to monogastrics; it is projected that the world will require a billion extra tonnes of grain to satisfy future food, feed, and fuel demands (IAASTD, 2009), which may be possible, but there are questions about the cropland that would be required, and thus there are real potentials to exploit synergies in mixed crop–livestock systems. Animal source foods are much more than an expensive and inefficient source of energy. But the animals convert low-biological-value protein foods that are less palatable and less nutrient-dense to high-biological-value foods that are highly palatable and nutrient dense (Caper, 2013).

Direct Contributions of Livestock to Nutrition Security

Poor people survive largely on diets based on starchy foods like cereals that fail to me*et* all their nutritional needs. The more people earn, the higher their consumption of nutrient-rich animal-source food. Consumption of meat and milk, driven by population increase, urbanization and rising incomes in developing countries, is forecast to increase faster than that for any crop product (IAASTD, 2009; Singh, 2014). With a growing middle class and a population growth rate of 1.3 percent per year, India has a growing demand for protein. For vegetarians that is met by pulses and oilseed crops. For non-vegetarians that includes poultry where production is growing about 10 percent a year. Per capita consumption of protein is still low compared to most developed countries and many developing ones (BAHS, 2014; Singh, 2014).

Milk: Milk is one of the best nutritious foods available to mankind. India's bovine herd continues to grow in response to strong demand for dairy products combined stocks estimated at 323.74 million head. India produces about 17 percent of the annual global milk output, 132.4 MMT of fluid milk, about 299 milliliters of milk per day per person (BAHS, 2014). However, the per capita availability of milk in India, the world's largest milk producer, is slightly more than the world average (FAOSTAT, 2015).

Meat: Broiler meat production was 3.6 million tons in 2014 (6% increase over 2013), fueled by escalating demand for animal protein and a rising preference for processed poultry products. India's per capita consumption of poultry meat is only 2.2 kg per annum in 2014; chicken is India's preferred non-vegetarian protein source (45% of meat). Buffalo, goat, pig, sheep and cattle contribute 19%, 16%, 8%, 7% and 5% of the production of meat, respectively. Poultry per capita consumption in 2014 is up 16% from 2010 while total consumption increased 23% for the same time period, due to a growing population (BAHS, 2014). Major drivers of consumption are: an expanding middle class, increasing employment levels and incomes, new demand for ready-to-eat products and the growing presence of affordable quick-service restaurants, and a general preference for poultry meat over other meats due to low prices and cultural and religious non-preferences for pork and beef. Among non-vegetarians, poultry, fish and mutton are the preferred meats, with poultry most likely to grow in demand as incomes increase. As dietary practices in India tend to prefer vegetarian and dairy-based sources are preferred protein sources, even among non-vegetarian consumers, it is unlikely that per capita consumption of meat and eggs will grow to levels seen in other countries. Though laws in India prohibit the slaughter of cattle for religious reasons, but slaughter is allowed for buffalo bulls and unproductive heifers. Much of India's beef (2.0 MMT) is from buffalo and increased demand for milk has led to a larger beef supply. In 2013, buffalo meat exports are forecasted at 2.15 million tons on a carcass weight equivalent basis, whereas Indian per capita consumption remains at 2 kilograms per person, reflecting a preference for pulses, dairy, and poultry (India Livestock and Products Annual, 2012).

Egg: Egg protein is one of the best protein sources available based on the composition of amino acids and their bioavailability (Iannotti *et al.*, 2014). India is one of the world's top producers of hen eggs, ranking 3rd behind China and the U.S. in 2011 (FAOSTAT, 2015). Egg production was 69,731 million eggs in 2012-13 (March-February), and the per capita availability of eggs has increased to 58 eggs per annum. However, Andhra Pradesh (33%) and Tamil Nadu (18%) produced the most number of eggs and there was variation in consumption pattern among different states. Animal-sourced foods are nutritionally dense sources of energy, protein, and various essential micronutrients and match particularly well with the nutrients needed by people to support normal development, physiological functioning, and overall good health. In contrast, plant based diets tend to be deficient in one or more essential amino acids, especially lysine, methionine, and threonine (Young and Pellett, 1994). Micronutrients (including iron, zinc, vitamin A, and calcium) also tend to be more bio-available in animal-source foods, and some, such as vitamin B_{12}, are found naturally only in animal-source foods (Naveena and Kiran, 2014). Animal-source foods provide several micronutrients simultaneously, which can be important in diets lacking more than one nutrient (Allen, 2005). Protein-energy malnutrition, iron-deficiency anemia, and vitamin A deficiency, all of which can be prevented if sufficient animal-source foods are included in the diet, have big impacts: these three diseases result in 17.4 million, 15.6 million, and 0.6 million disability-adjusted life years, respectively (WHO, 2009). Consumption of even small amounts of animal-source foods has been shown to contribute substantially to ensuring dietary adequacy, preventing under-nutrition and nutritional deficiencies (Neumann *et al.*, 2002; Naveena and Kiran, 2014), and having positive impacts on growth, cognitive function, and physical activity of children; better pregnancy outcomes; and reduced morbidity from illness (Neumann *et al.*, 2002; Sadler *et al.*, 2012). Micronutrients from animal-sourced foods may develop more competent immune systems and elicit better immune responses (Keusch and Farthing, 1986). With close to one billion of the world's poorest people relying on livestock for their livelihoods (FAO, 2012), it is tempting to assume that livestock-keeping households consume the animal-source foods they produce and that increasing productivity of livestock would impact positively on household nutrition (Boogaard and Moyo, 2015).

Indirect Effects of Livestock on Food Security

By generating cash incomes from the sales of animals, their products, or services, or through employment along animal-source food value chains, livestock in poor countries contribute to food security by providing income that can be used to purchase staple food (Boogaard and Moyo, 2015). It is estimated that livestock production and marketing are currently essential to the livelihoods of more than one billion people in Africa and Asia: one-seventh of humanity. Herrero *et al.*, (2013) found that dairy supports 124 million people in South Asia and 24 million in East Africa. The contribution of livestock to household income ranges widely, from 2% to more than 33% in a number of developing countries (Pica-Ciamarra *et al.*, 2011; Hermansen *et al.*, 2013). The massive increase in demand for livestock products witnessed over the past few decades has created equally significant opportunities for smallholder livestock keepers, but their distribution and demand vary from region to region (Herrero *et al.*, 2010). So for example, in urbanized economies, there may be less opportunities for smallholder provision of livestock commodities; but this also varies, with smallholders being far more competitive, for example, in the dairy sector, but far less likely to prosper for monogastric production (Tarawali *et al.*, 2011). In addition to directly providing cash-generating opportunities for livestock keepers, farm animals also create significant numbers of jobs and small business opportunities, many of them in rural areas where other income opportunities are limited. Livestock value chains represent a large and growing employment sector. They include farm-level production, input, and service industries to farmers; transportation of livestock and their products; and processing and marketing (Capper, 2013; McDermott *et al.*, 2013; Nampanya *et al.*, 2015).

Livestock and Agriculture

In mixed crop–livestock systems that produce 50% of cereals (Herrero *et al.*, 2010), livestock provides manure, contributes to land preparation, and provide ready cash to buy planting materials or fertilizer or to hire labor for planting, weeding, or harvesting. Livestock contributions can thus increase the area of land cultivated, the yields and productivity achieved, the feed produced from crop residues, and, through enhanced nutrient recycling, the sustainability of those farming systems (Yigrem *et al.*, 2015). Globally livestock manure supplies up to 12% of gross nitrogen input for cropping and up to 23% in mixed crop–livestock systems in developing countries (Liu *et al.*, 2010). Application of manure also improves the efficiency of inorganic fertilizers (Tittonell *et al.*, 2008). Use of manure is, however, influenced by economics, logistics, and regulations (FAO, 2011a), and there may be competition with other demands, such as for fuel. In contrast, in intensified, industrial livestock systems, where crop and livestock production enterprises are geographically separated, manure can become more of a liability than an asset (Gerber *et al.*, 2005). In many regions of rural India, draft power continues to contribute significantly to food production, but the number of draft animals is decreasing due to use of agriculture machineries (FAO, 2011a). In most of the mixed crop–livestock systems, the animal feed consists of mainly crop residues (Pattanaik *et al.*, 2010; Devendra and Leng, 2011). This enables animal source foods to be produced without competing with people for food. It is however debated whether to use crop residues as animal feed to get manure or directly use of crop residues as sources of organic matter to improve soils (Valbuena *et al.*, 2012). There is also an opportunity to develop food-feed crops (crops that can produce more and better quality crop residues as well as grain) (Pattanaik *et al.*, 2010; Capper, 2011; Capper and Bauman, 2013). Livestock is often the most important asset in poor rural households. They allow poor households to invest in land or small businesses, diversify their incomes, and become less poor and vulnerable, all of which enhance food and nutritional security (Ellis and Freeman, 2004; Yigrem *et al.*, 2015). Livestock can also provide a buffer in times when harvests fail or other disasters strike, thus smoothing out food availability. In many societies, poultry and small ruminants are often owned by women, who may also control any income obtained from their sale; this is more likely to be spent on their children or family's nutrition than if this income is controlled by men (Tangka *et al.*, 1999). Recent results show that improving women's access to inputs and services has the potential to reduce the number of malnourished people in the world by 100 to 150 million (FAO, 2011b).

Zoonotic Diseases and Food Safety

Livestock can also impact food security by transmitting diseases to people via vectors such as biting flies and through contaminated animal-source foods; these diseases limit productivity of people by reducing their ability to produce food themselves or to work to earn income to purchase food. With 13 major zoonotic diseases causing some 2.2 million deaths a year, mostly among poor and middle-income populations (Grace *et al.*, 2012b), the harm livestock cause to the nutrition and health of people is significant. There is need of strengthening the collaborations between veterinary and public health researchers and officials as well as imaginative new institutional arrangements for implementing risk-based assessments and practical solutions to human health threats from livestock (Randolph *et al.*, 2007).

Overconsumption of Animal-Sourced Foods

Overconsumption of animal-sourced foods can harm human health and well-being, impacting whole societies as well as individual households. Overconsumption of fatty red meats and hard cheeses, which have increased concentrations of saturated fats, can lead to cardiovascular disease, while overconsumption of processed meats, such as bacon and ham, has been associated with some cancers (Larsson and Wolk, 2012). Increased consumption of energy-dense meat, milk, and eggs also contributes to the global obesity epidemic leading to further complications (Tilman and Clark, 2014).

Livestock and Climate Change

Livestock plays a significant role in rural livelihoods and the economies of developing countries. In the long run, livestock production can impact negatively on food security through production of greenhouse gases (GHGs) that contribute to climate change. In tropical regions, climate change is expected to result in significant yield reductions, although in temperate regions, the impacts might be beneficial in places (Nelson *et al.*, 2009). Livestock contributes about 8.5 to 18% of CO_2 equivalents to anthropogenic climate change through carbon dioxide itself, mainly due to land use changes; methane emissions through enteric fermentation by ruminants; and nitrous oxide emissions, mostly from manure-handling practices (O'Mara, 2011). These emissions might be increased in the coming decades and in response; there will be increased pressure to increase efficiency of livestock production: more milk, meat, and eggs with fewer inputs and decreased GHG emissions per unit of production (Herrero *et al.*, 2013). Shifting to fewer, more productive animals of more productive breeds is one way to do this although doing so would require enhanced access to breeding, animal health and feed services, and inputs to keep these less hardy animals alive and productive (Tarawali *et al.*, 2011). Such an approach has "triple-win solutions", with synergies among productivity gains, environmental conservation, and poverty alleviation (Moran and Wall, 2011).

Schemes Facilitating the Livestock Sector

At present, the dairy industry's growth is led by strong consumer demand for milk protein, producers' interest in expanding production and government programs to increase the efficiency of milk production. The Ministry of Agriculture works with other agencies to set standards and issue sanitary permits for production and processing, provides assistance to farmer cooperatives and manages the Intensive

Dairy Development Program to increase milk production by 6 MMT per year over the next 15 years. Private sector investment has led to notable improvements in dairy management practices, including extension services, veterinary care, and improved genetics. A major pillar of the Government of India (GOI)'s livestock development strategy has been the subsidized public delivery of veterinary services. To improve the quality of these services, the Ministry of Agriculture's Department of Animal Husbandry, Dairying and Fisheries is implementing the Livestock Health and Disease Control program on a nation-wide basis, which aims to improve the diagnosis of a series of common diseases as said to be needed by Kaasschieter *et al.*, (1992). The National Dairy Development Board (NDDB), in partnership with the GOI and the World Bank, has developed a National Dairy Plan (NDP) in order to increase productivity of dairy animals and to provide rural milk producers with greater access to the organized milk-processing sector. The first phase of the plan, NDP 1, has a financial outlay of

416 million dollars (more than 20 billion rupees) and is being carried out between 2012 and 2017. NDP 1 will increase dairy production through improved breeding and feeding practices as well as improved extension and management services. It is also emphasizing on the expansion of India's dairy cooperatives, with development of community marketing systems and a formal, organized dairy economy/sector as a top priority. The Government of India has launched the National Mission for Protein Supplements in 2011-12 for taking up activities to promote animal-based protein production through livestock development, dairy farming, pig farming, goat rearing, and fisheries in selected blocks of the country. Other schemes named 'The Salvaging and Rearing of Male Buffalo Calves Scheme (SRMBC)' and 'The Utilization of Fallen Animals Scheme (UFA)' funded by the National Bank for Agricultural and Rural Development and launched to achieve a growth rate of 10 percent for the meat sector in the 11th Five Year Plan period. The SRMBC promotes the rearing of buffalo bull calves for meat production and develops linkages with export-oriented slaughterhouses. In addition, the GOI had initiated The National Project on Cattle and Buffalo Breeding (NPCBB) project to increase both the number of crossbred animals and in-milk animals (see http://dahd.nic.in/dahd/schemes.aspx).

Future Prospects

The UN Food and Agricultural Organisation (FAO) estimates that the world will have to produce ca. 60% more food by 2050 and we believe that animal protein production will grow even more–meats (poultry/swine/beef) will double, as well as dairy, and fish production will almost triple by 2050. Over the coming decades, population growth, urbanization, and income growth, especially in developing countries, will result in huge increases in demand for milk, meat, and eggs. Meeting that demand will place enormous pressure on the global food system. This has led some authorities to call for a global rebalancing: those who eat too little animal-source foods should eat more; those who eat too much should eat less (McMichael *et al.*, 2007). Making practical and implementable recommendations is a significant challenge (Westhoek *et al.*, 2011). The global livestock industry will have to considerably increase production in order to supply the population with animal-source foods, yet the industry must concurrently improve the three metrics of sustainability–economic viability, environmental stewardship and social responsibility (Erb *et al.*, 2012; Capper, 2013). Improving livestock productivity has positive sustainability implications as it reduces resource use and GHG emissions whilst improving economic viability. Productivity metrics that enhance sustainability include milk and meat yield, growth rates, feed efficiency, calving rate, parasite control and use of growth-enhancing technologies (Capper, 2013; Chagunda *et al.*, 2015; Nampanya *et al.*, 2015). Mixed crop–livestock farming systems currently produce most of the world's meat, milk, and staple crops. Addressing the role of mixed crop–livestock systems in the future, including issues such as efficiency of production as well as the complexities of market engagement, is crucial to address whatever trajectory of change these systems undergo in the coming decades if they are to contribute to food security in a way that is equitable, environmentally sustainable, economically viable (Capper, 2011; Capper and Bauman, 2013), and good for human health. As demand for animal proteins is increasing, Hoffman and Cawthorn (2014) highlighted that in addition to conventional livestock, non-traditional meat animals need to be given importance in areas where they are suitable for achieving global food security. Some of the livestock also decrease food supply by competing with people for food grains, especially grains fed to pigs and poultry. This in turn resulted in an increased grain prices thereby reducing human food security (Erb *et al.*, 2012). This circumstance argues for feeding more forages to livestock, particularly in the tropics where many livestock are reared on small farms. Recently, Rudel *et al.*, (2015) proposed the 'Livestock Plus' approach to help livestock production, where, farmers should intensify in sustainable ways the management of grasses, shrubs, trees, and animals. Effective Livestock Plus approaches take one of two forms: (1) simple improvements such as new forage varieties and animal management practices that spread from farmer to farmer by word of mouth, or (2) complex sets of new practices that integrate forage production more closely into farms' other agricultural activities and agro-ecologies. A recent study found that grass-based dairy production highly contributes to net food production, particularly if the amount of concentrates per kg milk is reduced (Ertl *et al.*, 2015).

References

Allen LH (2005) Multiple micronutrients in pregnancy and lactation: An overview. American Journal of Clinical Nutrition 81:1206S–1212S.

Basic Animal Husbandry and Fisheries Statistics (2014) Basic Animal Husbandry and Fisheries Statistics. Department of Animal Husbandry, Dairying and Fisheries. Ministry of Agriculture, Krishi Bhawan, New Delhi, India.

Boogaard BK and Moyo S (2015) The multi-functionality of goats in rural Mozambique: Contributions to food security and household risk mitigation. ILRI Research Report 37. International Livestock Research Institute, Nairobi, Kenya.

Capper JL (2011) Replacing rose-tinted spectacles with a high-powered microscope: The historical versus modern carbon footprint of animal agriculture. Animal Frontiers 1(1):26–32.

Capper JL (2013) Should we reject animal source foods to save the planet? A review of the sustainability of global livestock production. South African Journal of Animal Science 43(3): 233-246.

Capper JL and Bauman DE (2013) The role of productivity in improving the environmental sustainability of ruminant production systems. Annual Review of Animal Bioscience 1(1): 469-489.

Cawthorn DM and Hoffman LC (2014) The role of traditional and non-traditional meat animals in feeding a growing and evolving world. Animal Frontiers 4(4): 6-12.

Chagunda MG, Mwangwela A, Mumba C, Dos Anjos F, Kawonga BS, Hopkins R and Chiwona-Kartun L (2015) Assessing and managing intensification in smallholder dairy systems for food and nutrition security in Sub-Saharan Africa. Regional Environmental Change 1-11. doi: 10.1007/s12571-013-0247-y

Coleman-Jensen A, Rabbitt M, Gregory C and Singh A (2015) Household food security in the United States, 2014. Economic Research Report No. (ERR-194), USDA Economic Research Service. http://www.ers.usda.gov/publications/err-economic-research-report/err194.aspx (last verified on 16 Oct. 2015).

Das PK, Bhavani RV, Swaminathan MS (2014) A farming system model to leverage agriculture for nutritional outcomes. Agricultural Research 3(3):193-203.

De Cock N, D'Haese M, Vink N, Van Rooyen CJ, Staelens L, Schönfeldt HC, D'Haese L (2013) Food security in rural areas of Limpopo province, South Africa. Food Security 5(2): 269-282.

Devendra C, Leng RA (2011) Feed resources for animals in Asia: issues, strategies for use, intensification and integration for increased productivity. Asian-Australasian Journal of Animal Sciences 24(3): 303-321.

Ellis F, Freeman HA (2004) Rural livelihoods and poverty reduction strategies in four African countries. Journal of Developmental Studies 40(4):1–30.

Erb KH, Mayer A, Kastner T, Sallet KE, Haberl H (2012) The impact of industrial grain fed livestock production on food security: an extended literature review. Alpen Adria University Klagenfurt-Vienna-Graz, Austria.

Ertl P, Klocker H, Hörtenhuber S, Knaus W, Zollitsch W (2015) The net contribution of dairy production to human food supply: The case of Austrian dairy farms. Agricultural Systems 137, 119-125.

FAO (2009) The state of food and agriculture: Livestock in the balance. FAO, Rome. FAO (2011a) World livestock 2011—Livestock in food security. FAO, Rome. FAO (2011b) The fate of food and agriculture: Women in agriculture—Closing the gender gap for development. FAO, Rome.

FAO (2012) Livestock sector development for poverty reduction: An economic and policy perspective—Livestock's many virtues. FAO, Rome.

Gerber P, Chilonda P, Franceschina G, Menzi H (2005) Geographical determinants and environmental implications of livestock production intensification in Asia. Bioresource Technology 96: 263–276.

Grace D, Mutua F, Ochungo P, Kruska R, Jones K, Brierley L, Lapar L, Said M, Herrero M, Phuc P, Thao NB, Akuku I, Ogutu F (2012b) Mapping of poverty and likely zoonoses hotspots. Report to the Department for International Development. International Livestock Research Institute, Nairobi, Kenya.

Grace D, Olowoye J, Dipeol M, Odebode S, Randolph TF (2012a) The influence of gender and group membership on food safety: The case of meat sellers in Bodija market, Ibadan, Nigeria. Tropical Animal Health and Production 44 (1):S53–59.

Hermansen JE, Knudsen MT, Kristensen T (2013) Role of animal products in feeding the planet. In: Energy and protein metabolism and nutrition in sustainable animal production. Wageningen Academic Publishers 35-44.

Herrero M, Grace D, Njuki J, Johnson N, Rufino M (2013) The roles of livestock in developing countries. Animal 7(1): 3-18.

Herrero M, Thornton PK, Notenbaert A, Msangi S, Wood S, Kruska R, Dixon J, Bossio D, van de Steeg J, Freeman HA, Li X, Parthasarathy Rao P (2009) Drivers of change in crop–livestock systems and their impacts on agro-ecosystems services and human well-being to 2030. CGIAR Systemwide Livestock Programme. International Livestock Research Institute, Nairobi, Kenya.

Herrero M, Thornton PK, Notenbaert A, Wood S, Msangi, Kruska R, Freeman HA, Bossio D, Dixon J, Peters M, van de Steeg J, Lynam J, MacMillan S, Gerard B, McDermott J, Seré C, Rosegrant M (2010) Smart investments in sustainable food production: Revisiting mixed crop–livestock systems. Science 327:822–825.

IAASTD (2009) International Assessment of Agricultural Knowledge, Science, and Technology for Development Global Report. Island Press, Washington, DC. Iannotti LL, Lutter CK,

Bunn DA, Stewart CP (2014) Eggs: the uncracked potential for improving maternal and young child nutrition among the world's poor. Nutrition Reviews 72(6): 355-368.

Ingram J, Ericksen P, Liverman D (2010) Food security and global environmental change. Earthscan, London.

Joshi PK, Kadiyala S, Mahendra Dev S (2011) India's economy roars ahead but nutritional improvement is stalled. Global Food Policy Report. International Food Policy Research Institute, Washington DC, USA.

Kaasschieter GA, De Jong R, Schiere JB, Zwart D (1992) Towards a sustainable livestock production in developing countries and the importance of animal health strategy therein. Veterinary Quarterly 14(2): 66-75.

Keusch GT, Farthing MJ (1986) Nutrition and infection. Annual Review of Nutrition 6:131–154.

Kumar A, Ayyappan S (2014) Food security and public distribution system in India Agriculture Research DOI 10.1007/s40003-014-0115-9.

Larsson SC, Wolk A (2012) Red and processed meat consumption and risk of pancreatic cancer: Meta-analysis of prospective studies. British Journal of Cancer 106:603–607. Liu J, You L, Amini M, Obersteiner M, Herrero M, Zehnder AJB, Yang H (2010) A high-resolution assessment of nitrogen flows in cropland. Proceedings of National Academy of Sciences 107: 835–840.

McDermott J, Enahoro D, Herrero M (2013) Livestock futures to 2020: How will they shape food, environmental, health, and global security? Food Security and Sociopolitical Stability 201.

McMichael AJ, Powles JW, Butler CD, Uauy R (2007) Food, livestock production, energy, climate change, and health. Lancet 370:1253–1263.

Moran D, Wall E (2011) Livestock production and greenhouse gas emissions: Defining the problem and specifying solutions. Animal Frontiers 1(1):19–25.

Nampanya S, Khounsy S, Phonvisay A, Bush RD, Windsor PA (2015) Improving smallholder food security through investigations of carcass composition and beef marketing of buffalo and cattle in northern Lao PDR. Tropical Animal Health and Production 47(4): 681-689.

Naveena BM, Kiran M (2014) Buffalo meat quality, composition, and processing characteristics: Contribution to the global economy and nutritional security. Animal Frontiers 4(4), 18-24.

Nelson GC, Rosegrant MW, Koo J, Robertson R, Sulser T, Zhu T, Ringler C, Msangi S, Palazzo A, Batka M, Magalhaes M, Valmonte-Santos R, Ewing M, Lee D (2009) Climate change: Impact on agriculture and costs of adaptation. International Food Policy Research Institute, Washington, DC.

Neumann C, Harris DM, Rogers LM (2002) Contribution of animal source foods in improving diet quality and function in children in the developing world. Nutrition Research 22(1–2):193–220.

O'Mara FP (2011) The significance of livestock as a contributor to global greenhouse gas emissions today and in the near future. Animal Feed Science and Technology 166–167:7–15.

Pattanaik AK, Sharma K, Anandan S, Blummel M (2010) Food-feed crops research: a synthesis. Animal Nutrition and Feed Technology 10S: 1-10.

Pica-Ciamarra U, Tasciotti L, Otte J, Zezza A (2011) Livestock assets, livestock income and rural households. FAO, Rome.

Randolph T, Schelling E, Grace D, Nicholson CF, Leroy JL, Cole DC, Demment MW, Omore A, Zinsstag J, Ruel M (2007) Role of livestock in human nutrition and health for poverty reduction in developing countries. Journal of Animal Science 85:2788– 2800.

Rudel TK, Paul B, White D, Rao IM, Van Der Hoek R, Castro A, Boval M, Lerner A, Schneider L, Peters M (2015) LivestockPlus: Forages, sustainable intensification, and food security in the tropics. Ambio 44(7): 685-693.

Sadler K, Mitchard E, Abdi A, Shiferaw Y, Bekele G, Catley A (2012) Milk matters: The impact of dry season livestock support on milk supply and child nutrition in Somali Region, Ethiopia. Feinstein International Center, Tufts University, and Save the Children Addis Ababa, Ethiopia.

Singh RB (2014) Towards a food secure India and South Asia: making hunger history. Asia Pacific Association of Agricultural Research Institutions (APAARI), Available online at http://www. apaari. org/wp-content/uploads/2009/08/towards-a-food-secure-india making-hunger-history. pdf. DoA, 26.

Smith J, Sones K, Grace D, MacMillan S, Tarawali S, Herrero M (2013) Beyond milk, meat, and eggs: Role of livestock in food and nutrition security. Animal Frontiers 3:6-13.

Tangka FK, Jabbar MA, Shapiro BI (1999) Gender roles and child nutrition in livestock production systems in developing countries: A critical review (No. 27). ILRI.

Wu SH, Ho CT, Nah SL, Chau CF (2014) Global hunger: a challenge to agricultural, food, and nutritional sciences. Critical Reviews in Food Science and Nutrition 54(2):151– 162. Yigrem S, Markemann A, Abebe G, Ogutu JO, Piepho HP, Zárate AV (2015) Assessing the relative importance of dairy products to family nutrition in mixed crop-livestock production systems of Ethiopia. Food Security 7(5): 1003-1015.

2

Integrating Crops and Livestock in Indian Agricultural Systems What is the way forward?

Ashish Kumar and Bakul Rao
CTARA, IIT-Bombay, Mumbai, Maharashtra

Introduction

In the last two decades, there has been a significant change in the Indian society, not only in the terms of economics following the post 1991 reforms but also in the dietary and health sectors. There is an increasing demand for livestock products, as a result the farming systems are becoming more and more intensive. With the high input intensive agricultural practices on the one hand, the limitations in terms of environmental degradation, loss of biodiversity, health hazards to consumers, *etc.* are also on the rise which are acting as limiting factors to continue on the same path of intensification. To achieve sustainable intensification of agriculture, mixed crop–livestock systems, combining livestock and cash crops at farm level, are considered to be a good alternative (Russelle *et al.*, 2007; Wilkins, 2008; Ryschawy *et al.*, 2012). These practices benefit the environment by improving nutrient cycling (Hendrickson *et al.*, 2008). In the agriculture based states of India, about 50% of the income is from the crop–livestock systems (Deshingkar *et al.*, 2008). Mixed crop-livestock systems also generate higher economic efficiency in saving production costs through complementaries between crop and livestock (Wilkins, 2008). Apart from direct income by diversifying production, there is an added advantage of reducing risks with regard to market fluctuations (Russelle *et al.*, 2007).

The Indian agriculture has undergone major changes because of modernisation and intensification. An understanding of the changes leading to the decline in mixed farming systems may help Indian administration to preserve and promote them. Some of the policy and market pathways allow mixed crop–livestock systems to persist, whereas others lead to specialised farming systems. The analysis of cattle system dynamics has described changes in the past, and the underlying driving forces (Garcia-Martinez *et al.*, 2009). Thus, it is required to assess the diversity in farming systems and to elucidate the driving forces and the conditions involved under them. In developed countries, agrarian intensification and specialisation improved the productivity but it also had the added detrimental bearings on the environment and questioned the sustainability and economics of a huge number of farms (Wilkins, 2008). The chapter analyses the perspectives of mixed farming system in India and the future course of action to meet the impending demands.

Land holdings

India is a south-east Asian country, lies between latitudes 8° and 37° N and longitudes 68° and 97°. It is the seventh largest country in the world, and occupies a geographical area of 32.9 M km^2. Bestowed with the wide variety of biodiversity, Agriculture is the main occupation of the people and about 70% of the population is engaged in this activity. Livestock rearing is complementary to agriculture [FAO]. In agrarian economies, land, especially land redistribution plays a pivotal role in determining the practices, evolution and thus, the future perspectives and India is no exception to this. Indian agriculture is undergoing heavy stress as average land holding is decreasing day by day [Fig 1]. The growing population and division of the lands within the family reduces the average land holding and thus, there has been a significant shift in the farmers from the category of large and medium to the small and marginal ones [Fig. 2]. The majority of the farms in India are in the hands of small, marginal and semi medium farms accounting for more than 70% of the total land holdings [Fig. 3, Table 1]. With smaller land at disposal, there is a decrease in farmer's capacity to invest in land. With average land holding reduced, the cost of getting inputs and labourare is on the rise. So there has been a trend of a farmer migration from agricultural farming to the labour activities to earn his livelihood giving rise to the issues of informality.

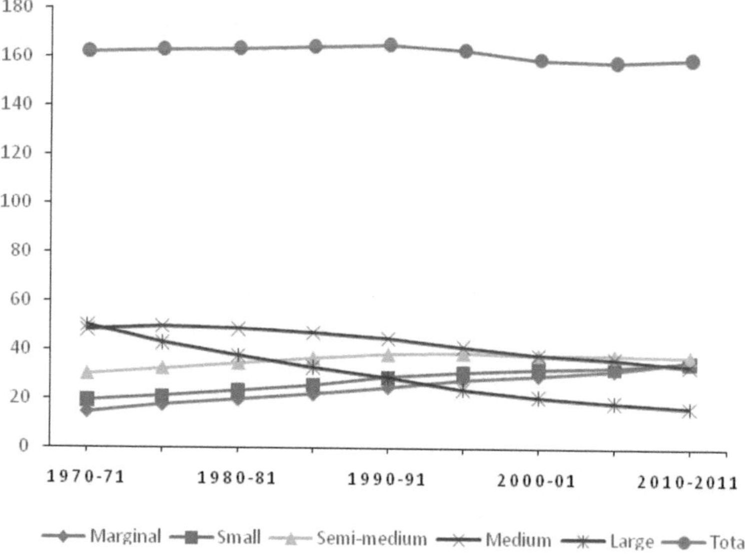

Fig. 1. Operated area in ha (million)

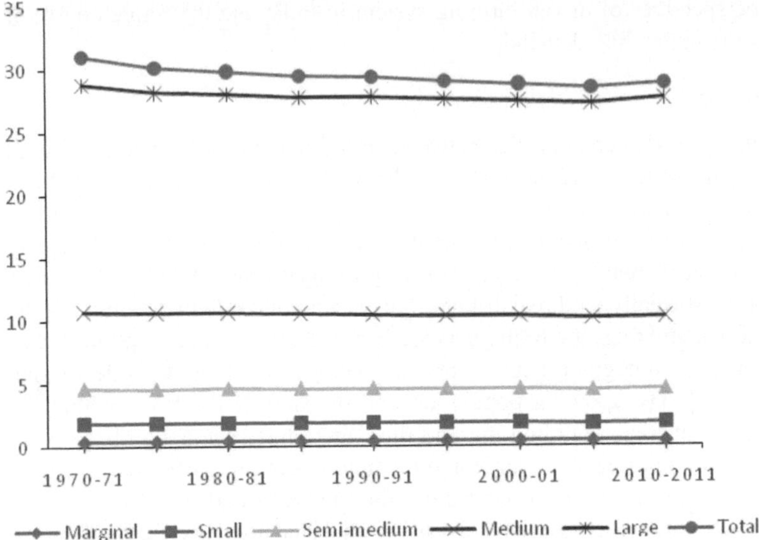

Fig. 2. Average land holding in India (in ha)

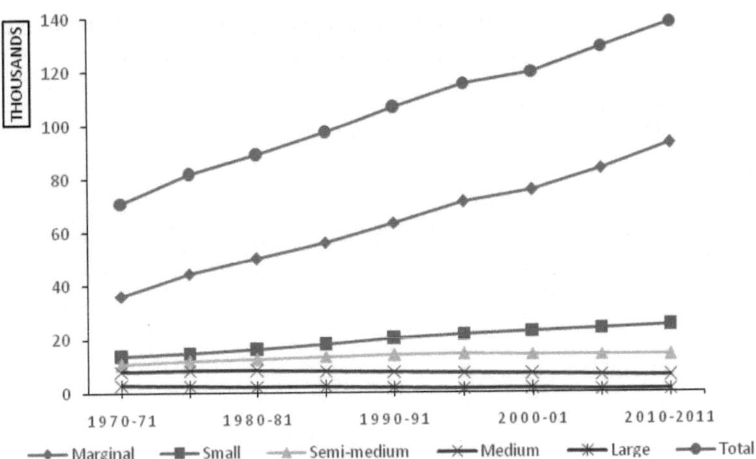

Fig. 3. Number of land holding in India

Table 1. Please provide caption

S. No.	Land holding (in ha)	Category
1.	< 1.0	Marginal
2.	1.0–2.0	Small
3.	2.0–4.0	Semi-medium
4.	4.0–10.0	Medium
5.	> 10.0	Large

*Classification as per the Agriculture Census, GOI.

The Livestock sector

Livestock sector is an important sub-sector of the agriculture of Indian economy. India is bestowed with large animal population ranking first in total cattle and goat population, third in sheep population [Fig. 4]. The animals in India are closely associated with the agricultural crops from ages forming an active part of not only society but economy as well. The share of the agricultural sector in total GDP declined from 34% in 1981–82 to 12.34% in 2010–11. The share of livestock in GDP declined also, but not as steeply as agriculture. It remained at 5–6% until 2000–01 and then gradually declined to 3.9% in 2010–11. However, the share of livestock in agricultural GDP increased consistently from 15% in 1981–82 to 27–28% in 2010–11. The paradigms of the Indian livestock sector are changing from mixed farming systems to the highly intensified animal husbandry systems. But still, the limiting factors of land holdings, multiplicity of stakeholders, *etc.* often restrict the sudden and frequent changes. One dimension of the livestock revolution is the intensification of the livestock practices, with production changing from being the traditional local multi-purpose activity to an increasingly market-oriented and vertically-integrated business (Delgado *et al.*, 1999; Steinfeld, 2002). The rate of returns from animal husbandry sector is on the rise. When the production of core agricultural crops are growing at a rate of 1.5-2% per annum, eggs and broilers are rising at a rate of 8-10% per annum (Mehta *et al.*, 2003). The rate of returns and growth is more in the poultry and small animals. The major contributors to production in the world's largest milk producer *i.e.*, India are small-scale production enterprises with a share of 70% and substantial quantities of livestock products are sold in informal markets (Costales *et al.*, 2010). There is an actual threat that large-scale intensive producers could undermine the viability of small-scale livestock production, thereby aggravating rural poverty (Steinfeld, 2002). While smallholders may continue to be competitive in the dairy sector, a more rapid switch to industrial systems is likely for pig and poultry production (Tarawali *et al.*, 2011).

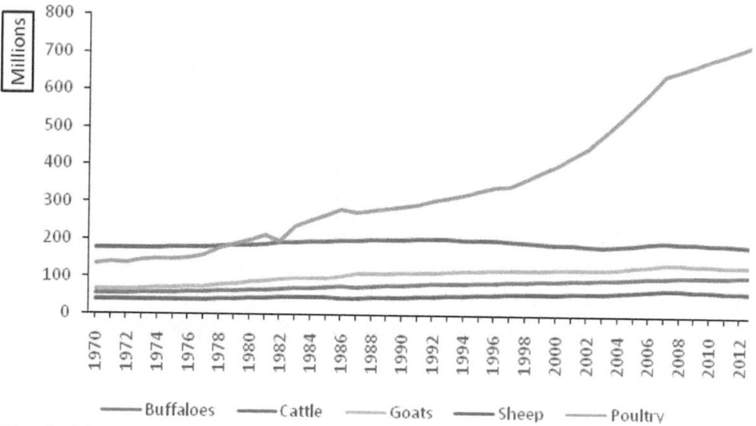

Fig. 4. Livestock sector in India

Farming system

The type of agricultural systems have direct impact on the environment (MA, 2005; Pretty, 2008; Kiers *et al.*, 2008; Place and Mitloehner, 2010). The increasing pressure on the agriculture system, the intensification is associated with the large use of pesticides and fertilizers, which can pollute water, air and natural ecosystems (Tilman, 1999). Naylor *et al.*, (2005) identified mixed farming, as an important alternative to reduce the negative impacts of agriculture. With the mixed farming systems the reconnection of livestock to the land can be established which can come up as a favourable alternative to the enduring advancement of mechanization agricultural practices (Herrero *et al.*, 2010). In mixed crop-livestock systems, animals can have multiple purposes besides the primary production of milk, meat, eggs and wool. Animals play the role as a capital stock, manure production, natural nutrient cycling of the animals along with providing the draught power in the smaller land holdings such as in India where mechanised farming with the tractors, *etc.* can be uneconomical. With the proper management in mixed farming, soil structure and organic matter can be efficiently preserved and improved for the degraded farms (Oomen *et al.*, 1998; Schiere *et al.*, 2002; Lantinga *et al.*, 2004; Watson *et al.*, 2005; Petersen *et al.*, 2007; Russelle *et al.*, 2007; Hendrickson *et al.*, 2008). Thus, this holds large promises for the development of sustainable agro ecosystems (Wilkins, 2008; Hilimire, 2011).

The way forward

From the evolutionary view there has been a considerable intensification of agriculture world-wide and India is no exception. This is mainly driven by economic growth, policies focussed at increasing food security, technology and a substitution of capital for labour. This led to the replacement of mixed farming practices with the monocultures. The livestock sector is specialised to varying degrees with the small animals and poultry sector at the higher levels as compared to the ruminants. The organised dairy sector is also swiftly moving towards industrial-style production systems. Such trends often raise questions on the sustainability aspects but on the other hand, there is increasing pressure to increase production to meet the demand for food in developing countries. With little opportunity to increase the limited resources, the higher production levels can be achieved by increasing productivity from the limiting resources, *i.e.*, intensifying production. A key question is, which form of intensification? Is there a future in specialisation and industrialisation or intensification of smallholder mixed systems? In the developed countries the intensification is driven by high working costs of labour, with capital being a substitute for the labour. The context of agriculture in the developing world such as India is different. Firstly, labour costs are much lower with a large unemployed population and limited employment opportunities outside agriculture with low literacy rates. With low labour costs in small-scale family farming systems, these can successfully compete with the larger farms. As reported in India, when family labour is not costed, the average profit per litre of milk produced is ₹2.45 for farms producing under 10 litres of milk per day which is much higher as compared to the ₹0.38 on farms producing over 150 litres per day (Delgado, 2008). The 50% of livestock feed is coming from the crop residues and this may increase to

70% by 2020 due to the limiting grazing areas and increasing livestock populations (NIANP, 2003; Ramachandra *et. al*., 2007). With the water scarcity leading the issues in India especially for the rural masses, the livestock water productivity is higher in mixed crop/livestock systems than mono-cropping (Singh *et. al*., 2004). For the mixed crop/livestock farmers the benefit from utilising manure are higher, as it can be applied to their own fields and the limited resources in transporting it from storage areas to fields. Considering the inherent potential of Indian cattle and with the better management in terms of feed and fodder, it is possible to double daily milk production in the country (Blummel *et. al*. 2009). With the new economic revolution on the turn and with new policy initiatives such as CSR, the involvement of the private sector can play a significant role with providing support at local, national and regional levels to ensure dynamic markets with well-established supply chains linking the farmers to the consumers with improved efficiency and returns (Hazell P, 2007) Thus, the small scale mixed systems in developing economies such as India have a significant role to play in terms of primary agricultural products both in agriculture and livestock, but also have significant multifactorial role in rural upgradation, employment generation, *etc*. as well.

Conclusion

The specialised cropping systems and the intensive livestock systems will play a significant role in feeding the future generations and the smallholder mixed crop/ livestock systems will not provide all the food that will be required. However, there is sufficient evidence to support the conclusion that small-scale mixed systems have a significant role to play in meeting the demands but also in rural development and upgradation. In some of the sub-sectors such as poultry, piggeries, *etc*. there has been a rapid evolution to intensive livestock systems and they have emerged as an industrial sector. But in the other sectors, like the ruminant sector (dairy) involving small, marginal farmers where much of the feed is still derived from crop residues, involving the family labour, the smallholder mixed systems will continue to play a vital role in providing food and employment. The challenges in the current scenario are to ensure the development and access of these farmers to the appropriate technologies and information for the sustainable productivity and incomes. This will require research that is focussed on the local needs and integrates it to the environmental issues of the society on the whole. The dynamic analysis of all the factors is required to be taken into consideration and the 'one-cause, one-solution' model is no longer going to achieve the ultimate goals to meet the future needs and substantiality goals. The unaltered foreign developmental models of the west can be replicated to a limited extent in a country such as India with its own rich biodiversity and socio-political issues and there is a need to develop own indigenous solutions to the problems. Thus, with the large population of farmers with marginal, small and semi-medium operational holdings owning about 87.7% of the livestock there is utmost need to develop this sector with the core objectives of inclusive growth and sustainability.

References

Blummel M, Anandan S, Prasad CC (2009) Potential and Limitations of By-product Based Feeding Systems to Mitigate Greenhouse Gasses for Improved Livestock Productivity. Diversification of Animal Nutrition Research in the Changing Scenario. 13th Biennial Animal Nutrition Conference. Animal Nutrition Society of India/National Institute ofAnimal Nutrition and Physiology, Bangalore.

Costales AC, Pica-Ciamarra U, Otte J (2010) Social consequences for mixed crop-livestock production systems in developing countries. In: Steinfeld H., Mooney H., Schneider F., Neville L., eds. Livestock in a changing landscape: Drivers, consequences, and responses. Island Press, Washington, DC, USA. 249–267.

Delgado CL, Narrod CA, Tiongco MM (2008) Determinants and Implications of the Growing Scale of Livestock Farms in Four Fast growing Developing Countries. Research Report 157. InternationalFood Policy Research Institute, Washington, DC.

Delgado C, Rosegrant M, Steinfeld H, Ehui S, Courbois C (1999) "Livestock to 2020 –The Next Food Revolution". Food, Agriculture and the Environment Discussion Paper 28. IFPRI/ FAO/ILRI.

FAO (2015) http://www.fao.org/ag/agp/agpc/doc/counprof/India/India.htm. Accessed on 10th Oct., 2015.

Hazell P, Poulton C, Wiggins S, Dorward A (2007) The Future of Small Farms for Poverty Reduction and Growth. 2020 Discussion Paper No. 42. International Food Policy Research Institute, Washington, DC.

Hendrickson JR, Liebig MA, Sassenrath GF (2008) Environment and integrated agricultural systems. Renew. Agr. Food Syst. 23, 304–313.

Herrero M, Thornton PK, Notenbaert AM, Wood S, Msangi S, Freeman HA, Bossio D, Dixon J, Peters M, van de Steeg J, Lynam J, Parthasarathy Rao P, Macmillan S, Gerard B, McDermott J, Seré C, Rosegrant M (2010) Smart investments in sustainable food production: revisiting mixed crop-livestock systems. Science 327: 822–825.

Hilimire K (2011) Integrated crop/livestock agriculture in the United States: a review. J. Sustain. Agric. 35: 376–393.

Kiers ET, Leakey RR, Izac AM, Heinemann JA, Rosenthal E, Nathan D, Jiggins J (2008) Agriculture at a crossroads. Science 320: 320–321.

Lantinga EA, Oomen GJM, Schiere JB (2004) Nitrogen efficiency in mixed farming systems. Journal of Crop Improvement 12: 437–455.

MA (Millennium Ecosystem Assessment) (2005) Ecosystems and Human Well- Being: Global Assessment Reports. Island Press, Washington, DC.

Mehta R, Nambiar RG, Delgado C, Subramanyam S (2003) Annex II: Livestock Industrialization Project: Phase II–Policy, Technical, and Environmental Determinants and Implications of the Scaling-Up of Broiler and Egg Production in India. IFPRI-FAO projecton Livestock Industrialization, Trade and Social-Health-Environment impacts in Developing Countries.

NIANP Feedbase (2003) National Institute for Animal Nutrition and Physiology, Bangalore 530–560.

Oomen GJM, Lantinga EA, Goewie EA, Van Der Hoek KW (1998) Mixed farming systems as a way towards a more efficient use of nitrogen in European Union agriculture. Environmental Pollution 102: 697–704.

Petersen SO, Sommer SG, Béline F, Burton C, Dach J, Dourmad JY, Leip A, Misselbrook T, Nicholson F, Poulsen HD, Provolo G (2007) Recycling of livestock manure in a whole-farm perspective. Livestock science 112(3):180-91.

Place SE, Mitloehner FM (2010) Contemporary environmental issues: a review of the dairy industry's role in climate change and air quality and the potential of mitigation through improved production efficiency. Journal of Dairy Science 93: 3407–3416.

Pretty J (2008) Agricultural sustainability: concepts, principles and evidence. Philosophical Transactions of the Royal Society B: Biological Sciences 363(1491): 447-465.

Ramachandra KS, Taneja RP, Sampath KT, Angadi UB, Anadan S (2007) Livestock Feed Resources in Different Agroecosystems of India:Availabilty, Requirement and Their Management. National Institute of Animal Nutrition and Physiology, Banglore.

Russelle MP, Entz MH, Franzluebbers AJ (2007) Reconsidering integrated crop livestock systems in North America. Agronomy Journal 99: 325–334.

Schiere JB, Ibrahim MN, Van Keulen H (2002) The role of livestock for sustainability in mixed farming: criteria and scenario studies under varying resource allocation. Agriculture, ecosystems & environment 90(2):139-153.

Singh OP, Sharma A, Singh R, Shah T (2004) Virtual water trade in dairy economy: Irrigation water productivity in Gujarat. Economic and Political Weekly 3492-3497.

Steinfeld H (2002) "Increasing Global Demand for Animal Products". In: Responding to the Increasing Global Demand for Animal Products: Programme and Summaries of an International Conference organised by BSAS, ASAS and MSAP, Merida. Mexico.

Tarawali SA, Herrero M, Descheemaeker K, Grings E, Blümmel, M (2011) Pathways for sustainable development of mixed crop livestock systems: Taking a livestock and pro-poor approach. Livestock Science 139: 11–21.

Tilman D (1999) Global environmental impacts of agricultural expansion: the need for sustainable and efficient practices. Proceedings of the National Academy of Sciences 96(11): 5995-6000.

Watson CA, Öborn I, Eriksen J, Edwards AC (2005) Perspectives on nutrient management in mixed farming systems. Soil Use and Management 21: 132–140.

Wilkins RJ (2008) Eco-efficient approaches to land management: a case for increased integration of crop and animal production systems. Philosophical Transactions of the Royal Society B: Biological Sciences 363(1491):517-525.

World Bank (1999) Indian Livestock Sector Review: Enhancing Growth and Development. The World Bank, Washington, D.C. and Allied Publishers, New Delhi.

3

Pig Production Attractive Entrepreneurship for Livelihood Security

Eaknath B. Chakurkar

Principal Scientist (Animal Reproduction) and Sectional In Charge Animal Sciences Section, ICAR Central Coastal Agricultural Research Institute, Old Goa-403402

Introduction

Meat has become an integral part of human food to meet the essential nutrients, like proteins. For a balanced diet, a good biological availability of meat is preferred in the modern day era. The per capita consumption of meat in India is only 14g per day as against the actual requirement of 125g. Non availability of quality meat and its exorbitant prices have restricted meat consumption. Increasing the meat production through intensive rearing of various meat animals will help to meet the ever growing demand of a balanced human diet. In the modern era and educational status social taboos are also getting relegated with need of quality proteins.

The very important role of pigs in human life is control of environmental pollution by scavenging the biological waste. Pig converts biological waste material to quality proteins in the form of pork. Pigs have a rapid growth rate, high reproductive efficacy, require comparatively less space, and can be reared on small scale in backyards or as commercial units. A major advantage of pig farming is that they can be fed on fibrous low quality agro byproducts and materials that are not suitable for human consumption leading to low production cost. Hence pig rearing can be a lucrative source of income for rural farmers in India.

Important aspects of pig production

Despite of above facts regarding pig rearing in India many youth from different states are coming forward to establish modern commercial pig units. These units are of two type one is breeding unit which maintains parent stock, produce the piglets and sale for fattening. Another group is the majority where piglets are purchased and fattened for pork. To increase productivity and profitability there is a need for improved pig husbandry like suitable breed, feeding practices, advanced technologies like breeding through Artificial Insemination sound diseases control and hygienic production can improve pig production of state as well as profit of individual farmers.

Among all the domestic animals, pigs are the most prolific animals with shorter generation intervals. A sow can be bred as early as 8-9 months of age and can farrow twice in a year. They produce 6-12 piglets in each farrowing. Pig products such as pork, bacon, ham, sausages, lard, *etc.* are increasingly in demand both for local consumption and for the export. Pig industry has a special significance as an enterprise in developing countries which raise pigs mainly by scavenging as traditional occupation in the rural areas.

Looking to the meager availability and tremendous demand of animal protein diet in India, it is felt that such demand could substantially be met by improving and multiplying pigs, mainly because of their prolificacy, faster growth, efficiency of feed conversion and shorter generation intervals. Efficiency and cost of production for a swine enterprise are directly associated with reproductive efficiency of the breeding herd.

Pig production status of India and scope

India contributes to 12 percent of the world livestock population with an alarming increase of livestock population at the rate of 2 million per annum (Mujumdar 2004). The availability of land for fodder production is restricted due to cultivation of commercial crops and rapid industrialization. In addition, lack of grazing land and ever increasing demand for green fodder is another constraint for rearing large animals such as cattle and sheep, goats, *etc.* In this scenario, small animals such as pigs, rabbits, poultry can support to meet the demand for animal protein requirements of the population.

In India, pig raising and the pork industry are in the hands of traditional pig keepers belonging to the lowest socio-economic strata with no means to undertake intensive pig farming with good foundation stock, proper housing, feeding and management. They are compelled to follow old and traditional methods with common village pigs, which could be designated as scrub animals. These animals usually produce litter of small size and inferior quality meat. The poor farmer is unable to provide any attention to their managerial practices and most of the time these animals are left loose to pick up feed stuff from waste areas of neighboring localities.

Scope

However, in spite of these drawbacks, the consumption of pork in the country has greatly increased in recent years. A number of piggeries have come up where pigs are reared on scientific lines and the manufacturing of pork products is carried out under modern conditions. The pig population has increased from 13.29 million in 1997 to 14.14 million in 2002–03 with an annual growth rate of 1.25 percent (17th Livestock census, 2003). As per 2012 census, the growth of crossbred pigs population is the indicating adoption of advances for better production.

Key points in pig production

Breeds, Nutritional management, Health management, Reproductive management, Marketing are the key points for profitable pig production.

Breeds

Breed of livestock plays a vital role in production as it decides acclimatization, growth rate, quality of meat, ability to utilize available foods, *etc.* Like all other species there are locally adopted pigs in all climatic zones of India but there are only three recognized breeds of pigs namely Megha Nihang, Ghungroo and Agonda Goan. Apart from these three breeds, many exotic breeds have been introduced like Large White Yorkshire, Duroc, Hampshire, Landrace, etc of which Large White Yorkshire is majorly adopted in many parts. For commercial purpose crossbred pigs will be beneficial as this will be a product of local breeds with some commercially viable high performing breeds like Large White Yorkshire.

Crossbred pig developed at ICAR-CCARI Goa

These are the pigs produced by crossing Agonda Goan female pigs with Large White Yorkshire males. These crossbred pigs have better growth rate and feed conversion efficiency. They do not require intensive care like pure exotic breed like large white Yorkshire. Reproductive parameters studied indicated that the age of puberty in crossbred females reduces as compared to Large white Yorkshire pigs. Age of puberty in the cross breed pigs ranged from 175 to 214 days and average age of puberty was 189.3 days. Age of maturity ranged between 203 to 233 days and the average age of maturity was 219.20 days. Average weight at puberty was 33.03 kgs whereas average body weight at maturity was 54.8 kgs. It was concluded that cross breeding has reduced the age of puberty and maturity than pure exotic breeds. Crossbred pig of Goa Local and Large White Yorkshire was successfully produced and performed well in intensive care as well as in farmers management conditions of Goa. Goa Local pigs have the growth rate of 100–120 g/ day and attain 30-40 Kg body weight after 8–9 nine months of rearing. While the crossbred pig Goa local X Large White Yorkshire has a growth rate of 450 g/ day and attains 80–90 Kg at marketing age. Thus by growing a crossbred pig, the farmer will get about 50 Kg additional body weight gain with low feed consumption, *i.e.*, about 4000 rupees per pig additionally.

Nutritional management

The successes of pig farming are dependent upon the efficient scientific feeding practices. In India, pigs are usually slaughtered at about 70kg body weight, which is generally achieved at six months of age. To meet the intensified pork production, properly balanced high quality ration must be provided to the pigs. Three types of rations are fed to the pigs before they reach the market weight *i.e.*, creeper/ starter, grower and finisher rations. The creeper/ starter feed is generally fed up to the attainment of 15-20 kg body weight, which is followed by grower feed up to the attainment of 50 kg body weight, and then followed by finisher feed up to the attainment of 70 kg body weight. However, in Goa most farmers feed their pigs with freely available food materials like hotel/kitchen waste, bakery waste, garbage from vegetable market, broiler offal, *etc.* It is suggested that these unconventional feeds should be fed as the partial replacement for the ingredients in standard ration to economize the pig production.

Water should be available for pigs of all ages 24 hours for normal physiology. Clean drinking water when available for all the times it helps to maintain all body activities optimum. watering nipples should be fixed in pigpens for this purpose.

Health Management

Like other livestock pigs also get sicknesses due to bacterial infections, viral infection and parasitic infestation. Many times stresses due to climate change or sudden change of feed or faulty food material causes illness in pigs. All the newly born piglets should be vaccinated at least against Swine fever at the age of 2 months. Vaccine against Pasteurellosis (Haemorrhagic septicaemia HS) and Foot and Mouth Disease vaccine like cattle is also preferred in pigs. Deworming in young pigs is essential, infection with roundworms can cause diarrhea, weight loss and death. Hence, the piglets should be dewormed regularly once every three months.

Reproductive management

Reproduction is a basic requirement of production. As pig is a litter bearing animal, litersize, liter weight and inter farrowing period decides the number of line animals produced during the unit period which is directly related to economics of pig production. For better reproduction, it is required to make use of advanced technologies in pig production. Artificial Insemination, Pregnancy diagnosis with Ultrasonography, care of pregnant sow and intensive care of litter before weaning is to be followed for the better pig production.

Artificial insemination

Artificial Insemination is a biotechnology where breeding is done without direct physical contact of male and female and semen is deposited in the female reproductive tract using catheter.

Need and Advantages of AI

Saving space and maintenance costs as we can decreases the number of boars, quick genetic progress in swine farm by using boars of higher genetic value through AI, production of same age and performance animal groups to slaughter is possible due to AI. Increase accuracy in genetic value evolution as, (a) A.I. boars generate more offspring, (b) Information measured by offspring and included in a selection index increases precision in the evaluation of measured characters and increase in the selection intensity, in order to obtain a higher number of births per boar by means of A.I., in comparison to natural mating. This leads to less selected boars. Control of sperm quality of boars, which are subject to various effects such as environment management and sanitary condition.

Advantages in health

The risk of sexually-transmitted infectious diseases is reduced as well as entrance of diseases-carrying animals is also reduced because there is no direct contact.

Synchronization of estrus

To get furrowing in a season when there is demand for the piglets is important from an economic point of view in the pig industry. For a commercial farm to get regular piglet production estrous synchronization as well as AI is required. For mass AI program. In fields also estrus synchronization is very much essential. This can be achieved with the technique of synchronization of estrus. To study the response of local non descript sows and Large White Yorkshire sows for synchronization, an experiment was designed. Prostaglandin F_2 alpha analogue (Dianoprest) was used for the synchronization of estrus in the sows at the dose of 7.5mg/animal and 10 mg / animal. The results indicated that synchronization of estrus was better in groups where 7.5 mg Dianoprost was given. Exhibition of estrous was as good as a natural estrous cycle. There was about 80 induction of estrous with a single dose schedule when sows were subjected for treatment in 10 days after weaning. In gilts, it was about 60percent with a single injection schedule. Conception rate after synchronization and AI was observed up to 70 percent.

Pregnancy diagnosis

Early and accurate identification of pregnant and non-pregnant sows and gilts improves reproductive efficiency in commercial swine farms. Numerous instruments and procedures are currently available for routine pregnancy diagnosis in sows like detection of return to estrus after mating, ultrasound and other laboratory methods and each method has its own advantages and disadvantages. Also, most tests which are available at present are unable to estimate litter size reliably in individual sows.

Ultrasonography: For these reasons, considerable effort is expended in developing a simple, accurate and inexpensive method of determining pregnancy soon after conception. The ideal method to diagnose gestation should allow a quick confirmation of pregnancy and should also be highly specific, sensitive and economic. Out of the various pregnancy diagnostic methods available in sows, trans-abdominal ultrasonography is being used commonly in Western countries as well as in India which is the most reliable method for early pregnancy diagnosis.

Marketing: Sale of product after produce is a major event in any entrepreneurship. Timely sale, quality of product decides the profit gain. Pigs should be marketed depending on local preferences like weight of pigs, fat content of pork and season. As an example in Goa state there is huge demand during the Christmas festive season. Pigs weighing 60-100kgs are generally preferred for pork as well as for the sausage industry. Therefore our production should be planned as per market demands.

References

Annual Reports ICAR Research Complex for Goa 2007-2013

Handbook of Swine artificial insemination Updated edition

KUBUS *S.A.C/E* 20. Pollgono Industrial EUROPOLIS 28230 Las Rozas de Madrid. Espana Reproduction in Farm Animals A text book By Sane et.al first Edition (1382).

Annual Reports of ICAR-CCARI Goa.

4

Role of Poultry for Livelihood Security in Northern India

Sandeep Saran

Principal Scientist (Agricultural Economics) and Head (PEAR), Central Avian Research Institute, Izatnagar-243122, Uttar Pradesh

Satyapal

Research Associate, ITMU, Central Avian Research Institute, Izatnagar-243122 Uttar Pradesh

Raj Narayan

Principal Scientist (Avian Genetics & Breeding), Central Avian Research Institute Izatnagar-243122, Uttar Pradesh

Introduction

India contributes about 5% to the world's eggs and 2.25% to chicken production (FAOSTAT, 2013). Indian Poultry Sector has been one of the fastest growing components of Indian economy with an annual compound growth rate of about 6% and 12% in egg broiler production, respectively. Poultry sector accounts for about 1% of the India's Gross Domestic Product (GDP) and 11.7% of the livestock GDP (*National Account Statistics*, 2013). With a turnover of over ₹600 billion, the sector provides employment to over six million people. The annual per capita availability has increased from 7 eggs in 1961 to 58 eggs in 2012; and poultry meat from 0.16 kg to 2.21 kg during the same period. However, the present availability levels are still far below the ICMR recommendations of 180 eggs and 11 kg meat per capita per annum. Ironically, consumption of poultry products has been highly skewed in favour of urban population. In fact, only 31% of the population residing in urban areas consumes 65% eggs and 70% of poultry meat and in a typical Indian village the egg consumption is not more than 10 eggs per capita per year. Despite higher prices of poultry products in rural areas, the penetrability and reach of poultry products have remained limited in rural India owing to fragmented markets and infrastructural bottlenecks. *Sekhon and Tejinder* (2007) have estimated that under a moderate growth scenario of 6% per annum in the Country's GDP the demand for meat and eggs is likely to shoot up to 9.7 and 15.32 MMT by 2021 and 2030, respectively. India would be easily able to meet this demand provided, the poultry egg and meat production continue to grow at the current levels.

India's Northern regions comprise the states of Himachal Pradesh (HP), Uttarakhand (UKD), Jammu & Kashmir (J&K), Punjab (PUN), Haryana (HAR), Rajasthan (RAJ) and Bihar (BHR). The states falling in the Indian Himalayan Region are sparsely populated as compared to other Northern states. These hilly regions are relatively less developed and are one of the most fragile and vulnerable ecosystems in the world due to their unique agro-ecological features and socio-economic conditions. The regions are characterized by winter and summer temperatures ranging 4°-7°C and 13°-18°C, respectively. The higher reaches are perpetually under snow and ice. The average annual rainfall exceeds 200 cm in the east but it is much less in the west. The positive attributes of this region are the niche advantages in the form of temperate climate for livestock and crop production as well as the nature-based farming tradition which still prevails. Notwithstanding the many hardships and the difficult terrain, local communities have created livelihood opportunities with great determination. On the other hand, the states such as UP and Bihar falling in Northern plains are densely populated. These states witness wide variations in annual temperature, rainfall and other weather parameters.

Table 1. Human population and density in Northern Indian states

States	Human Population (millions)			Density (per sq km)
	Male	**Female**	**Total**	
J&K	6.67	5.88	12.55	124
HP	3.47	3.38	6.86	123
UP	104.59	94.99	199.58	828
UKD	5.15	4.96	10.12	189
PUN	14.63	13.07	27.7	550
HAR	13.51	11.85	25.36	573
RAJ	35.62	33	68.62	201
BHR	54.18	49.62	103.8	1102
India	**623.72**	**586.47**	**1210.99**	**382**

Source: Census of India 2011, GOI.

The human population in the eight Northern states under reference together accounted for about 454.8 million (37.58%) of the country's population. UP and BHR together account for over 25% of the human population as per 2011 census data. HPis the most sparsely populated state followed by J&K, UKD and RAJ (Table 1). Population density in the states other than these states is more than that of the average population density of the country.

Table 2. Average size of holdings by size groups

					(Hectares)
States	**Marginal**	**Small**	**Semi-medium**	**Medium**	**Large**
J&K	0.35	1.40	2.68	5.43	22.34
HP	0.41	1.39	2.72	5.66	15.44
UP	0.39	1.40	2.72	5.52	15.01
UKD	0.44	1.43	2.71	5.45	23.11
PUN	0.61	1.38	2.64	5.74	14.75
HAR	0.46	1.47	2.87	6.09	17.95

					(Hectares)
States	**Marginal**	**Small**	**Semi-medium**	**Medium**	**Large**
RAJ	0.49	1.43	2.83	6.14	17.45
BHR	0.25	1.25	2.59	5.09	14.45
India	**0.38**	**1.42**	**2.71**	**5.76**	**17.37**

Source: Agricultural Census 2010-11, Dept. of Agri. & Coop., GOI

Table 3. Distribution of operational holdings by size group

					(%)
States	**Marginal**	**Small**	**Semi-medium**	**Medium**	**Large**
J&K	83.25	11.53	4.39	0.79	0.04
HP	69.78	18.17	8.83	2.87	0.34
UP	79.45	13.01	5.72	1.71	0.11
UKD	73.65	17.24	7.10	1.90	0.12
PUN	15.62	18.57	30.83	28.35	6.62
HAR	48.11	19.47	17.55	12.04	2.83
RAJ	36.46	21.94	19.38	16.36	5.86
BHR	91.06	5.86	2.56	0.50	0.02
India	**67.10**	**17.91**	**10.04**	**4.25**	**0.70**

Source: Agricultural Census 2010-11, Dept. of Agri. & Coop., GOI

A closer look at tables 2, 3 and 4 reveals that about 88-97% farmers have either small or medium land holdings in the Northern states with the exception of PUN and RAJ where such farmers account for about 34 and 58% holdings, respectively. A major proportion of total cultivated area is operated by marginal and small farmers in these states barring PUN, HAR and RAJ where distribution of land holdings is skewed towards medium and large farmers. Thus, the majority of farmers in these states have larger holdings as compared to those in Northern hilly states such as J&K, HP and UKD. Needless to emphasize that the majority of farmers these hilly states have meagre resources to sustain their livelihood.

Table 4. Proportion of area operated by size groups

					(%)
States	**Marginal**	**Small**	**Semi-medium**	**Medium**	**Large**
J&K	46.51	26.19	19.05	6.94	1.31
HP	28.52	25.53	24.21	16.43	5.31
UP	40.69	24.08	20.59	12.48	2.16
UKD	41.30	31.46	10.53	13.17	3.55
PUN	2.55	6.78	21.56	43.18	25.93
HAR	9.89	12.69	22.34	32.52	22.56
RAJ	5.86	10.23	17.86	32.73	33.33
BHR	25.83	22.91	27.27	14.58	9.39
India	**22.24**	**22.07**	**23.59**	**21.18**	**10.92**

Source: Agricultural Census 2010-11, Dept. of Agri. & Coop., GOI

As per 19th Livestock Census, India's poultry population was 729.3 million of which the eight Northern states accounted for merely 15.5% against 38% human population in these states. Whereas the poultry population in rural areas in the country has increased by 15% during 2012 over the previous census figures of 2007, the same in the urban areas has declined by over 25%. Another interesting observation has been decline of poultry population in 2012 as against 2007 census in the states like West Bengal (-39%), Tamil Nadu (-8%), Assam (-6%) and Odisha (-3.5%) and increase in poultry population in UP (114%), PUN (58%), HAR (49%) and BHR (11.5%). On the production front, the Northern states contributed only about 18% and 26% of the country's egg and poultry meat production. Among Northern states, the highest poultry population was reported in the state of HAR followed by UP, PUN, BHR and J&K (Table 5). Although HAR reported the highest poultry population, production and availability of poultry eggs and meat, the per capita availability figures appear to be inflated due to the fact that a sizable share of production from HAR is also channelized to neighboring state of Delhi. UP and BHR reported the least per capita availability of poultry eggs whereas HP reported lowest per capita availability of poultry meat. The availability of poultry meat and eggs in HAR and PUN was observed to be better than the country's average.

Table 5. Status of poultry in various Northern states

States	Poultry Population		Production		Availability	
	Rural (000 no.)	Urban (no.)	Eggs (Lakh no)	Meat* (000 t)	Egg/ person	Meat*/ person (g)
J&K	7490.5	783.2	6715	7.0	47	558
HP	1088.8	15.7	1069	1.0	16	146
UP	17185.6	1482.2	17074	175.0	8	877
UKD	4567.5	74.5	3079	2.0	31	198
PUN	15901.0	893.1	37911	79.0	137	2852
HAR	41735.6	1085.7	42343	324.0	168	12686
RAJ	7715.5	308.9	10335	19.0	15	277
BHR	12166.1	582.0	8372	37.0	8	356
India	**697895.3**	**31314.0**	**697307**	**2483.1**	**58**	2052

**2011-12*

Source: BAHS-2014; 19th Livestock Census Report, 2012 and Department of Animal Husbandry, J&K

Looking at the long term growth figures (table 6), it is evident that the poultry population has been increasing in the rural areas of all the Northern states except BHR, whereas sharp negative growth has been witnessed in the urban poultry population in most of the states except J7K, HP and UP. At all India levels also, it has witnessed a modest negative growth for the obvious reasons. Despite high growth in rural poultry population, the overall egg production in UKD has declined marginally, mainly due to negative growth in urban poultry population. The per capita availability of eggs has been consistently improving in all other states as indicated by positive growth figures.

The corresponding growth figures for meat availability also indicate significant improvement in meat availability in all the Northern states except for HP and UP. RAJ, PUN, HAR and UKD are among the high growth states in respect of per capita availability of poultry meat.

Table 6. Annual compound growth rate (2003-2012) (%)

States	Poultry Population@		Production	
	Rural	Urban	Eggs#	Poultry Meat$
J&K	5.02	5.64	1.44	3.07
HP	4.69	2.83	2.94	–4.76
UP	6.09	4.98	6.45	–1.78
UKD	11.67	–5.20	–0.44	16.78
PUN	6.37	–2.34	1.61	19.06
HAR	15.69	7.39	15.48	15.62
RAJ	4.00	–7.04	3.28	21.61
BHR	–1.13	–0.19	1.26	15.01
India	**5.66**	**–2.98**	**5.58**	**8.81**

Data source: @Livestock Census 2003, 2007, 2011
#2001-02 to 2012-13; $2007-08 to 2012-13;

Table 7. Distribution pattern of poultry in the Northern states (59th Round NSS)

States	No. of HH having Poultry per thousand HH		% share of land dedicated to poultry out of total land share for livestock farming	
	Rural	Urban	Rural	Urban
J&K	389	129	2.38	51.45
HP	37	10	0.00	0.00
UP	30	15	0.2	1.02
UKD	60	36	6.09	12.38
PUN	32	6	0.72	57.19
HAR	17	8	0.49	0.31
RAJ	40	7	0.09	1.37
BHR	53	23	4.00	20.93
India	**143**	**23**	**6.58**	**14.85**

Source: Livestock Ownership Across Operational Land Holding Classes in India, 2002-03, NSS Report No. 493 (59/18.1/1)

Poultry plays a significant role in the Northern states of the country as reflected by the proportion of households (HH) having poultry especially in rural areas (Table 7). Rural areas of J&K followed by UKD, BHR and RAJ have high concentrations of HH rearing poultry. Although except for J&K, the proportion of HH rearing poultry is much lower than the national average in rural areas. Similarly, the proportion of poultry keeping HH in urban areas of J&K and UKD is higher than the country's average. In HP, even the HH without any dedicated land resources have been rearing poultry. In other states, the share of land devoted to poultry in rural areas varies from negligible to over 6%. Urban HH in states like J&K, PUN and BHR allocated far more area to poultry out of the total share of land allocated for livestock (including poultry) as compared to the national average. The figures reflected the importance of poultry as means of livelihood in both rural as well urban areas in these states.

Table 8A. No. of HH having poultry per thousand HH across various land holdings (Rural)

States	Nil	<.002	0.002-.5	0.5-1.0	1-2	2-4	>4	Average*
J&K	40	0	274	424	239	99	132.5	389
HP	5	0	88	30	42	45	1000	37
UP	7	3	50	31	30	14	4	30
UKD	36	0	287	68	41	0	0	60
PUN	0	0	40	21	69	62.5	69	32
HAR	5	0	29	7	21	21	64	17
RAJ	4	22	83	74	25	17	9	40
BHR	26	89	100	42	56	34	90	53
India	**44**	**161**	**182**	**213**	**186**	**151**	**73**	**143**

Table 8B. No. of poultry per thousand HH across various land holdings (Rural)

States	Nil	<.002	0.002-.5	0.5-1.0	1-2	2-4	>4	Average*
J&K	119	0	11270	3840	8099	1773	4996.5	5523
HP	11	0	170	196	566	273	4000	193
UP	21	90	212	141	148	80	68	137
UKD	36	0	1280	1069	130	0	0	505
PUN	0	0	272	169	355	421	26543	1375
HAR	5	0	178	28	11615	42	116651	3613
RAJ	6	149	554	419	150	200	18	269
BHR	73	1048	554	363	487	215	809	328
India	**148**	**1128**	**1433**	**1866**	**1906**	**1268**	**2580**	**1232**

**Weighted;*
Source: Livestock Ownership Across Operational Land Holding Classes in India, 2002-03, NSS Report No. 493(59/18.1/1)

Table 8A further reinforces the importance of poultry rearing in the states. It is observed that even the landless households in all the Northern states (except PUN) have been rearing poultry, particularly in J&K, UKD and BHR, although the figure is lower than the national average. The proportion of HH keeping poultry in J&K across almost all the categories of land holding was very high as compared to the national average figures. Similarly, the number of poultry reared per thousand HH (Table 8B) was highest in J&K followed by HAR, PUN and UKD. It is also evident from these tables that the major proportion of poultry in these states is reared by marginal and small farmers. Thus, it is amply proved that (a) poultry can be reared even without dedicated land resources (b) that poultry can provide means of livelihood to the poorest of the poor.

The Value of Output (VoP) of output per capita from all agriculture and allied activities was highest in PUN followed by HP, HAR and J&K (Table 9). The per capita VoP from poultry rearing (egg production) was higher than national average in HAR, PUN and J&K. Other Northern states also derived reasonably high value of output from poultry activities *vis-à-vis* national average.

Table 9. Per capita value of output of various sub-sectors of agriculture (2010-11)

(₹per annum)

States	Total Agriculture	Total Livestock	Total Forestry	Total Fisheries	Agriculture and States Allied Activities	Eggs	Meat*
J&K	5273	247	2000	156	9903	87	451
HP	8309	299	2324	62	13681	19	171
UP	4096	1658	434	81	6269	7	186
UKD	4433	208	1847	15	8374	35	113
PUN	10773	5208	633	138	16752	162	710
HAR	84635	4234	604	110	13412	194	547
RAJ	4977	3476	891	23	9367	13	157
BHR	1742	1287	276	134	3439	12	172
India	**4758**	**197**	**689**	**347**	**7768**	**65**	**358**

* *Total meat of livestock*

Source: Director General, Central Statistics Office, Ministry of Statistics and Programme Implementation Govt. of India, New Delhi

Indian poultry industry has primarily been chicken oriented since its emergence. However, of late, India's poultry production portfolio has widened with the inclusion of diversified poultry species such as *Quail, Turkey, Duck, Guinea fowl* and more recently *Emu*. Chickens accounted for over 93% of the 729.3 million poultry population of the Country during 2011. In India, a number of poultry breeds, varieties and strains are available which are quite suitable for rearing poultry commercially as well as in rural set up under sub-optimal input regime.

Poultry Breeds

Although a number of poultry breeds were available in India, the Cobb 100 - a relatively older breed based on breeding stock imported from the United States and adapted to Indian climatic and disease conditions, owned by Venkateshwara Hatcheries (VH) currently accounted for 60-70% of all broilers in India. The nationwide infrastructure of VH supplied its stock to broiler operators, either as grandparents, parents, or DOCs, and also provided comprehensive veterinary services to its growers. At present, all broilers supplied by VH were Cobb 100. Another strain -Cobb 500, based on more recently imported breeding stock, has been reported to be under development, so was the case of Cobb 400 - based on cross between Cobb 500 and the acclimatized Cobb 100 strains.

Appendix-I provides details of some of the important Indian native breeds as also the strains, which were developed as a result of R&D in public sector for commercial exploitation and rural poultry farming purposes. Other breeds present in India included Ross (U.K.), Hybro (Netherlands), Hubbard (U.S.), Avian (U.S.), and Anak (Israel). Most of these breeds have entered only since 1995. Industry sources reported that the dominant role of the Cobb 100 breed and VH in the Indian broiler hatchery industry had both advantages and disadvantages for the growth of the broiler industry. On the technical side, the well-acclimatized Cobb 100 also proved to be a good *breeder's bird*, producing higher numbers of hatching eggs per parent, compared with other breeds. Besides, ready availability of chicks and veterinary support services from VH's widespread operations were other added advantages. The Cobb 100, however, was primarily a layer and, hence, provided a relatively low meat yield (75%), as compared to 77-78% from specialized broiler breeds. It remained to be seen as to how long it would take for the new breeds to become sufficiently acclimatized to Indian conditions to counter the hardiness and breeding advantages of the Cobb 100.

Poultry rearing in hilly regions

The primary reason for slow growth of poultry in the hill areas is extremes of climatic conditions, especially during winters. Housing for poultry in cold, arid climates is one of the most challenging tasks as requirement of optimum temperature of 25-35°C inside brooder and 15-20°C inside grower and layer houses is most difficult to achieve and required modifications in designs of traditional poultry houses.

The houses used for poultry in temperate hilly regions are above-ground mud walled poly sheds, semi-underground mud or stone walled houses, walls and sheds covered with plastic coated tarpaulin sheets and poultry houses kept in direct sunlight with provision for night shelter. According to Biswas *et al.*, 2010, fertility and hatchability were the main problems in the Himalayan region due to extreme cold conditions. Singh *et al.*, 2009 estimated economic potentials of free range indigenous fowl reared by rural women in Uttarakhand. The implications of research and extension agencies for further improvement and propagation of the *Giriraja* breed in the backyard poultry system were studied by Semmaran *et al.*, 2008. Mittal *et al.*, 2008 concluded that the strategy for mitigation of challenges of livelihoods and nutritional security in hilly regions may reduce migration and enhance the quality of life of people living in villages. The positive feature of hill districts was that they have enormous potential for high-value agriculture, livestock and poultry development. They suggested that the development strategy for Uttarakhand hills should be based on brand equity as Organic Green State to reap its benefits. This can be achieved by the goal of infrastructure development, agriculture diversification; poultry based livelihoods security.

The analysis based on the data collected from hill districts of Kumaon region for two production years, 2011–12 and 2012–13 revealed that farmers' access to critical inputs such as day-old chicks (DOCs) and feed played a key role in popularization of poultry based mixed farming systems. The government/private agencies promoting rural family poultry for women empowerment and poverty alleviation in the Kumaon Hills, emphasized on chicks brooding and trained a few Self Help Groups' (SHG) members to minimize chicks mortality during the early brooding phase by contract chicks-rearing. The DOCs purchased from the mother hatcheries were reared by the trained SHG members-turned-chick nursery-operators till 3-5 weeks. The grown up chicks were then sold to other SHG-members. This contractual model yielded a net profit of about 10% shared between SHG and the farmers in the ratio of 75:25. The farmers (SGH members) further reared the procured chicks in the backyard system in small flocks of 5-25 birds depending upon availability of open space and resources to procure them. Feed and chicks cost together accounted for 90% of the total cost of rearing. The adult male birds weighing about 3-4 kgs in 20-24 weeks were sold in the neighbourhood market whereas the female birds were reared for eggs. On an average, two batches of poultry were reared annually per family with a BC ratio of 2.94. The commercial broilers production in semi intensive systems appeared to have very thin profit margins primarily due to high input cost with a BC ratio of 1.10. Lack of finance, improper housing facilities, harsh climate and losses /damages to standing crops caused by free range poultry were the major impediments/constraints reported by the farmers in promotion of backyard poultry. Heavy mortality during the first 3-4 weeks of rearing of DOCs due to limited technical knowhow in respect of brooding was yet another major constraint in the backyard poultry system. However, the model of poultry farming prevalent in the hilly regions of Kumaon was quite successful and was in sync with the socio-economic status of the hill population which was essentially resource poor. The model was successful in addressing gender and equity issues also through women empowerment.

In most of the temperate regions the supplies of poultry egg and chicken is sourced from nearby production centres in the neighbouring states to fulfil the demand of hill regions. Besides demand and supply disequilibrium, high transportation and overhead expenses lead to limited poultry products availability and inflated prices in hilly areas further depriving the poor rural in remote hills. Thus, high prices of poultry products and limited availability in the hilly regions offer a great opportunity for the rural poor in these regions to adopt poultry as means of livelihood security and employment generation.

Challenges and Way Forward

Despite spectacular performance of the Indian poultry sector in the last few decades, poultry rearing in Northern states in general and hilly areas in particular have lagged due to the climatic, topographical and other associated constraints. Nutritional gaps at the grass root levels, trade liberalization under WTO, inequitably rising incomes, ever growing consumerism, depleting feed and other resources leading to escalation in feed prices and consequently in production cost, impending threats of climatic shifts and their impact on poultry including resultant predictable shortages of agro based feed ingredients and quality water as also growing consciousness for quality foods amongst consumers pose newer challenges. Besides, growing concerns for animal welfare, emerging and re-emerging poultry diseases and appropriate management of poultry waste to ameliorate its adverse environmental effects *etc.* are the added dimensions. Further, the whole array of poultry sector has been highly skewed and chicken centered eclipsing the growth potentials of other poultry species such as the duck, Japanese quail and turkey *etc*. which have been contributing significantly to the global poultry basket.

Poultry egg and meat are considered to be the cheapest source of animal protein. Hence, poultry may play a vital role in alleviating malnutrition among the rural poor and economically weaker sections. The need of hour is to think beyond conventional poultry production systems and to evolve innovative systems befitting the present demand to satisfy both qualitative and quantitative aspects of poultry production. Besides, linking production with national and international markets through suitable value chains is also of utmost importance to ensure viability of the production systems and revenue inflows.

References

Agricultural Statistics at a glance 2013, Ministry of Agriculture, Department of Agriculture and Cooperation, Directorate of Economics and Statistics, GoI, New Delhi.

BAHS (Basic Animal Husbandry Statistics) (2014) *AHSSeries13*,Ministry of Agriculture,Dept. of Animal Husbandry, Dairying and Fisheries,GoI, New Delhi.

Biswas A, Roy BG, Gogoi D, Ahmed M, Singh SB (2010) Poultry farming in the cold, arid Himalayan region of India. World's Poultry Science Journal 66(2): 297-308. Livestock Census-2012, 2007 and 2003, GoI.

Livestock Ownership across Operational Land Holding Classes in India, 2002-03, NSS Report No. 493(59/18.1/1), NSS 59th Round (January–December 2003),National Sample Survey Organization, Ministry of Statistics & Programme Implementation, Jan 2006, GoI.

Mittal S, Tripathi G, Sethi D (2008) Development strategy for the hill districts Uttarakhand. Working Paper No. 217. Indian Council for Research on International Economic Relations. Population Census 2011, Registrar General, GoI.

Saran S, Sasidhar PVK, Sastry KVH, Singh R (2005). Indian poultry industry: current scenario and future prospects- a review. Indian Journal of Animal Sciences 75(8): 992-998.

Semmaran M, Sasidhar PVK, Majumdar S, Chander M, Tripathi H (2008), Adoption behaviour of Giriraja backyard poultry by farmers in Karnataka. Indian Journal of Poultry Science 43(3): 343-345.

Singh B, Kumar S, Kaur N, Yadav SN (2009) Evaluation of external and internal egg quality traits of hill fowl reared under backyard system. Indian Journal of Poultry Science. 44(1): 25-29.

Singh CB, Dev C, Kumar D (2009) An economic analysis of free range poultry rearing in Garhwal Himalayas. Indian Journal of Poultry Science 44(1): 121-122.

5

Migratory Pastoralism Mainstay of Hill Livestock Farming Constraints and Future Prospects

P.K. Dogra

Dr. GC Negi College of Veterinary and Animal Sciences, CSK HP Krishi Vishvavidyalaya, Palmapur–176062, Himachal Pradesh

Varun Sankhyan

Dr. GC Negi College of Veterinary and Animal Sciences, CSK HP Krishi Vishvavidyalaya, Palmapur–176062, Himachal Pradesh

Sudesh Radotra

ICAR-Indian Veterinary Research Institute, Regional Station, Palampur-176061 Himachal Pradesh

Y.P. Thakur

Dr. GC Negi College of Veterinary and Animal Sciences, CSK HP Krishi Vishvavidyalaya, Palmapur–176062, Himachal Pradesh

Introduction

Pastoralism involving rearing of different livestock species makes significant contributions to the economy of developing countries, both in terms of providing employment and income opportunities and in supplying nutrition to rural poor. Pastoralism generally has a mobile aspect, and movement of animal herds in search of fresh pastures and water is a key feature qualifying pastoralism. The term *nomadic* is used when mobility is high and in irregular patterns; *transhumant* when there are regular back-and-forth movements between relatively fixed locations; and *sedentary* for the rest. Pastoralists inhabit zones where the potential for crop cultivation is limited due to steep terrain, extreme temperatures and low and highly variable rainfall. Within this unpredictable, vulnerable and dynamic environment, they have developed successful mechanisms of adaptation to maintain an ecological balance between themselves and the natural environment. Thus, pastoralism is a successful strategy to support a population on less productive land that adapts well to the environment. Transhumance is the seasonal migration of livestock and pastoralists between higher and lower pastures.

In Indian context, pastoralists can be defined as *"members of caste or ethnic groups with a strong traditional association with livestock-keeping, where a substantial proportion of the group derive over 50% of household consumption from livestock products or their sale*, and *where over 90% of animal consumption is from natural pasture or browse*, and *where households are responsible for the full cycle of livestock breeding"* (Sharma, Vijay Paul, 2003).

Nomadic pastoralism is a form of pastoralism where livestock are herded to find fresh pastures to graze. Strictly speaking, true nomads follow an irregular pattern of movement, in contrast to transhumance where seasonal pastures are fixed. However, this distinction is often not observed and the term nomads used for both. Pastoralism is a subsistence pattern in which people make their living by tending herds of large animals. The species of animals vary in different regions of the world, but they are all domesticated herbivores that normally live in herds and eat grasses or other abundant plant foods. Geographically, nomadic pastoralism is most prevalent in dry lands of Western India (Thar Desert) and in Deccan Plateau, as well as in mountainous regions of North India (Himalayas). The types of livestock raised under mobile, transhumant pastoral systems include buffaloes, sheep, goats, camels, cattle, donkeys, yaks, and even ducks.

Pastoralism in the Indian Himalayas

Pastoralism in the Himalayas is based on transhumance involving cyclical movements from lowlands to highlands to take advantage of seasonally available pastures at different elevations (Bhasin 1988). During summers, with snow melting in higher alpines, the pastoralists move up to these areas to graze their animals. After monsoon, they move down to occupy low altitude pastures for winter months. Movement of people and their livestock proceeds between previously earmarked sites, which become more or less regular seasonal encampments or bases.

Migratory pastoralism is common throughout the Himalayas from west to east. Some of the herding communities in the region include; goat and sheep herding Bakrawals of Jammu and Kashmir, buffalo herding *Gujjars* in Kashmir, parts of Himachal Pradesh and Uttar Pradesh, goat and sheep herding *Gaddis*, *Kanets*, *Kaulis* and *Kinnauras* in Himachal Pradesh, sheep herding *Bhotias* of Uttar Pradesh, yak herding

Sherpas of Khumbu, Nepal and lesser known communities in mountains of Bhutan, Sikkim and Arunachal Pradesh. All these herders follow a long-standing tradition of migrating up to alpine pastures of high Himalayas in summers and descending to the low-lying Himalayan foothills in winters. Some pastoralists in Himalayas are agro pastoralists and besides rearing animals they also cultivate land, although the major portion of their household income is drawn from pastoral activities. In addition, they also engage in a multitude of economic activities like handicrafts, trade and transport. For example, *Gaddis*, in Himachal Pradesh are known for their beautiful handicrafts; the embroidered caps made by *Gujjars* are also famous. The *Bhotias* are the most prominent trading community on the Indo-Tibet border and *Changpas* in Ladakh are involved in cross border trade with Tibet (Sharma, Vijay Paul, 2003).

Gujjars

The *Gujjars* derive their name from a Sanskrit term *Gurjara*. Historically, they were once dominant people in western India and gave the territory occupied by them the name Gujarat. For unknown reasons, the *Gujjars* migrated from western India and spread out all over the north-western part of Indian sub-continent and to some extent in central India. Cunningham (1871) describes their distribution to be in great numbers in every part of north-west India, and from the Peninsular Gujarat. *Gujjars* were once inhabiting eight provinces of Indian states; Delhi, Jammu and Kashmir, undivided Punjab (now consisting of Punjab, Haryana and Himachal Pradesh), the North West Provinces (now Pakistan), and other areas in and along the Himalayas. The contemporary *Gujjars* are known to raise sheep and goats as well as buffaloes. The small stock (sheep and goat) herders are known as *Bakarwal* and buffalo herders as *Gujjar* or *Dudh-Gujjar*. The *Bakarwal* inhabit the territory of Jammu and Kashmir whereas the buffalo-raising *Gujjars* are in Jammu, and sections of them have also moved in a south-east direction from Jammu and western Punjab to Himachal Pradesh and hills of Uttarakhand (Sharma, Vijay Paul, 2003). This movement has been caused by the depletion of grazing resources in Jammu and Punjab regions and also due to increase in both human and animal population.

Migration Pattern of Gujjar Community

The pastoral *Gujjars* of northern India practice transhumance and migrate with their households and livestock between summer and winter pastures. The base of their economic activities is keeping buffalo herds and they are specialized producers of dairy products that are sold in local towns. With the approach of summer months, when grass and other fodder as well as water becomes scarce in lower regions, the *Gujjars* take their herds to high-altitude pastures of Himachal Pradesh and Uttarakhand where grass is regenerated after snow. Winters are spent in the regions of Jammu, Punjab, lower districts of Himachal Pradesh and Uttar Pradesh (U.P.), and to the areas adjoining Rajaji National Park in U.P. Migration proceeds between predetermined sites along traditionally set routes and according to a more or less fixed timetable. The outward and inward journeys take about 15 to 20 days each.

Gaddis

The *Gaddis* live in northern India in the states of Himachal Pradesh, Uttar Pradesh and Punjab. Traditions say that *Gaddi's* ancestors originally came from Punjab and Uttar Pradesh, and fled from Muslim invaders of plains to Himalayan Mountains for refuge. Although shepherding is a key feature of the economic landscape of four districts of Himachal Pradesh–Kangra, Kullu, Kinnaur and Chamba- the main concentration is in Kangra and Dharamshala regions of Kangra district. The word *Gaddi* refers to a territorial group, or a special class of people who wear distinctive clothes. They travel and bear endless hardships in pursuit of their profession. However, in addition to herding sheep and goats, they are also becoming much more involved in farming. The recent trends towards settling in more hospitable climates have brought agriculture to the forefront of their economy and shepherding taking a secondary position.

Migration Pattern of Gaddi Community

Gaddis practice long distance herding of sheep and goats. Gaddis were earlier considered to be nomadic or semi-nomadic from Kangra valley but most Gaddis are now semi-nomadic and not nomadic, having permanent dwellings in Kangra valley from a government sedentarization programme. The *Gaddis* move from high pastures to low pastures during the year, leaving for the low hills and plains in October and returning to their fields in April. Following winter grazing in the Shivalik scrub forests, in early April, the herders begin to work their way northward, moving along the low mountain ranges that separate the Shivaliks from Dhauladhar. By early May, the Kangra *Gaddis* arrive in their villages, located on lower, southern slopes of the Dhauladhar range. They spend the next two months-grazing village forests and higher elevation forests of the Dhauladhar. The months of May and June are a particularly busy time in the *Gaddi* cultivation cycle because this is a time when the cultivators are required to harvest the winter crop and also to prepare the fields for the monsoon. In addition, the sheep and goats are penned for a number of nights on the freshly harvested fields thereby providing manure as fertilizer for the next crop. *Gaddi* shepherds spend summer in Lahaul and Spiti, and the Trans-Himalayan region north of Pir Panjal. Only a few herders do not move out, others migrate extensively. The access to summer pastures needs crossing of passes at high elevation, possible only once the winter snow has melted sufficiently. By the middle of June, the partial melting of the snow on Thamsar Pass allows herders to cross over into Bara Banghal region of Kangra district and make their way to nutritious forage of the alpine meadows (Saberwal, 1999).

By September, decreasing availability of forages forces the herders to begin their fall migration southward, including re-crossing of high passes and the descent to their own villages. During September, October and November the animals are grazed in forests of Chota Banghal region of Kangra district. By Mid- November, the herders begin to descend to their winter grazing grounds in Shivaliks. This journey lasts about a month, as the herder's wind their way across and along the gentle hills of Kangra valley until they come to scrub forests of the Shiwaliks. Many herders move further south to Hoshiapur, Punjab, stretching from Pathankot in the west to north of Ropar in the east. By December, the herders arrive at their winter grazing grounds.

Kinnauras

The people of Kinnaur in Himachal Pradesh have traditionally been referred to as *Kinners*, but the term *Kinnauras* is widely used. They live under harsh conditions, created by the inclement weather and climate. Kinnauras are the tribes inhabiting valleys between high mountains. Kinnaur district is a part of tribal belt in Himachal Pradesh that also includes the eastern part of Chamba and Lahaul Spiti districts. There are no reliable estimates of the size of Kinnauras. Flocks of sheep, goats and cows, yaks and horses are safety investments.

Migration Pattern of Kinnauras community

In summers, the flocks are driven to higher parts within Himachal borders. In winters, flocks are driven to foothill pastures around Dehradun (Uttrakhand). Nowadays, shepherds with their animals spend the winters also in Uttrakhand. As per tradition, Kinnauras hire shepherds from different parts of Himachal Pradesh and pay them clothes, shoes, basic foods (maize, salt, spices, ghee, *etc.*) and 7-8 animals (depending upon flock size).

Bhotias

Bhotias are sheep herding pastoralists and live in northern parts of Bhutan, Sikkim, and Nepal and along Indo-Tibetan border in Garhwal, Kumaon of Uttrakhand and Himachal Pradesh. They are a Mongoloid people who gradually moved off the Tibetan Plateau.

Bhuttias

Bhuttias are the most prominent pastoralists of the alpine regions of Lachung and Lachen valleys of northern Sikkim. They migrate to the lower forests of Mangan in the summer season.

Changpas

Changpas, in the south- eastern region of Ladakh are involved in cross border trade with Tibet. Their migration cycle is around various high altitude pastures of Rupshu plains in Changthang region of Ladakh (Sabharwal, 1996).

Monpas

Monpas live in Tawang and West Kameng districts of Arunachal Pradesh. They stay in the higher reaches of East Kameng and Tawang districts in the summer season and migrate to low lands around Tawang during the winter months.

Major Problems Experienced by Pastoralists

Government attitudes to pastoralists: In social evolutionary thinking, the nomadic lifestyle has traditionally been categorized as less civilized, less productive and more degrading than a settled lifestyle (Sabherwal, 1999). Due to problems of their cultural stereotyping, small population and migratory lifestyle, the Himalayan pastoralists are ignored in various policy-level decisions. Non-participation and ignorance of their rights and status have seriously marginalized these communities. Their political marginalization is visible across all Himalayan states where most of the pastoral groups are not vocal about their concerns. Most research conducted on Himalayan pastoralism is inclined more towards ecological concerns rather than taking a holistic view leading to a biased understanding. Many studies have concluded that the present knowledge of environmental degradation *vis-à-vis* livestock grazing by migratory Himalayan pastoralists is not sufficient and there is a need to rationalize and reinforce the existing knowledge. Studies elsewhere, from Poland to Tanzania to Mongolia, have shown that pastoralism can co-exist with, and contribute positively to, biodiversity conservation. However, no such study of the impacts of grazing on biodiversity conservation has been conducted in the Indian context.

Non-recognition of pastoral land rights: Local pastoral groups regard themselves as owners of pasture resources in Himalayas and follow traditional rules and regulations in distributing and managing these resources amongst themselves. The customary usage of forest resources or common lands is neither documented in government records nor officially recognized. There are instances where winter pastures of *Gaddi* pastorals in

Himachal Pradesh were allotted to landless people under some social welfare scheme ignoring the resource use and right to access of *Gaddi* pastoralists.

Population growth and land fragmentation

Owing to the growing human population in Himalayan region, land resources per household are decreasing along with subdivision and fragmentation of agricultural land. The data indicate that reduction in per capita cultivated land is as high as 46.7 percent within a decade in Central Himalayas.

Livelihood threats

1. **Reduced Pastures:** Across all the Himalayan states, the pastoral livelihoods are seriously threatened by the problem of shrunken pasturage. This decreasing availability of pasture resources has been due to misinformed conservation policies of the states and encroachment. Ever increasing human population, increased infrastructure and development in these areas have seriously reduced the size of available winter pasturage for pastoralists. Similarly, terrorist activities in areas bordering Jammu and Kashmir also affect summer pastures in the Himalayas. There are examples like Changthang pastures of Ladakh, Lachung valley pastures in Sikkim, the Tawang region of Arunachal Pradesh *etc.* The increasing agricultural activities in the high altitude regions of the Himalayas are also a threatening trend for Himalayan pastoralism.
2. **Disturbed Migratory Routes:** The migratory pastoralists in Himalayas travel long distances from low to high altitudes. On their way to summer or winter grazing lands, they halt at common lands of various villages, which is important for animal forage and their social relations with the agricultural communities. Himalayan states have gone through dramatic infrastructure and tourism development in the last few decades besides extensive road building, hydro power plants, hotels *etc.* across its length and breadth. As a result, pastoralists frequently have to alter their migratory routes and face problems of livestock being killed on roads, thefts and a constant pressure to move. There are instances where animals die of eating noxious weeds growing close to the roads or on degraded land.

Sedentarization

The Himalayan states of Himachal Pradesh and Uttarakhand have tried many times to settle their local nomadic communities against the very concept of migratory pastoralism. The non-supportive government policies had played an important role in decline of pastoral activities in the Himalayas. Further, the process of marginalization at cultural and policy level has seriously discouraged their upcoming generations to opt pastoralism as an occupation. The pastoralists feel that agriculture/horticulture provides a more secure future for their children as herding would become more and more difficult in future. For example, due to formation of Nanda Devi Biosphere Reserve and closing of Indo Tibet border for trade, the *Bhotia* pastoral population of Uttarakhand has migrated to lower regions permanently. Now many higher villages in Garhwal and Kumaon regions are vacant and there are no pastoral activities operational in these regions (Sabharwal, 2000). Similarly, the extensive army establishments in Jammu and Kashmir and Sikkim Himalayas have seriously affected the prospects of Himalayan pastoralism and there are many instances where the local pastoralists have switched over to daily wage labourers.

Production attributes of migratory goat and sheep husbandry, impact of certain improved management strategies en-route migration in Western–Himalayan region of Himachal Pradesh–a case study:

Sheep and goat rearing under the migratory system are generally associated with problems of poor nutrition, attack from predators, environmental extremes, high incidence of diseases and poor breeding methods. Understanding the processes and constraints associated with this migratory system is very relevant as more than 90% of the state's sheep and around 70% goat populations are reared under this system. Breeding and proper management are important aspects which could contribute significantly for improving production efficiency (Mandal, 2014). In view thereof, a study was undertaken to analyze the characteristics and trends in migratory goat and sheep husbandry, to identify the constraints of the migratory system and to assess the effect of improved management practices in adopted flock en route to develop effective technology intervention approaches for improving migratory production systems.

The study was conducted in sub-Himalayan ranges of Himachal Pradesh, India. The data of migratory flocks were collected through personal interviews by structured questionnaires. Four different migratory routes were selected in the entire state and 30-40 migratory farmers from each migratory route were interviewed. To understand the characteristics of migratory goat and sheep husbandry, after conducting the survey, four medium sized flocks, one from each migratory route, were adopted and monitored continuously during their migration for performance data. Among these four units, two were exclusive goat units and two mixed sheep and goat units. Reproductive and productive performances were studied using questionnaire and en route recordings. Various morpho-metric traits were measured along with body weight recordings at different age intervals, using fabricated weighing balance designed especially to suit migratory conditions. The data recording was done only for goats although various inputs were provided to all the flocks irrespective of the fact whether animals were included in the study or not. All the animals were identified by ear tagging. The baseline data on various productive and reproductive traits was generated. Thereafter, for studying the impact of improved practices and breeding management, strategic manage-mental and breeding inputs were provided to these flocks throughout the year for next three years along with data recordings. Every year 25-30 male goat kids were selected on the basis of three months body weights purchased and transferred to the institutional farm for further rearing up to age of their sexual maturity (one year). While at the institutional farm, these males were provided scientific management and screened for reproductive disorders. After attainment of sexual maturity, some superior males (on basis of body weight, average daily gain, breed confirmation and semen evaluation/reproductive screening) were supplied to adopted units as breeding input. The objective was to ensure buck rotation, screening for diseases (which can cause abortion through sexual transmission) and bring overall improvement. The flocks were monitored regularly during their entire route and performance was compared to base year. The primary or secondary data so generated was organized and subjected to statistical analysis. Descriptive statistics were computed and body weights were subjected to ANOVA using GLM (SAS version 9.2).

Flock and socio-economic characteristics: The data generated from the study and that collected from secondary sources revealed that the migratory goat and sheep husbandry was practiced by the *Gaddi* tribe. Different commissions were set up by the state government to regulate the land tenure and grazing permits by the tribes (Verma, 1996). The results of the survey are given in Table 1. On the basis of secondary data collected from various sources, the migratory flocks were classified under three categories *viz.* small flocks consisting of 100 animals, medium flocks of 200–350 animals and the large flocks having >350 animals.

Table 1. Socio- economic characteristics, flock structure and breeding management of migratory sheep and goat farmers

Particulars	**Flock**			
Flock Characteristic	**Small**	**Medium**	**Large**	**Overall**
Flock (No)/ Proportion of total	40 (40.8)	49 (50)	9 (9.2)	98
Total flock size	2477	7529	3416	13422
Average flock size (Mean ± SE)	64.5±2.72	153.7±6.36	379.6±15.45	136.9±10.49
Sheep (%)	56.51	56.71	59.25	57.44
Goat (%)	42.83	42.57	39.81	41.92
Others (dogs, ponies etc.)	0.65	0.71	0.94	0.76
Social characteristics				
Average family size (Mean ± SE)	5.53±0.22	5.74±0.27	6.89±0.91	5.76±0.18
Land holding (Mean ± SE)	8.87±0.95	7.25±0.88	9.94±1.03	8.15±0.60
Economic characteristics				
Income (all sources)/year, INR	53,625	57,143	71,111	56,990
Income (migratory farming/year)	26,875	36,120	43,333	32,959
Proportional income from migratory farming (%)	57.25	63.03	60.54	60.94
Breeding management				
Source of breeding buck				
Own Flock	24(60.0)	36(73.5)	7(87.5)	67(68.4)
Fellow farmer	6(15.0)	4(8.2)	0(0)	10(10.2)
Fairs/middleman	10(35.0)	9(18.3)	1(13.5)	20(20.4)
No of buck in flock	1–2	1–3	1–3	1–3
No of years buck used	3–4	4–5	4–5	4–5

Figure in parenthesis indicate the relative proportion of particular class compared to overall

The primary data generated through surveys revealed that the majority of flocks were medium sized (50%), followed by small flocks (40.2%) and larger sized flock (9.8%).

Due to various factors like ease of handling, shifting occupations, shrinkage of forest land and changing forest policies of the state, the farmers preferred medium sized flocks. Each flock had 3–4 ponies for carriage of loads during migration and 2-3 dogs (of distinct *Gaddi* breed) for watch and ward. Overall proportion of sheep, goats and other animals (ponies, dogs, *etc.*) was found to be 57.44%, 41.92% and 0.76% respectively. At present, the majority of flocks had goats and sheep in almost equal proportions but two to three decades earlier sheep used to be in majority. Exclusive goat flocks were also owned by some shepherds, which earlier were not the common practice. This could be attributed to the fact that during the last 10–15 years, the wool growth in the state had shown negative growth and wool remained no more lucrative to the farmers. On the other hand, due to consumer preference the demand for chevon has increased over the years as compared to mutton. In spite of reduction in proportion of sheep in migratory flocks, it still occupies a substantial proportion, albeit lower as compared to a decade earlier. In an earlier study, Singh *et al.*, 2006 reported that sheep and goats constituted 67.9% and 33.1% of a flock respectively in Kangra district, while present investigation revealed their contribution as 57.4% and 41.9% respectively.

This fact can be further corroborated from livestock census figures (19thlivestock census, 2012) which revealed similar trends in sheep and goat population. Over the last few censuses (Table 2), sheep and goat both showed decline in population, but the reduction in sheep was more marked than goat. Contrary to sheep, over the last 15 years, the goat population had shown positive growth during 2003–2007. The contribution of goats to the total livestock population remained more or less the same for past four livestock censuses, while sheep had shown a clear cut decreasing trend.

Table 2. Livestock population of studied area over period of 15 years

Census	Goat (millions)	Sheep (millions)	Total Livestock (TL) (millions)	Goat (%) of TL	Sheep (%) of TL	Sheep and Goat (%) of TL
16th census (1997)	1.17	1.08	5.22	22.41	20.68	43.10
17th census (2003)	1.13(–3.42)	0.93(–13.88)	5.21(–3.83)	21.68 (–3.25)	17.85–(16.58)	39.54(–8.26)
18th census (2007)	1.24(+9.73)	0.90(–3.23)	5.05(–3.07)	23.96(+10.5)	17.82(–0.02)	42.38(+7.18)
19th census (2012)	1.12(–9.67)	0.81(–10.00)	4.85(–3.96)	23.09(–3.63)	16.70(–6.28)	39.79(–6.11)
Annual change/ year (1997–2012)	–0.3%	–1.67%	–0.47%	+0.20%	–1.28%	–0.51%

TL: Total Livestock, Figure in parenthesis indicate percent change in particular category over the previous census

The average flock size for small, medium and large flocks observed in the present study was 64.5±2.72, 153.7±6.36 and 379.6±15.4 heads, respectively with an overall average of 136.9±10.49 animals. The overall average family size and land holding observed were 5.76±0.15 and 8.15±0.60 bigha, respectively. The flock size was found independent of family size and average land holdings, being more or less similar in different flock sizes. On an average, these farmers derived more than 60% of their income from migratory goat and sheep husbandry accounting to even 100% in some cases. The annual average income as per survey results was around ₹56,960 (876 USD)/ annum, which may be an underestimate as many times the farmers were reluctant to reveal actual income and disclose figures towards the lower side. Primary recording and subsequent economic analysis in the adopted and monitored flocks revealed that around ₹800 (12 USD) net profit per animal per year could be realized after counting for various losses in this production system. Accordingly, the farmers belonging to the medium category would earn between ₹1, 00,000–1, 20,000 (1540-1850 USD) per annum. The income reported in nomads of other parts of the country was comparatively lower (Suresh *et al*., 2013).

Breeding management: Farmer owned flock was the primary source (68.4%) of breeding buck (Table1) followed by bucks purchased from a middleman (20.4%) and only in limited cases (10.2%), the buck was purchased from fellow farmer's flock. Irrespective of flock size, the number of breeding bucks used at a given time in the flock usually ranged between 1- 3 while the majority of the flocks maintained 2 bucks only. These breeding bucks were found to be used continuously for 4-5 breeding seasons before their replacement. This practice was common in flocks of all sizes. Almost all farmers reported that they select male bucks either from their own flock or neighboring flocks, the selection was based on indigenous knowledge, traditional wisdom or certain myths that were passed from one generation to another. Major selection parameters were strong body conformation, white colour (black coloured buck and white buck with black patches were not selected), ear size (long pendulous ears are preferred over short ears). Similar breeding buck selection strategies based on traditional wisdom were also reported in Somali goats of Ethiopia (Gebreyesus *et al*., 2012). The buck: doe mating ratio was observed to be wide as farmers usually kept only one or two breeding bucks in their flocks. The periodical rotation of breeding buck was also not observed and bucks were used continuously for four to five breeding seasons or sometimes even more, which led to inbreeding in the flock. Female goat selection was usually not practiced and almost all the potential breedable doings were used for breeding. Occasionally few animals (old and suffering from some ailments) were culled by way of selling.

Seasonal feature of goat management: The main breeding season (Table 3) observed in migratory Gaddi goats was summer (March–May), with occasional breeding during winter (Sept-Oct). Generally, *Gaddis* preferred to harvest only one kidding per year. The season of mating and kidding favored only single kid crop per year so that while migrating up hills few young kids could be sold on the way back to lower and mid hill settlement and rest are reared for 3-4 months in upper hills to attain marketing weight and can be sold while migrating downhill in summer. Normally, the migration was completed in 1 to 2 months by travelling miles of distance in day time followed by rest at night. The migration is directed from lower to higher hills just before the onset of summers and from higher to lower hills before the start of winters. After migrating to upper or lower hills, animals were grazed for next 3-4 months at earmarked areas ranging from 10 to 25 km, having a permit to stay. The farmers camp around the specified grazing sites in open following shorter migrations of few miles from the camping site Normally the camping sites were far away from their permanent settlements. All routes and camping sites were so planned and executed that on a particular date during each year, these flocks could be spotted at the same place, which is repeated year after year. These route permits were inherited to the next generation since time immemorial.

Effect of improved management practices in adopted flock en-route: The study continued for four years to see the effect of intervention on production potential of migratory goat systems and results are summarized in Tables 4 and 5. The results revealed significant improvement in body weights at different ages in every unit every year, which could be attributed to imparting strategic manage-mental and breeding inputs. The differences observed between different units were not significant and almost all units revealed similar improvement trends. This further strengthened the findings of the study that with improved management strategy the production potential of migratory systems can be increased. Analysis of various reproductive parameters revealed continual improvement in population growth (5.5%), kidding rate, percent twin birth (10.92%) and decrease in the incidence of abortion/still birth (5.6%) over the years (Table: 3). The pre-weaning kid losses which are major losses in migratory husbandry showed substantial improvement (Table 3) over base year (39.42%) along with improvement in kid birth weight. This improvement might be attributed to improved management strategies. It can also be seen that adoption of better management practices and periodical monitoring of flocks helped in reducing kid mortality. The effect of introducing improved buck on flock performance could be visualized only after a span of 3–4 breeding seasons, although initial results are quite promising with reduction in abortion/stillbirth and improvement in birth weight. Acceptability of the breeding buck is very high among the flock owners and they are now having more accommodative approach to response to breeding management compared to initial phases of implementation of study, when they were reluctant to change their buck.

Table 3. Seasonal managemental features of migratory system sheep and goat production system

	Jan	Feb	Mar	Apr	May	Jun	Jul	Aug	Sep	Oct	Nov	Dec
Matings			**	***	***	**			*	*		
Kidding		*	*	*					**	***	***	**
Shearing												
Dipping		***	***						***			
Camping	***	***	*			*		*			**	***
Migration			*	***	**				***	***		
Vaccination												
Sale/ marketing			***	***	*	*	*	*		**	**	

**least common* ***moderately common* ****most frequent*

Constraints associated with migratory production system

Veterinary and institutional facilities: Although, state Department of Animal Husbandry ensured proper health care of migratory flocks and had established several dedicated institutions for the same, but these are limited to low and middle hills and are insufficient owing to very long and tedious migratory routes in tough topography (usually flocks migrates from lower hill about 350 m to inner Himalayan ranges up to 5000 m above MSL). Moreover, during summers the flocks climb to alpine pastures and it is difficult for these institutions to provide health care facilities at such remote places except in emergency situations.

Table 4. Body weight at different ages in the adopted flocks en-route migration

Factor	Weight(Kg)				
	Birth	3M	6M	9M	12M
Year					
2011–12	2.70±0.02(158)	14.91±0.39(178)	18.18±0.21(118)	21.16±0.34(142)	26.21±0.23(150)
2012–13	2.91±0.03(171)	14.88±0.13(235)	19.32±0.20(142)	23.65±0.16(128)	27.32±0.23(169)
2013–14	2.98±0.02(206)	15.03±0.13(209)	19.17±0.17(173)	23.57±0.12(163)	26.80±0.18(213)
	*	NS	*	*	*
Sex					
Male	3.08.03(218)	15.18±0.34(268)	20.15±0.32(84)	23.64±0.49(61)	28.67±0.52(54)
Female	2.72±0.03(317)	14.46±0.29(354)	18.19±0.23(349)	22.56±0.26(372)	26.40±0.24(478)
	*	NS	*	NS	*
Unit					
Unit1	2.88±0.05(176)	14.81±0.28(214)	18.76±0.36(172)	22.54±0.39(145)	26.88±0.49(173)
Unit II	2.88±0.06(120)	14.98±0.39(189)	19.25±0.43(113)	23.39±0.54(143)	26.54±0.61(159)
Unit III	2.85±0.04(97)	15.00±0.26(172)	19.02±0.39(115)	22.79±0.49(121)	26.65±0.51(169)
Unit IV	2.89±0.05(42)	14.92±0.36(47)	19.15±0.51(33)	23.70±0.56(24)	27.43±0.59(30)
	NS	NS	NS	NS	NS
Overall	2.88±0.02(535)	14.94±0.31(622)	18.95±0.18(433)	22.80±0.21(433)	26.80±0.21(532)

Attack of predators: One of the factors responsible for major losses during migration especially the young progeny was predation. Various predators including leopard, wolf and even occasionally they did direct marketing from the farmer. The price of a live animal was estimated by sex, size and body condition of animals and is subjected to individual assessment. Both survey and en-route monitoring revealed that sales by migratory farmers were subjected to suboptimal prices by the buyers. Ansari-Renani *et al.*, (2013) also reported similar marketing constraints in nomadic pastoralism in southern Iran. Another problem was marketing of milk; usually, sheep and goat milk is not a saleable commodity in the region. Only use of surplus milk was self-consumption or gifting to acquaintances who helped during migration by providing utensils, household items and even mobile charging facilities when farmers camp near village settlements. Very few farmers reported use of milk for making cheese or ghee. Similar marketing constraints have also been reported in neighboring Nepal in Himalayan region (Nepali *et al.*, 2007).

Conclusion

In spite of constraints, the migratory system is still sustainable being a low input system which effectively counterbalances its constraints and makes it a profitable venture. Moreover, the strong association of migratory systems with tribal populations and their cultural heritage will ensure its propagation as long as the entity of the tribe is maintained.

Many projects were undertaken by central and state agencies to ensure improvement both at managemental and genetic level but their effect would be visualized after some time.

Few farmers readily accept various extension messages developed for improvement of migratory goat husbandry and are reluctant to adopt strategies suggested, still preferring their indigenous wisdom and technical knowhow. Strong policies, trained human resources are required to ensure adoption of recommended strategies on a larger scale.

Sustainable migratory sheep and goat farming would be influenced to a greater extent by developing solutions for existing constraints, and it will require institutional and extension support. The majority of farmers are less adaptive to managemental interventions but effective extension messages aimed at increasing the profitability of migratory farming systems would eventually be accepted by the farmers. So there is a need to focus the research to identify those technologies which have potential for improvement along with good acceptability and adoption rate.

There must be some effective mechanisms to assess the effect of improved strategies which ultimately would require allocation of sufficient funds and maximizing the research contribution. The studies should focus on developing:

(a) Strategy to ensure optimum feeding including supplementary concentrate feeding of at least pregnant animals and breeding bucks during migration. (b) Management of rangeland and grazing area and formulation of new policies to minimize conflicts with the locals and forest officials during migration. (c) Characterization and estimation of nutritional potential/anti-nutritional effects of various types of fodder which animals consume during migration. (d) Recognition of chevon and mutton from migratory animals as brand in contrast to mutton and chevon from stall fed animals to fetch premium prices.

References

Angara- Renani HR, Rishkowsky B, Muller PJ, Momen SMS, Moradi S (2013) Nomadic pastoralism in southern Iran. Pastoralism: Research, Policy and Practice 3:11. Bhasin V (1988) Himalayan Ecology: Transhumance and Social Organization of Gaddis in Himachal Pradesh. Kamal Raj Enterprise, New Delhi.

Bhasin V (2013) Pastoralist of Himalayas. Journal of biodiversity 4(2): 83-113. Cunningham A (1871) Archaeological Reports, Vol. II. Cited in: The Tribes and Castes of North-Western India.

Jithendran KP (1998) Epidemiology of gastrointestinal nematodes in migratory sheep and goats in north west humid Himalayan region. Indian Journal of Animal Sciences 68(9): 894-96.

Kaul S, Singh DR, Kumar N (2004) Economics of migratory sheep-rearing backward areas of Rajasthan. J. Ind. Soc. Agric. Stat. 58(1):98. (Abstr.)

Mandal A, Karunakaran M, Ghosh MK, Dutta TK. Breeding strategies for sustainable goat farming in India. Research and Reviews. Journal of Dairy Science and Technology. 2014;3(1).

Misri B (1998) Migratory system of goat and sheep-rearing in Himachal Pradesh, India, In www.fao.org/ag/agp/agpc/doc/puplicat/tapafan3/32.doc.

Nepali MB, Tiwari MR, Sapkota S, Poudel HP, Acharya BR, Gautam S (2007) Marketing constraints to goats in the Western Hill of Nepal. Nepal Agriculture Research Journal. 8:95-102.

Saberwal VK (1999). Pastoral Politics - Shepherds, Bureaucrats, and Conservation in the Western Himalaya. Oxford University, New Delhi.1999

Sabharwal A (2000) Twice Unlucky- A study of Displaced High Altitude Tribal Communities in Central Himalayas. Down to Earth, January 2000.

Sharma VP, Köhler-Rollefson I, Morton J (2003) Pastoralism in India: a scoping study. Indian Institute of Management and League of Pastoral Peoples, Ahmedabad, India.

Singh DR, Kaul S, Sivaramane N (2006) Migratory sheep and goat production system: the mainstay of tribal hill economy in Himachal Pradesh. Agricultural economics research review 19(347-2016-16773): 387-398.

6

Animal Nutrition Technologies Farmers' Perception and Future Strategies

O.H. Chaturvedi, D. Sethi and S.M.K. Naqvi
ICAR-North Temperate Regional Station, Central Sheep and Wool Research Institute, Garsa-175141, Himachal Pradesh

Introduction

Advancement in agricultural research has increased productivity however, in recent years, poor linkage of research - extension services hampering the growth of agriculture sector. Firstly, the research problems are investigated without considering the priority of agricultural producers Secondly, knowledge generated at the agriculture research stations is not effectively transferred to the producers. Many studies have identified the weaknesses in the linkages between the research and extension institutions are the major reason for development of technology and its transfer. In most countries including our country, the communication between research and extension agencies is weak (USAID 1982, FAO 1984). Research-extension-farmer linkages are seen to be absent or weak in many instances. At the same time, there are duplications of efforts, with a multiplicity of agents attending to extension work without adequate coordination (Planning Commission, 2008). This ineffective linkage between research and extension has impeded the generation and transfer of technology appropriate for small-scale and resource poor farmers, particularly those who work in relatively low productive and heterogeneous agro-ecological areas (Ewell 1989). Problems in technology generation and transfer arise because these components are considered in isolation (World Bank 1985). According to a World Bank Report (1985), bridging the gap between research and extension is the most serious institutional problem for developing an effective research and extension system.

Delivery of meaningful extension is not so easy. Farmers living in widely dispersed communities can be difficult to reach. Farmers' information needs vary across locations, making extension challenging. Supply side rationing may be a problem in the sense that there are likely to be too few extension agents relative to the number of farmers. On the demand side, self-selection on the part of larger, more commercial farmers may bias outcomes. Extension service budgets may be inadequate. Issues of motivation, competence, performance and accountability of extension institutions and their agents may affect results (Anderson, 2007).

Four types of technologies have raised yields in agriculture and animal husbandry in the past: better crop varieties and livestock breeds, fertilizer and feed, mechanization, and chemicals underpinning crop protection and animal health. Knowledge and information constitute the necessary fifth ingredient for technical progress to take hold. Knowledge and information include agronomic and animal husbandry know how and data on such aspects as soil characteristics, the weather, and markets and prices.

Field situation

The land holding pattern and land utilization, as well as livestock keeping, are important pre-requisite for transferring the animal nutrition related technologies for improving the livestock production. Therefore, the socio-economic status and farming systems prevailing in dry zones of the country are discussed as under.

Socio-economic status of the farmers

Livestock production is source of subsidiary incomes for farmers in dry zones of the country due to low and irregular rainfall and lack of irrigation facilities. Annual rainfall of the rain fed area normally ranges from 20 to 50 cm. In the arid region of the country, land holding (acre) and proportion of holding (%) of marginal, small, medium and large farmers are 0.37 and 0.21, 3.60 and 5.05, 6.80 and 19.06 and 20.77 and 75.68, respectively. The proportion of irrigated land (%) with marginal, small, medium and large farmers of this region is 0.0, 21.25, 47.90 and 17.74, respectively while the overall irrigated land is 27.19%. The proportion of irrigated land is slightly lower in the area as compared to National figures (35%) because the area is typically semiarid and mostly rain fed (Chaturvedi *et al.*, 2002). Average family size in the area is 9.67 while it is higher in case of large farmers followed by marginal, small, medium farmers (Chaturvedi *et al.*, 2002). The percentage of people in agriculture (number of persons engaged and dependent on agriculture) is higher in case of large farmers followed by medium, small and marginal farmers. However, due to shortage of resources like land and agricultural inputs, marginal and small farmers work as agricultural labourers for their livelihood. Thus, agriculture (crop production and animal husbandry) seems main occupation for livelihood of 89.5 percent population (Chaturvedi *et al.*, 2002). The human: land ratio (human/acre) in semiarid eastern plane zone of the country is 1.37 while it is higher in case of marginal farmers followed by small, medium and large farmers (Chaturvedi *et al.*, 2002). The human to land ratio in semiarid eastern plane zone is similar to that exists in Bundelkhand region (semi-arid) of the country (Saran *et al.*, 2000).

Farming systems

In semiarid eastern plane zone of the country, the arable land under fodder cultivation is only 2.4 percent and most of the arable land is used for cultivation of maize, sorghum, pearl millet, cowpea, groundnut, sesamum, pigeon pea, green gram and black gram during *kharif* and mustard, chickpea, wheat, barley and vegetables during *rabi* season. Major fodder crops are sorghum, pearl millet and cowpea in *kharif* and lucerne, berseem, kasni, senji and oats in *rabi* season. In *zaid* hardly field crops are grown where the irrigation is available the small portion of land is utilized for fodder and vegetable production (Chaturvedi *et al.*, 2002). On the other hand, 4 percent of the arable land is under fodder cultivation in the country

With regard to requirement and availability of nutrients in our country, it is reported that there is a deficit of DM, DP and TDN to the tune of 27.5, 54.5 and 26.3 percent, respectively (Jakhmola and Misra 2000). In the arid region of the country, the average holding of livestock and ACU are 39.2 and 12.7 per ha, respectively. The average number of ACU are higher in case of large farmers followed by marginal, medium and small farmers. The livestock: land (ACU/acre) is higher in case of marginal farmers followed by medium, small and large farmers in arid region of the country (Saran *et al.*, 2000, Chaturvedi *et al.*, 2002, Chaturvedi *et al.*, 2008). Thus, it appears that large farmers keep more livestock compared to small, marginal and medium farmers because of larger family size and more manpower. The proportion of cattle, buffaloes, sheep and goats among the livestock in the arid region of India are 22.5, 17.1, 31.4 and 29.0 percent, respectively (Chaturvedi *et al.*, 2002). The proportion of large (cattle and buffaloes) and small ruminants was 39.6 and 60.4% indicating that among the livestock, sheep and goats have major contribution to the economy of the farmers of the arid region. Among the livestock, sheep husbandry fits in better with economical and climatologically choice matrix of the people in Rajasthan (Sirohi and Rawat 2000). The proportion of small ruminants is higher in case of marginal farmers followed by medium, large and small farmers in the arid region of Rajasthan. Sheep, goats, idle bullocks and non producing cattle are mostly grazed in mixed grazing on community/public rangeland for about 8–10 hours a day. The animals are grazed from 0600-1800, 0800-1700 and 0800–1700 hr during summer, rainy and winter seasons, respectively. Buffaloes are either stall fed or supplemented with dry roughage after grazing. Soaked oilseeds and their cakes, as well as concentrates mixed with wheat straw, sorghum or pearl millet *kadbi*, were also offered to the milch animals during the periods of green fodder scarcity. The rate of concentrate fed to milch cattle and buffaloes are 2.5–3.0 kg per animal per day (Chaturvedi *et al.*, 2002, Chaturvedi *et al.*, 2008). Similar amount of concentrate is also offered to working bullocks. Milch goats are provided concentrate @ 200–500 g per head per day. Sheep are reared exclusively on grazing, however, depending on season some greens are made available to them. The farmers rarely face the shortage of dry fodder while green fodder remains short due to socioeconomic status and agro-climatic reasons. The farmers poorly rear livestock in general and small ruminants in particular and they are not supplemented with concentrate mixture during critical stages of growth and advanced pregnancy. Although the goats are fed concentrate mixture during lactation while sheep are not fed concentrate mixture. This may be due to socio-economic status as well as lack of knowledge of improved and beneficial feeding practices. Under farmer's field conditions providing the supplement in the form of concentrate mixture @ 1–1.5% of the body weight to lambs is beneficial. The additional profit in terms of per Rupee spent was ₹1.42–1.74 due to supplementation (Chaturvedi *et al.*, 2000, Chaturvedi *et al.*, 2010). The biomass yield of the community rangeland utilized in mixed grazing is low (4.2 to 6.4 q DM/ha) which is insufficient to meet the nutrient requirement of ewes during late gestation. However, concentrate supplementation @ 1% of body weight to ewes during the period improved their production performance and growth rate of their lambs (Chaturvedi *et al*., 2001, Chaturvedi *et al*., 2011). Therefore, there is need to motivate the farmers for usefulness of supplementary feeding to sheep and goats during critical stages so as to boost the small ruminant production and thus maximum profit can be harvested.

Farmers' preference for adoption of available technology

Today, India stands at first position in milk production in the World. This has been achieved through generation of ambitious technology in the field of animal husbandry *viz*. improvement in breeds, improved feeding practices and health and management. Feeding livestock is an integral part of animal husbandry and it alone costs about 60-65 percent of the total cost of livestock production. Thus, it is an important part of livestock production while cost effectiveness of livestock production is considered. Farmers can economize the cost of livestock production and can increase their net returns through animal husbandry if they adopt nutrition related improved technologies. In view of deficit against the availability of nutrients in our country, the available feed resources have to be utilized efficiently by adopting the nutrition related technologies to bridge the gigantic gap between the availability and requirements of feed. The nutrition related improved technologies, which are transferable among the farmers for increasing the animal productivity at their farms.

1. Feeding of poor quality roughage after its urea treatment
2. Feeding of poor quality roughage after its urea-molasses-mineral enrichment
3. Feeding of cost effective pellet feed/complete feed blocks
4. Supplementation of concentrates during critical physiological stages *viz*. growth, advance pregnancy and lactation.
5. Regular supplementation of minerals and salts
6. Feeding of chaffed fodders

The all above technologies have their usefulness but the farmers' perception of adoption is detailed as under.

Farmers prefer a technology that provides visible profits with minimum inputs. For example, use of hybrid varieties in place of *desi* varieties in case of crop production provides high yield and thus substantial return. Similarly the improved varieties of fruits and flowers are preferred for higher profit. On the other hand, feeding of urea treated or urea-molasses-mineral enriched straw gives less return that is invisible. Therefore the farmers are reluctant to adopt these technologies but farmers become very much interested in adopting these when there is scarcity of good quality feeds and fodders. Thus, farmers also keep their minds open for adopting the need-based technologies. Farmers also rear improved breeds of livestock to get more income, although only those farmers adopt this who are resourceful. However, in case of technology related to health management, it hardly matters for the farmers that whether or not they are resourceful, if they understand that by this treatment of the disease or by this prophylactic measure, the productivity and life of the animal can be sustained then the farmers adopt the technology related to health management. However, if the animals are unproductive and unhealthy in case of small ruminants and not being cured by minimum inputs, then farmers often sell such animals for slaughter. On the other hand, in case of large ruminant farmers spent money on treatment as much as they can. Farmers are reluctant to adopt the technology related to reproduction *i.e.*, A. I. It happens so because of obvious reasons. Besides this, farmers also consider simplicity of the technology during its adoption. On the basis of magnitude of profit and nature of handling, farmers' preference for adopting the technology can be ranked as under:

1. Heavy profit and simple
2. Moderate profit and simple
3. Less profit and simple
4. Heavy profit and complex
5. Moderate profit and complex
6. Less profit and complex

Farmers' perception/ feedback to nutrition related technology

Farmers are very much concerned about the cost effectiveness of the technology because of their socio-economic status and lack of resources. For example, concentrate supplementation during various physiological stages is profitable but purchase of readymade concentrate mixture or preparation of cost effective concentrate mixture at the farm place itself depends upon the availability of resources. Further, preparation of concentrate mixture is not an easy task for all kinds of the farmers because it requires proper training under the supervision of animal nutritionist. Improvement of poor quality crop residue through urea treatment or urea molasses enrichment is useful during scarcity. However, urea treatment is a time consuming work and requires higher quantity of water while the infrequent availability of molasses and mineral mixture are the major problems that exist with these technologies. Farmers' perception regarding mineral supplementation of livestock is good in improving the general health and productivity of their livestock but the infrequent availability of the mineral mixture or mineral bricks are the problem for not widely adopting this technology.

Inputs like mineral mixture or mineral bricks, complete feed blocks, readymade concentrate mixture, molasses *etc.* should be made available within the periphery of 4-5 km. Similarly, the infrequent availability of complete feed pellets/ blocks and less technical knowledge of these materials among the farmers make them reluctant to adopt these technologies.

Status of application of technology/practice by farmers

Farmers are very much concerned about the cost effectiveness of the technology because of their socio-economic status and lack of resources. Farmers are convinced that improvement of poor quality crop residue like straw/stovers through urea reatment or urea molasses mineral enrichment is useful for enhancing the production performance of the ruminants especially during scarcity. However, urea treatment is a time consuming and requires higher quantity of water hence these are the constraints for adopting the urea treatment of poor quality roughage. Infrequent availability of molasses and mineral mixture are the major problems that exist with the adoption of urea molasses mineral enrichment of straws and *kadabis*. Landless, marginal and small farmers are reluctant to adopt these technologies due to resource crunch whereas resourceful farmers are not adopting due to cumbersome technologies. Most the farmers allow their ruminants for grazing and supplement their animals besides the grazing. Thus, in this feeding system the role of poor quality roughage is secondary. Even during scarcity of grazing and green fodder, farmers prefer feeding of poor quality roughage and concentrate supplementation because of simplicity and easy handling. Farmers prefer feeding of straws of pearl millet, sorghum, paddy, barley and wheat in the form of *Sani i.e.*, mixing it with water and little quantity of concentrates. *Sani* is being adopted by the farmers since ages as it improves palatability and nutrient utilization. Farmers are reluctant to feed newer feed resources such as mustard straw because of poor feeding value. Instead of feeding mustard straw to animals, farmers prefer to sale mustard straw to buyers using it for other purposes *viz.* fuel, briquetting, packaging materials *etc.* Farmers adopt supplementation of concentrates during active phase of growth, late gestation and early lactation. However, there exists a gap in rate of supplementation due to socio-economic status of the farmers. Regular supplementation of mineral mixture is not being practiced by the farmers due to lack of knowledge about benefits of feeding and distant availability. Government agencies giving subsidies on chaff cutters being purchased by the farmers. Since farmers experience themselves the wastage of fodders fed un-chaffed. Hence, most of the farmers usually chaff their fodders before feeding them to their animals.

Lesson learned

Improvement of poor quality roughage especially straw is cumbersome and labour intensive in nature. Marginal and small farmers have poor facilities to adopt the technology. The returns by adopting this technology are negligible *i.e.*, not visible. This technology may prove adoptable if the agencies are established for treatment of straw at village level. Similarly, preparation of pellets or complete feed blocks is also cumbersome and requires heavy input. Farmers are short of resources to adopt this technology. Further, farmers are economically poor and short of knowledge about benefits of feeding concentrate pellets and complete feed block. These technologies can be adopted by the farmers if pellets and complete feed blocks are made available to them at cheaper rate in their vicinity. Farmers should be made aware of the benefits of mineral supplementation to their animals as well as chaffing of the fodders for feeding to animals.

Future strategies

Agricultural research findings are of little use if farmers do not adopt these. Unfortunately, the only effect of such research is to produce an interesting article in a scientific journal or a report that lodges on shelves in the library. Hence research must be related to farmers' problems if it is to be adopted by the farmers for improving their production (Van Den Ban 1994). Traditionally, the resource poor farmers had a lack of power and the organizational ability to pressure the research systems to meet their needs. Their access to research information is limited, and the pressing concerns of their daily existence make it very difficult for them to focus on long-term technological changes. Most of the developing countries are concerned about rural poverty, malnutrition, unsustainable agricultural production and urbanization. Part of the problem is due to lack of effectiveness of agricultural research. Further, the research being conducted is not relevant to the farming situation. This lack of relevance of research is due to poor linkages between the research and its clients *i.e.*, farmers and extension. Thus the linkages between agricultural research institutes, farmers and extension subsystems are vital for successful technology generation and transfer. Direct links with farmers, developed through on-farm research, ensure relevance and rapid feedback. Linkages with extension agencies ensure impact on wider dissemination of location specific technologies. The effectiveness of transfer of technology (TOT) is greatly influenced by the linkages between and among research, extension, client and input subsystems that are actively engaged in agricultural development (Kunju 1992). The absence of these linkages leads to unresponsiveness, irrelevant technologies that result in poor adoption or non-adoption. It is estimated that only 30 percent of the transferable technology has been disseminated among the farmers. Following are the points that are essential for technology generation and transfer.

1. Strong linkages between and among research, extension, client and input subsystems should be developed.
2. Comprehensive communication and extension of transferable and adoptable technologies by various extension media among the clients are required. The communication may be direct (group discussion, demonstration, showing video films *etc.*) or indirect (technology prescription and slogans on television and radio, newspaper and magazine *etc.*).
3. Traditional technology that is disappearing with the changing scenario should be disseminated among the farmers.
4. The materials to be used in a technology should be easily available and also at a cheaper rate.
5. Training of the farmers for specific technologies should be strengthened through on-campus and off-campus trainings.

It is relevant here to note that the five 'E' principles *i.e.*, economical, energy saving, equity, employment and eco-friendly, should be applied in technology generation that makes it efficacy for adoption point of view.

References

Anderson JR (2007) Agricultural Advisory Services, Background paper for the World Development Report 2008, Agriculture and Rural Development Department, World Bank, Washington, D.C.

Chaturvedi OH, Bhatta R, Sankhyan SK, Karim SA (2010) Nutrient utilization and production performance of lambs grazing on community rangeland with and without concentrate supplementation. Indian Journal of Animal Sciences 80: 693-696.

Chaturvedi OH, Mishra AS, Karim SA, Jakhmola R C (2000) Effect of supplementary feeding on growth performance of lambs under field conditions. Indian Journal of Small Ruminants 6: 110-112.

Chaturvedi OH, Mishra AS, Santra A, Karim SA Jakhmola RC (2001) Effect of supplementary feeding during late gestation on production performance of ewes grazing on community rangeland. Indian Journal of Animal Sciences 71: 714-17.

Chaturvedi OH, Sankhyan SK, Mann JS and Karim SA (2008) Livestock holding pattern and feeding practices in semiarid eastern region of Rajasthan. Indian Journal of Small Ruminants 14: 224-229.

Chaturvedi OH, Sankhyan S K, Mann JS, Karim SA (2011) Production performance of ewes grazing on community rangeland supplemented with concentrate during late gestation and early lactation. Indian Journal of Animal Sciences 81: 531-533.

Chaturvedi OH, Tripathi MK, Mishra AS, Verma DL, Rawat PS, Jakhmola RC (2002) Land as well as livestock holding pattern and feeding practices of livestock in malpura taluk of semiarid eastern plane zone. Indian Journal of Small Ruminants 8: 143-146.

Ewell P T (1989) Links between on- farm research and extension in nine countries. ISNAR, The Hague.

F A O (1984) *Agricultural Extension*: A Reference manual, 2nd ed. Food and Agricultural Organisation, Rome.

Jakhmola RC Misra AK (2000) *Feeding Strategies Using Unconventional Feeds*. In: Proceedings of III Biennial Conference of Animal Nutrition Association held at CCSHAU, Hisar, India from 7-9 November. Pp.83-98.

Kunju OAR (1992) Transfer of agricultural technology: Structural and functional linkages- a case of improved rice varieties. Concept publishing company, New Delhi. Planning Commission (2008) Eleventh Five Year Plan (2007-2012), Vols. I&III, Government of India, New Delhi.

Saran S, Singh RA, Singh R, Rani SI, Singh K K (2000) Feed resources for rearing livestock in Bundelkhand region of Uttar Pradesh. *I*ndian Journal of Animal Sciences 70: 526-29.

Sirohi Smita, Rawat PS (2000). Resource use efficiency in sheep farming: A case study of district Tonk, Rajasthan. Indian Journal of Small Ruminants 6: 42-47.

USAID (1982) *AID experience in agricultural research: a review of project evaluations*. United States Agency for International Development, Evaluation Discussion Paper, No.13. Van den ban AW, Hawkins HS (1994) *Agricultural Extension*. Longman Scientific and Technical Co. New York. Pp.26-33.

World Bank (1985) Agricultural research and extension: an evaluation of the World Banks' experience. The World Bank, Washington D C., USA.

7

Role of Prebiotics in Gastrointestinal Health and Function

A.K. Samanta, Sohini Roy, C. Jayaram, A.P. Kolte, Manpal Sridhar S. Senani and A. Dhali

Feed Additives and Nutraceuticals laboratory
ICAR-National Institute of Animal Nutrition and Physiology, Adugodi Hosur Road, Bengaluru–560030. Karnataka

Introduction

The livestock occupies a significant niche in the social fabric of the Indian subcontinent from the dawn of civilization. During the initial days of civilization, animals served human society in many ways. The livestock is not only producing high biological value products *i.e.*, milk, meat but also provide manure for maintaining soil health, draught power for crop production, wool and fiber for apparel industry, low cost means of transport in rural and desert areas, companion for sports and of course a "readily disposable asset" for any kind of emergency expenditure. Hence, livestock represents one of the major driving forces for the growth of the rural economy. As a result, the livestock industry becomes one of the niche sectors of the national economy to propel faster growth along with securing the livelihood of millions of people. During the twentieth century, balanced ration was the key focal point of animal nutrition research either for enhancing the productivity or managing the livestock economy through interventions of knowledge in the areas of improvement of poor quality roughages, bypass protein, bypass fat, mineral supplements, complete feed blocks, vitamins, area specific mineral mixture, feed additives such as antibiotics, ionophores, hormones *etc.* However, during the beginning of the twenty first century, several issues appeared pertaining to the livestock sector such as feed quality and safety, designer animal products, healthy animal products, ecological treatment for digestive disorder, organic animal production, residues of antibiotics, hormones and heavy metals in accordance with the consumer preference and awareness. In the light of concerns on "transfer of antibiotic resistance genes from animal to human", several nations have imposed bans on application of antibiotics as feed additives. Keeping in view the above perspective, research is underway around the world to find alternatives to antibiotics to guard the gastrointestinal of animals without compromising productivity or product quality of livestock. Under such circumstances, prebiotic is receiving greater attention in India and abroad as gastrointestinal health guards in order to produce safe and healthy animal products after due consideration to the environment, animal welfare, consumer awareness and public health.

Concept of prebiotic

Although beneficial effects of consuming fermented milk amongst Bulgarian farmers for higher longevity was realized as early as 1905 by E. Metchnikoff, but the novel concept of prebiotic came into light only during the mid-nineties of the previous century. Accordingly, prebiotic is defined as "a non-digestible food ingredient that beneficially affects the host by selectively stimulating the growth and or activity of one or a limited number of bacteria in the colon" (Gibson and Roberfroid, 1995). It was realized that the definition of prebiotics is more or less similar to the definition of dietary fiber except the selective stimulation by the former. With the growing interests and intense research and development activities on prebiotic, it was proposed to revisit its definition and suggested to exclude the word 'non-digestible'. The updated definition of prebiotic encompasses as "a selectively fermented ingredient that allows specific change, both in the composition and or activity in the GI microflora that confers benefits upon host well being and health" (Gibson *et al.*, 2004). Later on, the concept of prebiotic was suggested as "non-viable food components, ingredients or supplements that selectively modulate the microbiota of the digestive ecosystem, thus conferring benefits upon host well being and health" (Roberfroid, 2007). During the same period, FAO constituted a committee to look into the aspects of prebiotic. According to FAO (2007), "a prebiotic is a non-viable food component that confers a health benefit on the host associated with modulation of microbiota". Further, an attempt has been made to broaden the site of action of prebiotics such as skin, oral cavity and female genital tract in addition to its fundamental action at the GI tract (Pineiro *et al.*, 2008). However, the proposers of the prebiotic concept opposed the philosophy of broadening its application sites such as vagina and skin and wanted to restrict once again to the gastrointestinal microflora only. Accordingly, the accepted definition remains closer to the original concept as it was proposed during mid nineties of previous century and it defines prebiotic as "a selectively fermented ingredient that results in specific changes in the composition and /or activity of the gastrointestinal microbiota thus conferring benefit(s) upon host health" (Gibson *et al.*, 2010). It sounds emphasis was given on prebiotics keeping in view its application in human beings only. Therefore, the following criteria were suggested later on for a molecule/ substrate to qualify as prebiotic keeping in view the digestive system of both ruminants and non-ruminants (Samanta *et al.*, 2007, 2013, 2015).

- Indigestible by animals own gastric or pancreatic enzymes
- Selectively utilized by so called beneficial gut microflora (exception several rumen bacteria ferments prebiotics)
- Plant source or produced by enzymatic action
- Non-absorption from the epithelial surface of gastrointestinal tract
- Protects structural and functional integrity while passing through either acidic or alkaline pH of gastrointestinal tract
- Exhibit its potentiality even at minute concentration

- Remains intact while undergoing physical action of digestion process *i.e.*, mastication, chewing, mixing with several fluids etc
- Presence of chemicals bonds that is inaccessible to harmful gut microflora
- No residue problems
- Non-carcinogenic
- Its fermentation should not lead to generating metabolites of toxic nature
- Easy to mix with other feed ingredients or micronutrient mixture

Historical evidence of prebiotic consumption in India

Gut microflora have been co-evolved along with human evolution to perform several health-promoting functions and prevent the body from the adverse effects of enteric pathogens. Diet plays a great role to maintain the composition of gut microflora. Albeit the concept of prebiotic has been introduced recently, the consumption of prebiotic through diverse food materials has been reported from the beginning of human civilization. Historical evidence suggested that ancient population Indus valley civilization was well informed about the importance of prebiotic rich agricultural crops (Samanta *et al.*, 2011). Evidence suggested that the major cereals during Indus valley civilization include wheat, barely in addition to some lentils and tubers. Nutritional analysis revealed that wheat crop stores the carbohydrates in the form of fructan (a prebiotic) in addition to its higher content of beta glucan. The other food items of the Indus valley population included milk, meat, fish, fruits and dates. Today, it is well known that milk is one of the important sources of galactooligosaccharides (GOS), which have an immense role in maintenance of gut health and function (Boehm and Stahl, 2007). This substantiates that our ancient Indian population was consuming enough quantities of prebiotics through their routine diets during the periods of Indus valley civilization (Pokharia, 2008, Samanta *et al.*, 2011). The present day scientists are attempting to mimic the similar line of dietary schedules for augmenting gut health and to keep away from the degenerative diseases. Research findings indicated that more than 36,000 plant species store the carbohydrate fractions in the form of inulin or fructans (Hendry, 1987). Therefore, it is ample clear that our ancient Indian population was regularly consuming the prebiotic at higher levels than the modern Indian population through their selected dietary ingredients.

Commonly used prebiotic

Even though it is not mentioned in the definition of prebiotic in its chemical form, the prebiotic essentially belongs to the class of carbohydrate compounds. Essentially, prebiotics are indigestible carbohydrate compounds (mainly short chain oligosaccharides; except tagatose) which can be produced either by enzymatic reactions or synthesized from plant biomass through a series of processes including extraction, precipitation, isomerization, hydrolysis, catalysis, etc (Table 1). Currently many prebiotic compounds are available and most popular among them are inulin, fructooligosaccharides, xylooligosaccharides, galactooligosaccharides, soya oligosaccharides, arabino-xylooligosaccharides, pectin oligosaccharides, mannan oligosaccharides, arabinogalactans and tagatose.

Table 1. List of prebiotics and their source

Name of prebiotic	Source/ raw materials	Method of production
Inulin	Chicory root, onion, garlic, bamboo shoots, Jerusalem artichoke, banana, leek *etc.*	Extraction
Fructooligosaccharides	Sucrose	Enzymatic catalysis (fructosyl transferase)
	Inulin	Enzymatic hydrolysis (Inulinase)
Galactooligosaccharides	Lactose	Enzymatic (Beta galactosidase)
Xylooligosaccharides	Corn cobs, corn husks, wheat bran, rice barn, sugarcane bagasse, wheat straw, rice straw, almond shell, peanut shell *etc.*	Autohydrolysis, mild acid hydrolysis, enzymatic (xylanase)
Pectin oligosaccharides	Cell walls of fruits and vegetables like apple pomace, citrus peels, sugar beet pulp, potato fibers, sunflower head	Mild acid hydrolysis, enzymes (endo-polygalacturonase, exopolygalacturonase *etc.*)
Arabionogalactans	Leek seeds, carrots, ryegrass, carrot, radish, black gram beans, pears, wheat, tomato, ragweed, sorghum, bamboo grass, coconut meta and milk, larch tree *etc.*	Natural secretion of Acacia plants, water extraction, enzyme application.
Mannan oligosaccharides	Guar seed, locust bean, tara gum, tuber of konjac, copra meal, coffee seed, yeasts cell walls *etc.*	Steam, microwave irradiation, thermal hydrolysis, mild acids, enzymatic (mannase).
Tagatose	D-galactose	Enzymatic (L-arabinose isomerase)
Arabino-xylooligosaccharides	Wheat barn, Psyllium husks	Enzymatic (xylanase)

Effect prebiotics in ruminants

The encouraging results of prebiotics on human health especially the gut microbial ecology have prompted the livestock researchers to explore its potentiality on different livestock species. Presently frugal information is available on the potential effects of prebiotics in ruminant animals. All the rumen hemicelluloses degrading bacteria are capable to utilize the xylooligosaccharides as growth substrate (Cotta and Whitefield, 1998). These are *Butyrovibrio fibrisolvens*, *Eubacterium ruminantium*,

Ruminococcus albus etc. Under in vitro fermentation system, it was noticed that there was reduction of total gas production by 8 to 10% following addition of inulin in roughage based total mixed ration without any adverse effects on either dry matter digestibility or total volatile fatty acid production (Samanta *et al.*, 2012). The rumen pH is unaltered (6.7), when galactooligosaccharides is given to the Holstein cows maintained on orchard grass silage or alfalfa silage (Santoso *et al.*, 2003). Mwenya *et al.*, (2005) also did not notice any significant changes of rumen pH in steers when fed the galactooligosaccharides; however, recorded significantly higher oxidation reduction potential. The rumen ammonia nitrogen concentration is slightly lower in galactooligosaccharides supplemented Holstein cows and steers, which might be due to the utilization of ammonia for microbial protein synthesis in the rumen (Santoso *et al.*, 2003, Mwenya *et al.*, 2005). Lower rumen ammonia nitrogen concentration in sheep is also observed in sheep as a result of prebiotic supplementation, which may be due to the suppression of ammonia producing bacteria (Mwenya *et al.*, 2004).

Though the total rumen volatile fatty acid concentration (10–12 mEq/100 ml rumen liquor) is not much affected by the prebiotics supplementation (Samanta *et al.*, 2015a), but the proportion of individual volatile fatty acids are altered (Mwenya *et al.*, 2005). The lower ratio of acetate to propionate in cows supplemented with galactooligosaccharides during 1st and 6th hours after post feeding perhaps indicated suppression of methane production. Loss of energy in the form of methane is significantly lower in steers maintained on high concentrate diets containing galactooligosaccharides (2.2 vs.2.4 MJ/100MJ Gross Energy intake). This may be a result from stimulation of *Bifidobacteria* that increase the propionate production at the expense of acetate (Mwenya *et al.*, 2005). Therefore, methane emission (liters/day) is reduced by 11% in galactooligosaccharides supplemented diets of dairy cows. Similarly, methane production is also reduced by 10% in sheep as a result of galactooligosaccharides incorporation. The inclusion of inulin in the milk replacer of pre ruminant calves diet leads to significantly higher body weight gains and better feces consistency (Kaufhold *et al.*, 2000, Verdonk and Leeuwen 2004). Inclusion of the soy carbohydrates in the di*et al*so tended to increase the endogenous flow of nitrogen at the terminal ileum (Verdonk *et al.*, 1998). It is postulated that this increase might be caused by fermentation in the small intestine increasing the flow of bacterial nitrogen to the large gut. Inulin-type fructans may play a role in creating and maintaining a desired, stable microflora in the rumen, small and large intestine of pre ruminant calves.

Effect prebiotics in non-ruminants

Swine

Pigs are exposed to many kinds of stressors from growth to maturity. During such circumstances, there is breach in the gut microbial homeostasis as a result of changes in gut microflora composition. Presently the European Union has banned the use of antibiotics in feed and some countries are considering banning it as feed supplements. Under such circumstances, prebiotics either derived from plant or synthesized through the action of microbial enzymes could occupy the vacuum of antibiotics for improving the productivity of livestock keeping in mind the residue problems of antibiotics, development of cross resistance as well as consumer awareness. Administration of oligofructose results in a higher number (1.68×10^{10} vs. 4.85×10^{9} CFU/g fecal contents) of *Bifidobacteria* on the 6th day of consumption (Howard *et. al.*, 1995). In an effort to see the potentiality of prebiotic inulin on recovery from diarrhoea induced by cholera enterotoxin at the age of three weeks piglets, the population of *Lactobacilli* is significantly higher in both caecum (9.3 vs. 7.7 $\log_{10}$ CFU per gram) and at colon (9.3 vs. 8.3 $\log_{10}$ CFU per gram) following supplementation of 9.5 g of oligofructose (Oli *et al.*, 1998). On the other hand population of harmful bacteria *i.e.*, *Enterobacteria* is reduced significantly at both caecum (6.2 vs. 7.4 $\log_{10}$ CFU per gram) and colon (6.2 vs. 8.5 $\log_{10}$CFU per gram) in piglets consuming oligofructose. Recently, the present authors undertook an experiment to see the potentiality of prebiotic as an alternative to antibiotics in grower pigs. The study revealed significant changes in the microbial abundance based on operational taxonomic units (OTUs) among the groups (Samanta *et al.*, 2015c). Presumptive identification of organisms was established based on the fragment length of OTUs generated with three restriction enzymes (MspI, Sau3AI and BsuRI). The abundance of OTUs representing *Bacteroides intestinalis*, *Eubacterium oxidoreducens*, *Selonomonas sp.*, *Methylobacterium sp.* and *Denitrobacter* sp. was found significantly greater in inulin supplemented pigs. In contrast, the abundance of OTUs representing pathogenic microorganisms *Atopostipes suicloacalis* and *Bartonella quintana str. Toulouse* was significantly reduced in inulin supplemented pigs. The OTUs were found to be clustered in two major phylotypes; inulin and control-tetracycline (Chikkeruer *et al.*, 2014, Samanta *et al.*, 2015b).

The pig waste is associated with malodor owing to being contributed by several microbial metabolites namely short chain fatty acids, phenols, indoles, sulfides *etc.* Supplementation of chicory inulin in the diets of pig resulted in a significant decrease of ammonia concentration in both caecum and colon. Supplementation of prebiotics also enhanced both dry matter and organic matter digestibility at ileum (Houdijk *et al.*, 1997).

Poultry

The microflora of the poultry gut is presumed to play multidimensional roles including digestion, metabolism, pathogen exclusion, immune stimulation, vitamin synthesis *etc.* Under *in vitro* culture system, it is established that *Salmonella* serotype does not grow in the presence of oligofructose as sole source of energy, while so called beneficial microflora namely *Lactobacillus lactis*, *Entercoccus faecium* and *Pediococcus* grow well because of their ability to produce enzymes capable to break down the osidic bonds present in prebiotics (Oyarzabal and Conner, 1995). Therefore, it is noteworthy to incorporate prebiotic for overcoming *Salmonella* in chickens. Inclusions of oligofructose in the diets of chicks enabled substantial reduction in *Salmonella* colonization at the gastrointestinal tract (Bailey *et al.*, 1991, Fukata *et al.*, 1999).

Supplementation of inulin as prebiotics in the diet of layers and broiler birds improved the growth performance (Yusrizai and Chen, 2003, Verdonk and Leeuwen, 2004). Contradictorily, some of the research endeavors fail to get a positive response on growth performance following inulin supplementation in birds (Ortiz *et al.*, 2009). The variability in the effectiveness of inulin may be ascribed to several factors namely level of inclusion, type of diet, animal individuality, degree of hygiene *etc*. The dietary inclusion of graded levels of inulin has no significant effect on the relative weight and relative length of the duodenum, jejunum, ileum and ceca of poultry birds (Yusrizai and Chen, 2003, Ortiz *et al.*, 2009).

Inulin, being a prebiotic, is not digested by the birds own gastric or pancreatic enzymes but utilized by the specific group of microflora namely bifidobacteria and lactobacilli at the large intestine for production of various short chain fatty acids and lactic acids (Samanta *et al.*, 2010). The production of fatty acids at the large intestine leads to lowering of luminal pH. Acidic pH is found to increase mineral solubility and facilitates higher mineral absorption. In this respect butyrate is more effective than acetate for enabling higher Ca absorption. Recently it has been established that supplementation of xylooligosaccharides (0.5% of diet) generated from either corn husks or green coconut husks results into an increased population of beneficial microflora and a decreased population of pathogenic microflora at ceacum in broiler birds (Jayapal *et al.*, 2014). Further, the supplementation of xylooligosaccharides in broiler birds also ensures favorable blood biochemical profile in terms of cholesterol and triglycerides.

Mechanism of action of prebiotic

The prebiotic supplementation in animals exhibits beneficial effects to the animals either production of improvement of product quality through following actions:

- Selective stimulation of beneficial gut microflora
- Enhanced production of short chain fatty acids
- Increased mineral absorption
- Immune stimulation
- Inhibition of Harmful pathogen
- Lipid metabolism

Advantages of prebiotics

The primary aim of livestock production is to deliver safe and healthy food for the human population keeping in mind public health, consumer awareness and demand, environmental issues and animal welfare. On the other hand, increase in the incidence of human infections by antibiotic-resistant bacteria leads to the banning of antibiotic applications in food animal production. The ban on antibiotic application has heightened existing searches for alternatives to antibiotics that give similar or enhanced production qualities as highly reliable as the antibiotics currently provided to food animals. Functional foods, especially the prebiotics are effectively recognized as useful dietary adjuncts to manipulate the gut microflora towards healthy balance (Samanta *et al.*, 2012a). As most of the prebiotics are derived from plant sources, these are safe and possibly have adverse effects. The major advantages of prebiotics are as follows (Samanta *et al.*, 2007):

- Biological origin
- Low energy value
- Stimulate the growth and activity of beneficial gut microflora
- Reduces the population of harmful gut microflora
- Enhances mineral absorption
- Non-carcinogenic
- Enhances nitrogen utilization
- Alters rumen acetate to propionate ratio for directing less methanogenesis
- Modulate immune system
- No residual effect
- Reduces triglycerides in blood

Market potential of prebiotics

Prebiotics are gaining a huge popularity within the functional food market as they can offer an array of benefits. As the future outlook for the prebiotics market is highly encouraging and demand driven, several nutraceuticals manufacturers are on the way to capitalize the market to fulfill the growing demands. According to recent market research, the prebiotics demand is expected to reach USD 4.5 billion in 2018 with an annual growth rate of 10 -12%.

Future perspective

As the research findings on prebiotics will continue to accumulate, the concept of prebiotic will be more clear, enabling classification of certain biomolecules where the evidence is currently sparse or absent. Moreover, a better understanding of structure to function relationship of prebiotic along with the identification of the metabolic profile of target microorganism will help to determine the specific health attributes of the prebiotic. Future research should focus on cost effective production of prebiotic coupled with establishment of mechanisms of action through advanced scientific knowledge. The regular effective doses of prebiotic also need to be evaluated. In the present day, most popular targets of prebiotic are lactic acid bacteria and bifidobacteria. However, by increasing our knowledge about gut microbial diversity using different molecular approaches, other bacteria can also be identified as a target for a specific prebiotic. Further research on prebiotic should also focus on the immunological and other disease related aspects.

References

Bailey JS, Blankenship IC, Cox NA (1991) Effect of fructooligosaccharides on salmonella colonization of the chicken intestine. Poultry Science, 70: 68 (suppl.): 167.

Boehm G, Stahl B (2007) Supplement: Effects of Probiotics and Prebiotics Oligosaccharides from Milk. The Journal of Nutrition, 137: 8475-8495

Chikkerur J, Jayapal N, Samanta AK, Kolte AP, Senani S, Prasad CS (2014) Monitoring gut microflora changes by T-RFLP analysis in grower pigs supplemented with prebiotics. Proceedings of 2nd Annual Conference of Probiotic Association of India and International Symposium on "Probiotics and microbiome: Gut and beyond, held at New Delhi. Pp 91.

Cota MA, Whitefield TR (1998). Xylooligosaccharides utilization by ruminal anaerobic bacterium *Selemonas ruminantium*. Current Microbiology, 36: 183-189

FAO (2007) Food and Agriculture Organization Technical Meeting on prebiotics. www.fao.org/ag/agn/agns/index_en.stm

Fukata T, Sasai K, Miyamoto T, Baba E (1999) Inhibitory effects of competitive exclusion and fructooligosaccharides, singly and in combination on Salmonella colonization of chicks. Journal of Food Protection, 62: 229-233

Gibson GR, Roberfroid MB (1995) Dietary modulation of the human colonic microbiota: introducing the concept of prebiotics. Journal of Nutrition, 87: S287-S291

Gibson GR, Probert HM, Rastall RA, Roberfroid MB (2004) Dietary modulation of the human colonic microbiota: updating the concept of prebiotics. Nutrition Research Review, 17: 259-275.

Gibson GR, Scott KP, Rastall RA, Tuohy KM, Hotchkiss A, Dubert-Ferrandon A, Gareau M, Murphy EF, Saulnier D, Loh G, Macfarlane S, Delzenne N, Ringel Y, Kozianowski G, Dickmann R, Lenoir-Wijnkoop I, Walker C, Buddington R (2010) Dietary prebiotics: Current status and new definition. IFIS Functional Foods Bulletin, 7(1): 1–19.

Hendry G (1987) The ecological significance of fructan in a contemporary flora. New Physiology, 106: 201-216.

Houdijk JGM, Hartemin, R, Van Laere KMJ, Williams BA, Bosch MW, Verstagen MWA Tamminga S (1997) Fructooligosaccharides and trans-oligosaccharides in weaner's pig diets. In: Proceedings of International symposium "Non-digestible Oilgosaccharides: healthy food for the colon" Pp 69-78, Wageningen, The Netherlands.

Howard MD, Gordon DT, Pace IW, Garleb KA, Kerley MS (1995) Effects of dietary supplementation with fructooligosaccharides on colonic microbiota populations and epithelial cell proliferation in neonatal pigs. Journal of Pediatric gastroenterology Nutrition, 21: 297-303.

Jayapal N, Sondhi N, Chikkerur J, Samanta AK, Kolte AP, Senani S (2014) Xylooligosaccharides from green coconut husks. Proceedings of Global Animal Nutrition Conference held at Bengaluru from 20th to 22nd April, 2014. Pp 106.

Kaufhold JN, Hammon HM Blum JW (2000) Fructooligosaccharides supplementation effects on metabolic, endocrine and hematological traits in veal calves. Journal of Veterinary Medicine Series A 47: 17-29.

Mwenya B, Santoso B, Sar C, Gamo Y, Kobayashi T, Arai I, Takahashi J (2004) Effects of including beta 1,4 galactooligosaccharides, lactic acid bacteria or yeasts culture on methanogenesis as well as energy and nitrogen metabolism in sheep. Animal Feed Science and Technology, 115: 313-326.

Mwenya B, Sar C, Santoso B, Gamo Y, Kobayashi T, Morikawa R, Takura K, Umetsu K, Kogawa S, Kimura K, Mizukoshi H, Takahashi J (2005) Comparing the effects of beta 1,4 galactooligosaccharides, and L-cysteine to monensin on energy and nitrogen utilization in steers fed a very high concentrate diets. Animal Feed Science and Technology, 118: 19-30.

Oli MW, Petschow BW, Buddington RK (1998) Evaluation of fructooligosaccharides supplementation of oral electrolyte solutions for treatment of diarrhea. Digestive Disease Science, 43: 138-147.

Ortiz LT, Rodriguez ML, Alzueta C, Rebole A, Trevino J (2009) Effect of inulin on growth performance, intestinal tract size, mineral retention, and tibial bone mineralization in broiler chickens. British Poultry Science, 50: 325-332.

Oyarzabal OA, Conner DE (1995) In vitro fructooligosaccharides utilization and inhibition of Salmonella spp. by selcetd bacteria. Poultry Science, 74: 1418-1425.

Pineiro M, Asp NG, Reid G, Macfarlane S, Morelli L, Brunser O, Tuohy K (2008) FAO Technical meeting on prebiotics. Journal of Clinical Gastroenterology, 42: S156– S159.

Pokharia AK (2008) Paleoethnobotanical record of cultivated crops and associated weeds and wild taxa from Neolithic site, Tokwa, Uttar Pradesh, India. 2008, Current Science, 94: 248-255.

Roberfroid M (2007) Prebiotics: the concept revisited. Journal of Nutrition, 137: 830S-837S.

Samanta AK, Kolte AP, Chandrasekharaiya M, Thulasi, Sampath KT, Prasad CS (2007) Prebiotics: The rumen modulator for enhancing the productivity of dairy animals. Indian Dairyman, 59: 58-61.

Samanta AK, Senani S, Kolte AP, Sridhar M, Jayapal N (2010) Application of prebiotics in poultry. Agrovet Buzz, Vol. III (3): 38-42.

Samanta AK, Kolte AP, Senani S, Manpal Sridhar, Jayapal N (2011) Prebiotics in ancient Indian diets. Current Science, 101: 43-46.

Samanta AK, Senani S, Kolte AP, Sridhar M, Bhatta R, Jayapal N (2012) Effect of prebiotic on digestibility of total mixed ration. Indian Veterinary Journal, 89: 41- 42. Samanta AK, Senani S, Kolte AP, Sridhar M, Sampath KT, Jayapal N (2012a) Production and in vitro evaluation of xylooligosaccharides generated from corn cobs. Food and Bioproducts Processing, 90: 466-474.

Samanta AK, Jayapal N, Senani S, Kolte AP, Sridhar M (2013) Prebiotic inulin: Useful dietary adjuncts to manipulate the livestock gut microflora. Brazilian Journal of Microbiology, 44(1): 1-14.

Samanta AK, Jayapal N, Chikkerur J, Roy S, Kolte AP, Senani S, Sridhar, M (2015) Xylooligosaccharides as prebiotics from agricultural by-products: Production and applications. Bioactive Carbohydrates and Dietary Fibers, 5: 62 -67.

Samanta AK, Sharath B, Jayapal N, Kolte AP, Senani S, Sridhar M, Prasad CS (2015a) Comparison between probiotic and prebiotic on rumen metabolites and microbial population in lambs. Indian Veterinary Journal, 92: 11-13.

Samanta, Ashis Kumar, Jayaram C, Jayapal N, Sondhi N, Kolte AP, Senani S, Sridhar M, Dhali A (2015b) Assessment of Fecal Microflora Changes in Pigs Supplemented with Herbal Residue and Prebiotic. PLoS ONE, 10(7): e0132961

Samanta AK, Chikkerur J, Roy S, Kolte AP, Senani S, Sridhar M (2015c) Metagenomic analysis of hindgut microflora of pigs supplemented with feed additives. Proceedings of 9thBiennial Animal Nutrition Association Conference. Pp 115.

Santoso B, Kume S, Nonaka K, Gamo Y, Kimura K, Takashi J (2003) Influence of beta galactooligosaccharide supplementation on nitrogen utilization, rumen fermentation, and microbial nitrogen supply in dairy cows fed silage. Asia Australian Journal of animal Sciences, 26: 1137-1142.

Verdonk, J.M.A.J. and Leeuwen, P, Van. 2004. The application of inulin-type fructans in diets for veal calves and broilers. In Inulin and oligofructose Feel good Factors for health and well-being, 4th Orafti Research Conference, Paris, February 12 –13, 2004. pp 50-51.

Verdonk JMAJ, Beelan GM, Jansman AJM, Huisman J (1998) Effect of soya carbohydrate fractions on the ileal digestibiity and endogenous flow of nitrogen in veal calves. Pp 341-343. In: Recent advances of research in antinutritional factors in legume seeds. Ed: AJM Jansman, GD Hill, J Huisman, AFB Vander Poel. Wageningen, The Netharlands.

Yusrizai Y, Chen TC (2003) Effect of adding chickory fructan in feed on broiler growth performance, serum cholesterol, and intestinal length. International Journal of Poultry Science, 2: 214-219.

8

Modern Biotechnological Tools for Augmenting Livestock Production and Health

Dharmendra Kumar, Naresh L Selokar, P S Yadav

Animal Physiology and Reproduction Division, ICAR-Central Institute for Research on Buf aloes, Hisar-125001, Haryana

Introduction

The modern biotechnologies (animal cloning, stem cells, and transgenesis) have contributed immensely to increasing livestock productivity, particularly in developed countries, and could help to alleviate poverty and hunger, reduce the threats of diseases and ensure environmental sustainability in developing countries. A wide range of biotechnologies are available and have already been used in developing countries in the animal science disciplines, *i.e.*, animal reproduction, genetics and breeding; animal nutrition and production; and animal health. In animal reproduction, genetics and breeding, artificial insemination (AI) has perhaps been the most widely applied animal biotechnology, particularly in combination with cryopreservation, allowing significant genetic improvement for productivity as well as the global dissemination of selected male germplasm. Complementary technologies such as monitoring reproductive hormones, oestrus synchronization and semen sexing can improve the efficiency of AI. Embryo transfer provides the same opportunities for females, albeit on a much smaller scale and at a much greater price. Biotechnologies in animal health are used to increase the precision of disease diagnosis as well as for disease control and treatment. The Biotechnology Industry Organization claims that the genetic engineering of animals in agriculture offers ''tremendous benefit to the animal by enhancing health, well-being and animal welfare'' (Gottlieb and Wheeler 2008). Further, improvements are still needed in product composition and production efficiency, especially in growth, disease resistance, and reproduction. In this regard, transgenic animals stem cells, cloning and other emerging biotechnologies will have important roles in producing more and higher quality animal food.

Animal cloning: faster way to produce superior animals

Cloning technology is already being used commercially in some parts of the world for the replication of elite breeding animals, mostly cattle and also pigs, which are used to produce animals farmed for food production (Suk *et al.*, 2007). The birth of Dolly in 1996, the first animal cloned from an adult cell was not universally celebrated. Critics of biotechnology worried that genetically modified livestock would fill the supermarket with identical copies of someone's idea of unnatural perfection. Up to 2004, about 1500 calves had been produced through somatic cell nuclear transfer (SCNT), mainly in Europe, North America, Japan and New Zealand, but also in South America and Asia (Heyman, 2005). China produced the first cloned buffalo in 2004 and India followed suit in February 2009 world's first cloned buffalo calf through the handmade/hand-guided cloning technique. With this advancement, India has entered an era of buffalo cloning, an important dairy and meat animal, through a simplified technique. After the birth of the first cloned buffalo, subsequent work on this approach which led to the birth of offspring produced using ear skin-derived somatic cells (Shah *et al.*, 2009), embryonic stem cells (George *et al.*, 2011), semen derived somatic cells (Selokar *et al.*, 2014) and recently, urine-derived somatic cells (Madheshiya *et al.*, 2015) as nuclear donors, or that produced from a vitrified–warmed cloned embryo (Saha *et al.*, 2013). In addition to faster multiplication of domestic buffalo populations, scientists currently use this technology to conserve and manage population of endangered species, specially the Bovidae family such as Wild buffalo (*Bubalus arnee*), belongs to the Bovidae family and is found in India, Nepal, Bhutan, Cambodia and Thailand. In central India, wild buffaloes are only found in the Indravati Tiger Reserve Udanti, Chhattisgarh. In Udanti Wildlife Sanctuary only ten buffaloes, including eight male and two female are left; hence there is an urgent need to restore their population. In this regard, Saini *et al.*, (2015) reported that successful cloning of wild buffalo through production of cloned calf using somatic cells from wild buffalo and recipient oocyte from domestic buffalo. Although the technology still has relatively low success rates and there seem to be substantial problems with the welfare of some of the cloned animals, cloning is used both within basic research and the biomedical sector. The next step seems to be to implement cloning in the agricultural production system and several animals have been developed in this direction. In the agricultural sector, cloning can be used as a tool within farm animal breeding.

Stem cells towards veterinary clinical/therapeutic application

The generation of stem cells was initiated in mouse but gained importance because of clinical reasons in humans, however, their establishment is gradually increasing every day in domestic animals like pig, sheep, goat, dog, cat, horse, cow or buffalo for purposes such as the creation of models of human genetic diseases and cell transplantation therapies. The established stem cell lines would be useful in the precise genetic engineering of these animals for improved production traits and products, for disease resistance and biopharming (Seamark, 1994). However, ES cell lines could be used to accomplish these latter goals, either through chimera technology already well-established in producing genetically modified mice (Wells *et al.*, 2003), or by improving the efficiency of somatic cell nuclear transfer technology that is currently used in the production of genetically engineered ungulates (Donovan *et al.*, 2005; Wall *et al.*, 2005). Here, we present state-of-the-art of stem cells in domestic animals and their clinical and therapeutic prospects in livestock production and health. In veterinary science research has been conducted on horses, dogs and cats for development of stem cell-based treatments of wide range of injuries and diseases such as myocardial infarction, stroke, tendon and ligament damage, osteoarthritis, osteochondrosis and muscular dystrophy in large animals, as well as humans (Assmus *et al.*, 2002; Murphy *et al.*, 2003; Sampaolesi *et al.*, 2006; Taylor *et al.*, 2007). Stem cells offer tremendous potentials for accelerating and improving tissue healing. In fact, stem cells isolated from embryos as well as various tissues such as bone marrow, adipose tissue, testicular tissue, etc have been used in various livestock species, for therapeutic purposes (Table 1). In veterinary practices, mesenchymal stem cells-based approaches are currently used for the treatment of tendon, ligament, or cartilage/joint injuries in horses or dogs. The first therapeutic application of stem cell-based therapy was performed in horse to treat equine suspensory ligament desmitis by Herthel (2002). Stem cell-based treatments for ligament injury, tendon injury, osteoarthritis, osteochondrosis, and sub chondral bone cysts have been commercially available to practicing veterinarians to treat horses since 2003 in the United States and since 2006 in the United Kingdom (todaysveterinarypractice.com). Similar kind of treatment for tendon and ligament injury and osteoarthritis in dogs has been available for veterinarians in the United States since 2005. The efficacy of these treatments has been shown in double-blind clinical trials for dogs with osteoarthritis of the hip and elbow (Nixon *et al.*, 2008). However, few research-based reports documented the use of stem cells to enhance fracture repair and future application may include therapeutic use in cardiovascular, gastrointestinal, or neuroendocrine body systems. Besides this, ESCs, iPS cells, and cord blood derived cells are also beginning to be investigated in the laboratory but have not yet been applied to the clinical scenario (Fortier and Travis, 2011). Stem cells are thought to mediate repair via five primary mechanisms: (1) providing an anti-inflammatory effect, (2) homing to damaged tissues and recruiting other cells, such as endothelial progenitor cells, that are necessary for tissue growth, (3) supporting tissue remodeling over scar formation, (4) inhibiting apoptosis, and (5) differentiating into bone, cartilage, tendon, and ligament tissue (Yamada *et al.*, 2004; Csaki *et al.*, 2007). The last two decades have seen a surge of interest in the research and clinical availability of stem cell treatments. Innovative techniques of cell and tissue processing, based on tissue engineering, have been developed. Cell expansion and tissue reconstruction through ex vivo cultures are core processes used to produce engineered tissues with sufficient structural integrity and functionality (Kino-Oka and Taya, 2009).

Table 1. Clinical and therapeutic applications of stem cells in livestock species (Kumar *et al.*, 2011, Yadav *et al.*, 2012).

Species	Problem addressed	Source of stem cells used for treatment	Outcome/remark about treatment	References
Equine	Suspensory ligament desmitis	Bone marrow aspirate from sternum	improved return to athletic function rates over conventional therapies	Herthel, 2002.
	Tendon injuries	Culture-expanded bone marrow mesenchymal stem cells	Favourable effects on tissue organization and composition of injured tendons and ligaments 90% of treated horses successfully returned to pre-injury athletic function and race horses suffered no re-injury of the superficial digital flexor tendon after 2 years whereas all of the horses of a control population suffered from re-injury	Schnabel *et al.*, 2009; Crovace *et al.*, 2010
	Wound healing	High-density platelet-rich plasma with adipose-derived stem/stromal cells	Effective tissue regeneration in acute and chronic wound defects	El-Sharkawy *et al.*, 2007
	Acute cartilage injury	Bone marrow mesenchymal stem cells	Overcome the cartilage injury in femur bone	Wilke *et al.*, 2007
Goat	Osteoarthritis	Bone marrow mesenchymal stem cells	Modulation of local T cell-mediated response and enhanced tissue regeneration	Murphy *et al.*, 2003
	Testis xenografting	Spermatogonial stem cells	Supported spermatogenesis	Honaramooz *et al.*, 2002
Sheep	Osteoarthritis	Bone marrow mesenchymal stem cells	Enhanced regeneration of cartilage and meniscus	Murphy *et al.*, 2003
	Testis xenografting	Spermatogonial stem cells	Supported spermatogenesis	Zeng *et al.*, 2006

(Contd.)

Species	Problem addressed	Source of stem cells used for treatment	Outcome/remark about treatment	References
Canine	Osteoarthritis	Adipose derived stromal vascular fraction cells	Improvement in the hip joint and elbow joint	Black *et al.*, 2007; Black *et al.*, 2008
	Testis xenografting	Spermatogonial stem cells	Supported spermatogenesis	Abrishami *et al.*, 2010.
	Dilated cardiomyopathy, spinal injuries and diabetes	ESCs	Improved after treatment symptoms	Tecirlioglu and Trounson, 2007
Pigs	Testis xenografting	Spermatogonial stem cells	Supports spermatogenesis	Honaramooz *et al.*, 2002

Transgenic animal and its impact

A transgenic animal is one that has integrated a gene or DNA sequence (a 'transgene'), which has stably incorporated the transgene into its germ-line and is able to pass the transgene on to its offspring. The methodologies used to produce transgenic livestock such as pronuclear injection, sperm-mediated DNA transfer, embryonic stem cells, recombinant retroviruses, and nuclear transfer "Cloning" have been reviewed earlier in detail (Wall 2002, Wheeler & Walters 2001; Wheeler *et al.* 2003) and that aspect will not be covered in this chapter. There are many potential applications of transgenic methodology to develop new and improved strains of livestock. Practical applications of transgenics in livestock production include enhanced prolificacy and reproductive performance, increased feed utilization and growth rate, improved carcass composition, improved milk production and/or composition, modification of hair or fiber, and increased disease resistance. Development of transgenic farm animals will allow more flexibility in direct genetic manipulation of livestock (Wheeler *et al.*, 2003, Kues and Niemann, 2011). Genetic modification of livestock will enhance animal welfare by producing healthier animals. Animal welfare is a high priority for anyone involved in the production of livestock. The application of transgenic methodology should provide opportunities to genetically engineer livestock with superior disease resistance. One application of this technology is to treat mastitis, an inflammation of the mammary gland, typically caused by an infectious pathogen(s). Mastitis causes decreased milk production. Transgenic dairy cows that secrete lysostaphin into their milk have higher resistance to mastitis due to the protection provided by lysostaphin, which kills the bacteria *Staphylococcus aureus*, in a dose-dependent manner (Donovan *et al.*, 2005). Lysostaphin is an antimicrobial peptide that protects the mammary gland against this major mastitis-causing pathogen. Recent progress has produced prion-free (Richt *et al.*, 2007) and suppressed prion livestock (Golding *et al.*, 2006). Prions are the causative agents in bovine spongiform encephalopathy (BSE) or 'mad cow disease' in cattle and Creutzfeldt-Jacob disease (CJD) in humans. This is only a partial list of organisms or genetic diseases that decrease production efficiency and may also be targets for manipulation via transgenic methodologies. Apart from these advances in transgenic technology provide the opportunity either to change the composition of milk or to produce entirely novel proteins in milk (Table 1). The improvement of livestock growth or survivability through the modification of milk composition involves production of transgenic animals that: (1) produce a greater quantity of milk; (2) produce milk of higher nutrient content; or (3) produce milk that contains a beneficial 'nutriceutical' protein. The major nutrients in milk are protein, fat, and lactose. By elevating any of these components, we can impact the growth and health of the developing offspring. Cattle, sheep, and goats used for meat production can benefit from increased milk yield or composition. These applications of transgenic technology could lead to improved growth and survival of offspring.

Table 2. Expression of human proteins through transgenic animal in mammary gland.

Protein Expressed	Species Where Expressed	Promoter	Reference
Lysozyme	goat	Bovine αs1-casein	(Maga *et al*., 2006)
Lysostaphin	cattle	Ovine β-lactoglobulin	(Wall *et al*., 2005)
Bovine β and κ casein	cattle	Bovine β-casein	(Brophy *et al*., 2003)
IGF-I	pig	Bovine α-lactalbumin	(Donovan *et al*., 2001)
α-lactalbumin	pig	Bovine α-lactalbumin	(Bleck *et al*., 1998)

References

Abrishami M, Abbasi S, Honaramooz A (2010) The effect of donor age on progression of spermatogenesis in canine testicular tissue after xenografting into immunodeficient mice. Theriogenology, 73:512-522.

Assmus B, Schächinger V, Teupe C, Britten M, Lehmann R, Döbert N, Grünwald F, Aicher A, Urbich C, Martin H, Hoelzer D, Dimmeler S, Zeiher AM (2002) Transplantation of progenitor cells and regeneration enhancement in acute myocardial infarction (TOPCARE AMI). Circulation, 106(24): 3009-17.

Black LL, Gaynor J, Adams C, Dhupa S, Sams AE, Taylor R, Harman S, Gingerich DA, Harman R (2008) Effect of intra articular injection of autologous adipose derived mesenchymal stem and regenerative cells on clinical signs of chronic osteoarthritis of the elbow joint in dogs. Veterinary Therapeutics, 9: 192-200.

Black LL, Gaynor J, Gahring D, Adams C, Aron D, Harman S, Gingerich DA, Harman R (2007) Effect of adipose-derived mesenchymal stem and regenerative cells on lameness in dogs with chronic osteoarthritis of the coxofemoral joints: a randomized, double-blinded, multicenter, controlled trial. Veterinary Therapeutics, 8: 272-284.

Bleck GT, White BR, Miller DJ, Wheeler M B (1998) Production of bovine α-lactalbumin in the milk of transgenic pigs. Journal of Animal Science, 76: 3072–3078.

Brophy B, Smolenski G, Wheeler T, Wells D, L'Huillier P, Laible G (2003) Cloned transgenic cattle produce milk with higher levels of bcasein and k-casein. Nature Biotechnology, 21: 157– 162.

Crovace A, Lacitignola L, Rossi G, Francioso E (2010) Histological and immunohis to chemical evaluation of autologous cultured bone marrow mesenchymal stem cells and bone marrow mononucleated cells in collagenase-induced tendinitis of equine superficial digital flexor tendon. Veterinary Medicine International, 250978.

Csaki C, Matis U, Mobasheri A, Ye H, Shakibaei M (2007) Chondrogenesis, osteogenesis and adipogenesis of canine mesenchymal stem cells: a biochemical, morphological and ultrastructural study. Histochemistry and Cell Biology, 128(6): 507-20.

Donovan D M, *et al.*, (2005) Engineering disease resistant cattle. Transgenic Research 14: 563-567.

Donovan SM, Monaco MH, Bleck GT, Cook JB, Noble MS, Hurley WL, Wheeler MB (2001) Transgenic Over-Expression of Bovine α-Lactalbumin and Human Insulin-Like Growth Factor-I in Porcine Mammary Gland. Journal of Dairy Science 84: E216–E222.

El-Sharkawy H, Kantarci A, Deady J, Hasturk H, Liu H, Alshahat M. VanDyke TE (2007) Journal of Periodontology, 78: 661-669.

Fortier LA. Travis AJ (2011) Stem cells in veterinary medicine. Stem Cell Research and Therapy, 2: 9.

George A, Sharma R, Singh KP, Panda SK, Singla SK, Palta P, Manik R, Chauhan MS (2011) Production of cloned and transgenic embryos using buffalo (*Bubalus bubalis*) embryonic stem cell like cells isolated from in vitro fertilized and cloned blastocysts. Cell Reprogramming, 13(3): 263-272.

Golding MC, *et al.*, (2006) Suppression of prion protein in livestock by RNA interference. PNAS (USA) 103, 5285-5290.

Herthel DJ (2002) Suspensory desmitis therapies. Proc 12th ACVS Symp, 165-167. Heyman Y (2005) Nuclear transfer: A new tool for reproductive biotechnology in cattle. Reproduction Nutrition Development, 45: 353 - 361.

Honaramooz A, Snedaker A, Boiani M, Scholer H, Dobrinski I. Schlatt S (2002) Nature, 418: 778-781.

Kino-Oka M, Taya M (2009) Recent developments in processing systems for cell and tissue cultures toward therapeutic application. Journal of Bioscience and Bioengineering, 108: 267–276.

Kues WA, Niemann H (2011) Advances in farm animal transgenesis. Preventive Veterinary Medicine, 102(2):146-56.

Kumar D, Anand T, Yadav PS, Sethi RK (2011) Clinical and therapeutic application of stem cells in domestic animals. Indian Journal of Comparative Microbiology, Immunology and Infectious Diseases 32(1&2): 1-5.

Madheshiya PK, Sahare AA, Jyotsana B, Singh KP, Saini M, Raja AK, Kaith S, Singla SK, Chauhan MS, Manik RS, Palta P (2015) Production of a Cloned Buffalo (*Bubalus bubalis*) Calf from Somatic Cells Isolated from Urine. Cellular Reprogramming, 17(3): 160-9.

Maga EA, Shoemaker CF, Rowe JD, Bondurant RH, Anderson GB, Murray JD (2006) Production and processing of milk from transgenic goats expressing human lysozyme in the mammary gland. Journal of Dairy Science, 89: 518-524.

Murphy JM, Fink DJ, Hunziker EB, Barry FP (2003) Stem cell therapy in a caprine model of osteoarthritis. Arthritis & Rheumatology, 48: 3464-3474.

Nixon AJ, Dahlgren LA, Haupt JL, Yeager AE, Ward DL (2008) Effect of adipose derived nucleated cell fractions on tendon repair in horses with collagenase-induced tendinitis. American Journal of Veterinary Research, 69:928-937.

Richt JA, *et al.*, (2007) Production of cattle lacking prion protein. Nature Biotechnology, 25: 132-138.

Saha A, Panda SK, Chauhan MS, Manik RS, Palta P, Singla SK (2013) Birth of cloned calves from vitrified-warmed zona-free buffalo (*Bubalus bubalis*) embryos produced by hand made cloning. Reproduction, Fertility and Development, 25(6): 860-865.

Saini M, Selokar NL, Raja AK, Sahare AA, Singla SK, Chauhan MS, Manik RS, Palta P (2015) Effect of donor cell type on developmental competence, quality, gene expression, and epigenetic status of interspecies cloned embryos produced using cells from wild buffalo and oocytes from domestic buffalo. Theriogenology, 84(1):101-108.

Sampaolesi M, Blot S, D'Antona G, Granger N, Tonlorenzi R, Innocenzi A, Mognol P, Thibaud JL, Galvez BG, Barthélémy I, Perani L, Mantero S, Guttinger M, Pansarasa O, Rinaldi C, Cusella De Angelis MG, Torrente Y, Bordignon C, Bottinelli R, Cossu G (2006) Mesoangioblast stem cells ameliorate muscle function in dystrophic dogs. Nature, 444(7119): 574-9.

Schnabel LV, Mohammed HO, Miller BJ, McDermott WG, Jacobson MS, Santangelo KS, Fortier LA (2007) Platelet rich plasma (PRP) enhances anabolic gene expression patterns in flexor digitorum superfi cialis tendons. Journal of Orthopaedic Research, 25:230-240.

Seamark RF (1994) Progress and emerging problems in livestock transgenesis: a summary perspective. Reproduction, Fertility and Development, 6: 653-657.

Selokar NL, Saini M, Palta P, Chauhan MS, Manik R, Singla SK (2014) Hope for restoration of dead valuable bulls through cloning using donor somatic cells isolated from cryopreserved semen. PLOS One, 9(3): e90755.

Shah R, George A, Singh MK, Kumar D, *et al.*, (2009) Pregnancies established from handmade cloned blastocysts reconstructed using skin fibroblasts in buffalo (*Bubalus bubalis*). Theriogenology, 71: 1215–1219.

Suk J, Bruce A, Gertz R, Warkup C, Whitelaw CBA, Braun A, Oram C, Rodríguez-Cerezo E, Papatryfon I (2007) Dolly for dinner? Assessing commercial and regulatory trends in cloned livestock. Nature Biotechnology, 25: 47- 53.

Taylor SE, Smith RK, Clegg PD (2007) Mesenchymal stem cell therapy in equine musculoskeletal disease: scientific fact or clinical fiction? Equine Veterinary Journal, 39: 172-180.

Tecirlioglu RT, Trounson AO (2007) Embryonic stem cells in companion animals (horses, dogs and cats): present status and future prospects. Reproduction, Fertility and Development, 19: 740-747.

Wall RJ, Powell A, Paape MJ, Kerr DE, Bannermann DD, Pursel VG, Wells KD, Talbot N, Hawk H (2005) Genetically enhanced cows resist intramammary Staphylococcus aureus infection. Nature Biotechnology, 23: 445–451.

Wall RJ (2002) New gene transfer methods. Theriogenology, 57: 189-201. Wells DN, Laible G, Tucker FC, Miller AL, Oliver JE, Xiang T, Forsyth JT, Berg MC, Cockrem K, L'Huillier PJ, Tervit HR, Oback B (2003) Coordination between donor cell type and cell cycle stage improves nuclear cloning efficiency in cattle. Theriogenology, 59(1): 45- 59.

Wheeler MB, Walters EM (2001) Transgenic technology and applications in swine. Theriogenology, 56: 1345-1369.

Wheeler, M. B. *et al.*, (2003) Transgenic animals in biomedicine and agriculture: outlook for the future. Animal Reproduction Science, 79: 265-289.

Wilke MM, Nydam DV, Nixon AJ (2007) Enhanced early chondrogenesis in articular defects following arthroscopic mesenchymal stem cell implantation in an equine model. Journal of Orthopaedic Research, 25: 913-925.

Yadav PS, Mann A, Singh J, Kumar D, Sharma RK, Singh I (2012) Buffalo (*Bubalus bubalis*) fetal skin derived fibroblast cells exhibit characteristics of stem cells. Agricultural Research, 1: 175–182.

Yamada Y, Ueda M, Naiki T, Takahashi M, Hata K, Nagasaka T (2004) Autogenous injectable bone for regeneration with mesenchymal stem cells and platelet-rich plasma: tissue engineered bone regeneration. Tissue Engineering, 10: 955-964.

Zeng W, Avelar GF, Rathi R, Franca LR, Dobrinski I (2006) The length of the spermatogenic cycle is conserved in porcine and ovine testis xenografts. Journal of Andrology, 27: 527-533.

9

Techniques of Boar Semen Collection, Preservation and Artificial Insemination

S. Naskar
ICAR-IVRI Eastern Regional Station, 37, Belgachia Road. Kolkata-700037, W.B.

Introduction

During the last decade, there has been a dramatic increase in use of artificial insemination (AI) by commercial swine producers in many European countries. Till 1990, less than 7% of sows & gilt in the USA were bred by Artificial Insemination. Today, over 70% of the animals are bred by AI. Maybe in a couple of years all swine producers will probably utilize this technology.

In India, it is still in infant stage. Some research work has already been done in scattered ways in various Research Institutes but it is still in the four walls of the laboratory. Some Govt. farms have been doing AI in swine with liquid semen.

Pig is the most important livestock in all Northeastern Hill States and there is no superior indigenous germplasm available in this region. Productivity of local pigs is very low. All through, improvement programmes had undertaken in different state Govt. farms, Central Govt. farms through upgrading with the help of suitable exotic pig breeds like Hampshire, Large Black, and Large White Yorkshire *etc.* Superior germplasm was distributed to farmers for better productivity. But, improvement till date is not impressive due to lack of superior germless, high feed cost, lack of breeder farmers and lack of incentives to the poor farmers. Maintenance of breeding boar for small farmers is very expensive not only in individual capacity but also on community basis. So, AI is the only tool for quicker, safer, quicker and economic why out for swine improvement like cattle.

The semen collection area and dummy sow

Semen can be collected from boar in two different ways. It can be collected from the boar while mounting on an estrus sow/gilt. In this method there are problems like (1). The boar may be too large to be supported by smaller females. In that case, a female can't bear the weight of male. (2). Some females may begin to walk around the pen making and it is difficult to collect the semen (3). It is difficult to get estrus females every now and then. (4). Sometimes females may disallow a particular male.

So the preferred approach is to collect semen from a boar trained to mount a dummy sow. Dummy sow should be located in an isolated semen collection room or pen that measure at least 10 ft × 10 ft and has a non-stick floor. Rubber breeding mats provide excellent footing. Once the boar is in semen collection area, should not be provided feed and water *etc.* The room or pen should provide a means of escape for the producer in the event a boar becomes hostile.

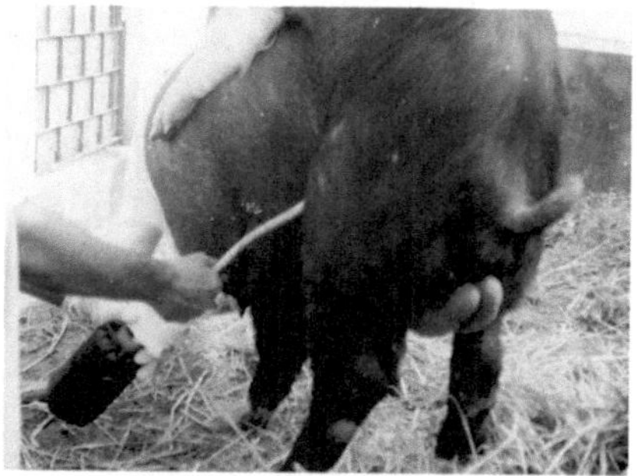
With the help of estrus sow

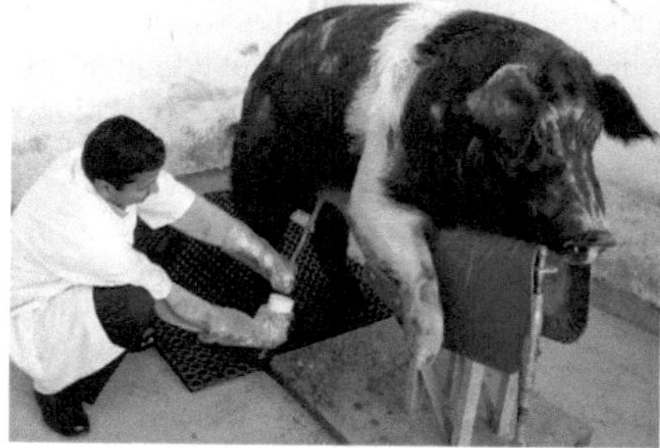
With the help Dummy sow

Training the Boar

Ideally, the boar should be trained between 8 to 10 months of age although older boars used for natural service may also be adopted for collection in dummy sow. The key word for training a boar for collection is patience. To begin, the boar is moved to the collection room or pen three times at daily intervals, with the purpose of getting the animal acquainted with dummy sow. Boar, being trained should be exposed to the dummy sow immediately after collection of semen from an already trained boar. Many boars mount the dummy sow during one of the first few training sessions. A boar that does not mount after two or three exposures to the dummy sow can be tricked by sprinkling of semen from another boar. This technique is necessary only until the boar has been trained to mount. Another option is letting the boar mount, but not breed, a sow that is in estrous and in the same area as the dummy sow. After removing the sow by letting her exit near the dummy sow, the boar may be stimulated to mount the dummy sow. Alternatively, the sow in estrus is penned or caped near the head of the dummy sow.

A trained person can also allow mounting a sow that is in estrus and is standing parallel to the dummy sow and the trainer can begin collecting semen and after approximately two minutes, have an assistant gently push the boar over onto the dummy sow while the collection continues. The sow in estrus is then removed from the room.

The administration of lutalyse hormone ($PGF_2\alpha$) enhances the libido in boars display mounting and mating behaviour. It is also reported that it increased the volume and total number of sperm cells in the sperm rich fraction of ejaculates (Hashizyme and Niwa, 1984)

Semen Collection

Before attempting to collect semen from boar, clip the long hairs on the sheath because it interferes with the collection process. During the collection process, patience is again very much important. Allow the boar to mount and make a few copulation thrusts, intend the penis and display an erection the corkscrew end of the penis is grasped with a bare or gloved hand. If gloves are used that should not be latex because chemicals on these types of gloves are spermicidal. After a few moments, the boar will cease thrusting and begin to ejaculate. Rhythmic pulsation should be given during collection and semen should be collected into a thermos or sterilized bottle which should be protected with a jacket to prevent cold shock. The gel traction should be filtered out of the ejaculate during collection using sterilized gauge put into boucher funnel. The grip on the penis should not be loosened during ejaculation which on an average requires 7–10 minutes.

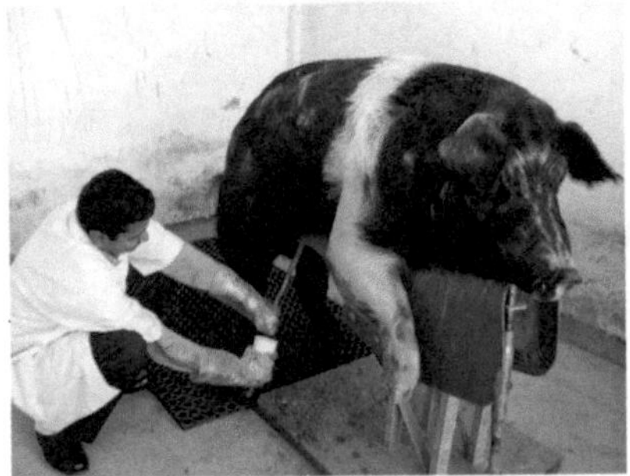

Gloved Hand Technique

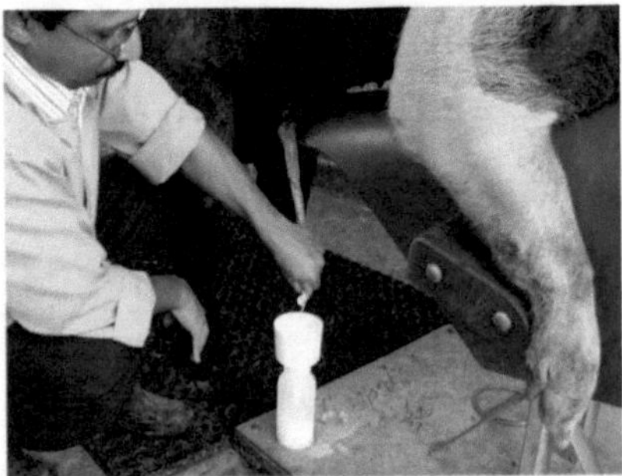

Bare Hand Technique

Evaluation of Boar Semen Quality

The boar ejaculates semen in fractions. The first fraction of an ejaculate is the pre sperm fraction. This fraction contains fluid from the prostate gland and amounts to 25-30 ml. This fraction serves to flush urine and bacteria out of the boar's urethra and is typically discolored and foul smelling.

The second phase of the ejaculate is the sperm–rich fraction. This part is usually 40–100 ml and contains 80–90% of the total sperm. The third fraction is the largest by volume (80 to 200 ml) and is typically sperm poor. It is often discarded in order to prevent over dilution of the sperm rich fraction. The last fraction is the gelatinous phase and is 25–30 ml in volume. Except for the first fraction, all phases are collected through a filter to remove the gelatinous materials that originated from the boar's bulbo-urethral gland. During natural service, it functions to effectively seal the ejaculate volume inside the female uterus. All ejaculates have to meet minimal quality control standards in order to assure that reproductive efficiency is not limited by boar's semen fertility when using AI. In general, ejaculates from boars that are healthy and collected at proper intervals should easily meet the minimally acceptable criteria. However, since factors such as stress, diseases and environmental factors can significantly reduce the quality of a boar ejaculates, several criteria for acceptance of an ejaculate can help to prevent economic loss that results from lower conception rate and reduced litter size. Routine evaluation of ejaculates is:

Volume

Semen is commonly collected in containers that allow for determination of volume. Otherwise, it can be measured by measuring cylinder and it varies from 50–250 ml depending on breeds.

Color

Semen ejaculates should also be evaluated for color. The ejaculate should normally be milky to chalky in appearance. A pink color indicates the presence of blood and may suggest an injury or a urinary Infection. A yellow–tinged ejaculate may indicate that some urine was inadvertently collected, and therefore the ejaculate should be discarded. Good quality semen ejaculates should not have a strong or offensive odor. A strong odor indicates the presence of preputial fluid.

Consistency

A visual assessment of the opacity or consistency is an indication of the number of sperm cells, less transparent samples, therefore, contains more sperm cells. The sperm rich fraction is creamy in appearance and allows little light to pass through. The sperm poor fractions are more watery in appearance, are more transparent and have fewer cells. Ejaculate turbidity is another indicator for sperm cell numbers. It appears when the sample is gently rotated and a swirling motion can be seen in the liquid.

Gross motility

It can only be performed with a microscope. A warned slide and samples will allow for fair assessment of mortality. Low power is usually sufficient (20x) to see the entered sample vigorously in motion. Semen mobility decreases during storage, the minimum motility during initial evaluation of semen should be higher than 80%.

Semen concentration

Sperm concentration can be counted with the help of haemocytometer (Cell Counting Chamber). This can also be done through a spectrophotometer.

Live, dead and abnormal spermatozoa

Estimation of live spermatozoa and abnormality percentage is very much important with respect to fertility point of view. Normally, semen samples with 60% live percent sperm should be used for AI with abnormality percentage of 10–15%.

Table 1. Physical and Morphological characteristics of boar ejaculates of different genetic groups.

S. No.	Physical attributes	Genetic group		
		Hampshire	Cross Bred 75%	Cross Bred 50%
1.	Average volume (ml)	215.52 ± 21.35	190.15 ± 28.11	163.74 ± 40.38
2.	Color	Creamy white	Creamy white	Creamy white
3.	Consistency	Thin milky	Thin milky	Thin milky
4.	Initial motility	88.75 ± 9.63	84.60 ± 7.15	82.35 ± 8.35
5.	Live spermatozoa (%)	91.18 ± 6.16	90.65 ± 8.25	85.60 ± 10.18
6.	Dead spermatozoa (%)	8.82 ± 2.16	9.35 ± 2.46	14.40 ± 2.38
7.	Abnormality (%)	15.75 ± 0.23	15.96 ± 0.16	24.54 ± 0.28
8.	Sperm Concentration (million/ml)	290.15 ± 30.26	240.68 ± 35.95	230.45 ± 38.20
9.	pH	7.30 ± 0.05	7.32 ± 0.05	7.33 ± 0.04

Table 2. Various abnormalities of boar spermatozoa

S. No.	Types abnormalities	Genetic Group		
		Hampshire	Cross Bred 75%	Cross Bred 50%
1.	Head	1.25 ± 0.65	1.35 ± 0.46	2.17 ± 0.59
2.	Mid piece	1.45 ± 0.17	1.58 ± 0.26	2.78 ± 0.23
3.	Tail piece	4.86 ± 0.54	3.84 ± 0.67	6.59 ± 0.41
4.	Proximal droplets	3.48 ± 0.64	3.84 ± 0.67	7.99 ± 0.41
5.	Distal droplets	4.71 ± 0.23	4.96 ± 0.16	5.01 ± 0.26
6.	Total	15.75 ± 0.27	15.96 ± 0.16	24.54 ± 0.28

Dilution and preservation of Boar Semen

Extender function allows for making multiple inseminations from a single ejaculate of a superior animal. It also provides temperature protection for sperm while reducing the metabolic rate of sperm cells in cool storage. The extender functions to provide membrane stabilization in cool temperature, energy sources for sperm metabolism, pH buffering from sperm cell waste, ions for membrane and cell balance and antibiotics to prevent the growth of microbes that can cause diseases and compete for nutrients. Various extenders are available for preservation of boar semen under liquid state.

The extenders preferably used are BTS (Belt Ville thawing solution), Modena and Zornobsa. There are commercial extenders available also like BTS -49, X-cell, safe cell and safe cell plus, androhap *etc.* All these commercial extenders are for long term preservation (3–5 days). Similarly BTS and Modena are also used for long term preservation and Zornobsa is for short term (2-3 days) preservation.

Table 3. Composition of different extenders

S. No.	Composition	BTS	Modena	Zornobsa
1.	D–glucose (g)	18.56	13.75	5.75
2.	Tri Sodium citrate	30.0	3.45	58.25
3.	Sodium EDTA (g)	0.65	1.175	1.175
4.	Sodium carbonates (g00	0.60	0.50	0.875
5.	Potassium chloride (g)	–0.375	–	–
6.	Citric acid (g)	–	1.45	2.05
7.	Tris (g)	–	2.825	3.5
8.	Cysteine (g)	–	–	0.035
9.	Gentamycine sulphate (μg)/ml	150	150	150
10.	Double distilled water (ml)	500	500	500

Dilution of the ejaculate is generally done depending upon the sperm concentration for successful fertility. Usually one billion sperm per dose should be kept for better conception rate. The dilution ratio varies from 1:1–1:5 which is more common. Excessive dilution sometimes reduces motility and increases sperm abnormality especially tail abnormality. Both dilutor and samples should be kept in a water bath and the temperature should be similar prior to dilution. Before final dilution, dose has to be calculated. Generally 90–100 ml liquid/ fresh semen is used for AI with sufficient numbers of progressive motility spermatozoa. After final dilution, it has to be packed in a pouch/cachette or kept in a bottle for A.I.

Preservation of boar semen in liquid state

Diluted semen can be preserved for 3–4 days with a progressive motility of precisely 50 percent at 18 °C. Report indicated that the best temperature to preserve semen at liquid states is 18 °C to 20 °C. whereas, below 18 °C and above 20 °C reduced the motility of spermatozoa. Increases in temperature above 20 °C enhance the metabolic activity of spermatozoa which reduces the viability and motility in a longer period of preservation.

Table 4. Progressive sperm motility at different temperature

Temperature range	0 Hr	24 hrs	48 hrs	72 hrs	96 hrs
5 °C	80.28 ± 0.68	20.45 ± 1.08	10.46 ± 0.91	6.38 ± 0.80	4.89 ± 2.42
15 °C	80.86 ± 0.71	68.33 ± 0.91	57.42 ± 2.99	37.73 ± 2.99	32.86 ± 1.73
18 °C	80.74 ± 1.35	75.59 ± 1.33	69.24 ± 1.45	69.24 ± 2.52	53.04 ± 2.87
20 °C	79.94 ± 1.20	74.10 ± 0.93	67.37 ± 2.31	58.39± 3.83	51.53 ± 3.17
22 °C	81.04 ± 1.83	73.08 ± 1.03	65..65 ± 2.51	55.39 ± 3.86	44.41 ± 4.15
24 °C	81.60 ± 1.06	70.19 ± 1.54	59.61 ± 2.68	50.20 ± 2.23	40.28 ± 2.53.
26 °C	80.12 ± 1.17	65.14 ± 1.52	50.05 ± 1.86	40.03 ± 4.24	38.18 ± 2.52
28°C	81.20 ± 0.94	64.37 ± 1.68	42.69 ± 1.33	36.21 ± 1.72	37.20 ± 2.10
30 °C	80.26 ± 0.96	61.78 ± 0.97	40.24 ± 0.78	32.84 ± 1.97	31.06 ± 1.77

Table 5. Progressive motility of spermatozoa at controlled and room temp.

Extender	18 °C				Room temperature (19 °C to 26 °C)			
	24	48	72	96	24	48	72	96
BTS	76.36 ± 3.50	69.09 ± 3.49	61.36 ± 3.50	53.09 ± 3.57	70.90 ± 3.40	62.27 ± 3.46	55.00 ± 3.17	47.72 ± 3.37
Modena	72.86 ± 4.78	66.43 ± 4.37	60.06 ± 4.39	49.57 ± 4.40	65.00 ± 4.26	55.71 ± 4.34	49.29 ± 3.98	41.42 ± 422
Zornobsa	68.57 ± 4.78	62.41 ±4.74	57.14 ± 4.53	45.42 ± 5.25	60.00 ± 4.58	50.75 ± 4.54	41.43 ± 3.52	32.36 ± 4.47

Artificial Insemination

Artificial insemination (AI) in swine is not a new technique. There are reports as early as the 1930s of collecting semen for insemination. One of the disadvantages of AI is that it may require a higher level of management than some natural service. There is a greater chance of human error associated with A.I. than with natural services when a boar naturally mates a sow, the semen is not subjected to severe changes in the environment and is generally deposited into the female more than once during a period that spans the optimal time for fertilization. In contrast, many environmental changes are possible when semen is collected, diluted transported and deposited artificially.

The insemination must be done correctly and at the optimal times. Sanitation of the equipments is an important consideration in all AI Procedures. Nowadays, disposable materials are mostly used for AI.

The greatest advantage of AI is that it permits to make use of superior genetic material a minimal cost than some natural service system. Purchasing semen allows genetic diversity which can be used to optimize crossbreeding systems on smaller farmers and increases genetic progress. This can be achieved without the expenses of purchasing and maintaining a simple superior boar. Moreover, good boars can be used more extensively than those used for natural service, because AI increases the numbers of insemination per ejaculate.

To obtain a high conception rate and litter size, estrous detection must be done carefully and without fail.

Swine estrous cycle

The estrous cycle in the pig averages 21 days but ranges from 17 to 25 days. The first day of standing heat, when the female is receptive to the male and to be mounted, is referred to as day 0. The two or three days that female is sexually receptive is termed as *estrus.* The female may or may not exhibit other visual signs, including mounting or attempting to ride other females, swollen, red vulva, mucous from vulva, "popping" of the ears and increased vocalization and activity. In gilts, estrus may last only a day or two, while a sow may be in estrus for three days. The ovulation occurs 23–48 hours after the onset of estrus, this event is extremely variable.

Detecting estrus

Estrous detection in an AI system is vital to the success of each breeding. The procedure must be accurate in estimating the onset of estrus. Trice daily estrous detection can be more effective than once daily detection, though it requires more labour and time. For better detection, perform estrous detection first in the morning and in the evening time. Check the animals when they are not frustrated, distressed or disturbed. Sometimes a mature boar is necessary to induce the female in standing reflexes for AI. This is more important for gilt.

Timing

Timing of artificial insemination is most important for maximizing pregnancy rates and litter sizes in swine. The most critical factor is ensuring that insemination with fertile semen occurs 12 to 18 hours before the moment of ovulation. The sperm inseminated require time in the female reproductive tract to reach the site of fertilization and time to gain the ability to bind and penetrate an egg (capacitation). Once the sperm reach the site of fertilization (within 30 minutes to 8 hours after deposition), they will attempt to fertilize an egg if one is present and they are capable. If the eggs are not present, then sperm will bind to the surface of the female oviduct and wait until ovulation occurs and hormones signal their release from the surface of the female tract. Once ovulated, the window for fertilizing the egg is approximately, 8–12 hours.

Method of Insemination

Before using the semen, 3 evaluations should be done.

Clear the vulva of the female before AI.

Lubricate the tip of the spirette or catheter using non-spermicidal lubricant or a few drops of extended semen. Avoid getting lubricant in the opening of the spirette/catheter.

Gentle guide the spirette/catheter, with the tip pointed up, through the vagina to the cervix. The bottle of the diluted semen is not attached to the spirette/catheter at this time. Keep the tip pointed up to reduce the chance of coming into contact with the bladder, which could cause a backflow of urine to the catheter. If this happens, use a new catheter because urine kills sperm. This is the primary reason that the bottle of diluted semen should not be connected to the spirette/catheter until the cervix has been entered. Not connecting the bottle at this point also avoids exposing the semen unnecessarily to extremes of light or temperature. When using catheter system instead of the bottle, it is common practice to attach the cochette before inserting the spirrete/catheter because great dexterity is required.

- Use counterclockwise rotation to insert the spirette into the cervix. Resistance can be felt by gently pulling back on the spirette. A foam-tipped catheter is not always inserted into the cervix, but usually is positioned up against the cervix.
- Gently invert the bottle of diluted semen two to three times to mix the semen. Attach the bottle to the end of the spirette and discharge the semen slowly. A gentle squeeze to start the process may be needed. After that the semen should be allowed to be taken by uterine contraction.
- When all the semen has deposited into the female, remove the spirette by rotating it clockwise while gently pulling.
- A new catheter/spirette should be used for each time of insemination to eliminate the possibility of transmission of disease.
- Keep the female in quiet surroundings for 30 minutes. Distress at this time may disrupt semen transport and fertilization.

References

Hashizume T, Niwa T (1984) Effect of administration of prostaglandin F2 on the properties of sperm rich fraction of boar semen. Japanese Journal of Animal Reproduction, 30: 182-189.

Levis DG (1989) Artificial Insemination of swine. Nebraska Co-operative Extension. EC 89-264.

Naskar S, Khan MH, Das A, Hassin D (2006) Physical and morphological characteristics of boar semen of different genetic group. Indian Veterinary Journal, 83: 798-799.

Naskar S, Khan MH, Das A, Bordoloi RK (2006) Study on preservation of boar semen at different temperature in liquid state. Indian Veterinary Journal 83: 737-740.

10

Food and Feeding Strategies in Freshwater Aquaculture

G.H. Pailan and B.K. Mahapatra

ICAR-Central Institute of Fisheries Education, Kolkata Centre, 32 GN Block Sector-V, Salt lake, Kolkata 700091, West Bengal

Introduction

The concept of feeding system of different aquatic components of the aquaculture is not simple like that of domestic animals where feed, feeding and the animals can be observed closely and manipulated at once. In case of aquaculture both biotic and abiotic factors play an important role in feeding as well as the growth of the animal. Factors like water temperature, dissolved oxygen, light intensity, *etc.* regulate the intake of feeding, its digestion and assimilation. Conditioning factor, feed conversion rate, survival rate, percent weight gain, daily weight gain, specific growth rate are some of the parameters used routinely to monitor the effects of feeding on growth performance of the fish.

In aquaculture, supplementary feed is provided in conjunction with the available natural food such as plankton, periphyton, benthic organisms, aquatic plants *etc.* Aquaculture is a feed-based industry, with artificial feed accounting for major expenditure exceeding 60% of total operational cost. In India, freshwater aquaculture is mainly carp-based, which accounts for about 89% of total aquaculture production (Ayyappan and Jena, 1998). Successful and sustainable aquaculture depends upon the provision of nutritionally adequate, eco-friendly and economically viable artificial feeds. Effective utilization of feed depends upon many factors such as acceptability of the feed, its digestion, assimilation *etc.* apart from other rearing management protocols.

Artificial feeds need to be formulated and manufactured to provide all the required nutrients at adequate levels for optimum growth, immunity and reproduction. Faulty nutrition leads to poor growth and nutritional disease and due to poor condition, increased susceptibility to infection. The production of nutritionally balanced diets for fish requires efforts in research, quality control and biological evaluation.

Food and feeding habit

Fishes feed on a wide range of food materials and obtain their nourishment from plants as well as animals. Depending upon the number of food items consumed by fish, they may be called stenophagic (feeding on a few different types of food) or euryphagic (feeding on a variety of foods). Various kinds of protozoans, micro-crustaceans, microscopic invertebrates, larvae and eggs of various animals form the food of fishes. Among the larger animals eaten by fish are the annelid worms, snails, mussels, crustaceans, insects, insect larvae, small fishes, tadpoles and even frogs. Some species consume unicellular and filamentous algae, and parts of higher aquatic plants. Some species depend exclusively on zoo- and phytoplankton and are called plankton feeders.

Food eaten by various species of fish has been divided into four categories *viz.* basic, secondary, incidental and obligatory food.

1. The main food is also called basic food. This is the natural food taken and preferred by a fish under favourable conditions.
2. Secondary food is consumed by the fish when available.
3. Incidental food enters the gut by chance along with other items and is rarely seen in the gut contents.
4. Emergency or obligatory food is ingested by the fish to survive under unfavourable conditions when the basic food is not available.

Fry and fingerlings have different feeding habits than the adults. They possess a small and short intestine and usually prefer zooplankton consisting of microscopic animals, protozoans, rotifers, cladocera and crustacean larvae. These are easily digested than the phytoplankton.

Feeding habits

Generally, fishes are described as carnivorous, herbivorous or omnivorous. However, only a few can be strictly classified as carnivorous or herbivorous as the availability of plant or animal material determines whether it will be eaten by a particular species or not. Besides these, some species fed entirely on plankton and form a separate group called the plankton feeders. Some specialize in only one type of food and are referred to as insectivorous, crustacean feeders, mollusk feeders, larvivorous, piscivorous *etc.*

Carnivorous: Several species fed mainly on animals, which constitute a high percentage of their food (more than 75%). Their food consists of crustaceans, insects, their larvae, mollusks, smaller fishes and tadpoles.

Herbivorous: Many fresh water species feed mainly on plant material and their food consists of filamentous algae and parts of higher aquatic plants. The gut content of these fishes when analyzed is found to consist of 75% or more plant material and 1-10% of animal matter.

Omnivorous: A number of species fed on a mixed diet, *i.e.*, both plant and animal matter and cannot be categorized as carnivorous or herbivorous. The food of these species consists of algae, parts of higher plants, rotifers, insects and their larvae, crustaceans, bryozoans.

Plankton feeders: Some species of fishes fed on zoo- and phytoplankton and have evolved an efficient filtering mechanism for obtaining food. These species can be either omnivorous or carnivorous.

Detrivores: The fishes that largely fed on detritus *i.e.*, a mixture of sediments, decaying organic matter and bacteria as their food.

Surface, column and bottom feeders

Freshwater fishes can also be divided into three groups based on ecological zone (niche) they occupy for feeding. These are surface feeders, mid or column feeders and bottom feeders. Food composition and feeding habits of some important finfish and freshwater prawns are given in Table 1.

Table 1. Food composition and feeding habits of some important fin fish and freshwater prawn

Species	Food	Feeding habit
L. rohita (Rohu)	Unicellular and multicellular algae, decaying higher plants, debris, detritus and mud	Herbivorous/column feeder
L. calbasu (Calbose)	Pieces of algae, decaying higher plants, vegetable debris, detritus and mud	Herbivorous/bottom feeder
C. mrigala (Mrigal)	Algae, decaying plant and animal matter, detritus and mud	Omnivorous/bottom feeder
C. catla (Catla)	Unicellular algae, microscopic plants, rotifers, protozoans, larvae of insects and crustacean	Plankton feeder/surface feeder
L. bata (Bata)	Algae, microscopic plants, higher plant material, detritus, mud	Herbivorous/bottom feeder
H. molitrix (Silver carp)	Unicellular algae, rotifers, protozoans, decaying vegetation	Plankton feeder/surface feeder
C. idella (Grass carp)	Aquatic vegetation, various weeds	Herbivorous/column feeder
C. carpio (Common carp)	Algae, macro-vegetation, insects, crustaceans, their larvae	Omnivorous/bottom feeder
C.batrachus (Magur)	Aquatic insects, worms and their larvae, other crustaceans	Omnicarnivores/bottom feeder
H. fossilis (Singhi)	Aquatic insects, worms and their larvae, other crustaceans	Omnicarnivores/bottom feeder
P. hypophthalmus (Pangus)	Aquatic insects, worms and their larvae, other crustaceans	Omnicarnivores/bottom feeder
S. trutta fario (Brown trout)	Animal matter, aquatic insects, worms and their larvae, other crustaceans	Carnivores/bottom feeder
O. mykiss (Rainbow trout)	Animal matter, aquatic insects, worms and their larvae, other crustaceans	Carnivores/bottom feeder

Species	Food	Feeding habit
M. rosenbergii (Freshwater prawn *or scampi)*	Larvae prefer zooplankton mainly minute crustaceans and very small worms, post larvae and adults are omnivorous and mainly feed upon algae, aquatic plants, mollusks, aquatic insects, worms and other crustaceans	Omnivorous/Bottom feeder

Nutrient requirement

Each fish species has specific nutritional requirements *i.e.*, requirement for protein, energy, vitamins, minerals *etc.* which are essential for growth, reproduction and other normal physiological functions. A deficiency of one or more of essential nutrients resulted in a reduced performance, occurrences of disease or even death. These nutrients may come from artificial feed or natural food. To achieve the maximum rate of performance the fish must receive the entire essential nutrient in liberal and balanced quantities. There may be other objectives in feeding programme such as holding fish at a certain desired size for a long period, pigment enhancement, reproductive purposes *etc.* under these conditions a nutritionally balanced diet is still important. To formulate the high-quality, eco-friendly and cost-effective fish feed with all the required nutrients in a proportionate ratio, precise knowledge of the quantitative dietary requirement of nutrients for fish is essential.

Protein

Protein forms the most important and the most expensive component of the diet and helps in tissue building *i.e.*, growth. Therefore, the amount of protein in the diet should be limited to that which is needed for growth, tissue repair *etc.* A continuous dietary supply of protein is essential because it cannot be stored, rather a continuous breakdown and synthesis takes place through the protein turnover process. Gross protein requirements are highest in initial feeding fry and that they decrease as fish size increases. To grow at the maximum rate fry must have a diet in which nearly half of the digestible ingredients consist of balanced protein, which is decreased to several folds with increasing age of fish and prawn raised at standard environmental temperature.

Estimated dietary protein requirements of some important fish species are given in Table 2.

Table 2. Estimated dietary protein requirement of some important fish species

Species	Crude protein level in diet (%)
Cyprinus carpio	38–40 (young and brood stock) 30–33 (adult)
Ctenopharyngodon idella	38–40 (young and brood stock) 30–33 (adult)
Hypophthalmichthys molitrix	37–42 (young and brood stock) 30 (adult)

(Contd.)

Species	Crude protein level in diet (%)
Labeo rohita	40–45 (young and brood stock) 28–30 (adult)
Catla catla	40–45 (young and brood stock) 28–30 (adult)
Cirrhinus mrigala	40–45 (young and brood stock) 28–30 (adult)
Clarias batrachus	40–52 (young) 28–32 (adult)
Macrobrachium rosenbergii	35–40 (young and brood stock) 28–30 (adult)

Essential amino acids (EAA)

The protein quality is influenced primarily by amino acid composition. The amino acids are the building blocks of proteins; about 23 amino acids have been isolated from natural proteins. Ten of these are indispensable for fish and prawns (Table 3). The fish is incapable of synthesizing amino acids and must therefore obtain these from the diet. Generally information on protein requirement will be of limited value unless optimum needs of 10 essential amino acids are known.

Table 3. Essential amino acids requirements of some important fish

EAA (% of Protein)	Rohu	Catla	Mrigal	Common carp	Catfish	Fresh water Prawn	Rainbow trout
Arginine	4.8	5.8	5.3	4.3	4.3	3.7	5.0
Histidine	2.5	2.3	2.1	2.1	1.5	0.7	1.8
Isoleucine	2.4	3.0	2.8	2.5	2.6	0.6	2.0
Lysine	6.2	5.7	5.9	5.7	5.1	3.2	4.5
Leucine	3.7	4.6	4.3	3.3	3.5	1.0	3.5
Methionine*	3.6	2.9	3.2	3.1	2.3	1.2	2.8
Phenylalanine**	3.7	4.0	4.0	6.5	5.0	1.7	4.5
Thereonine	5.0	4.3	4.1	3.9	2.0	1.6	2.0
Tryptophan	1.0	1.1	1.0	0.8	0.5	0.5	0.5
Valine	3.6	3.8	3.5	3.6	3.0	2.1	3.2

The amino acid requirement of grass carps and silver carps are slightly lower than Indian major carps.

Factors affecting protein requirements

1. Size of fish: Fish like land animals have higher protein requirements during their early life than later phase of growth.
2. Physiological function: less protein is needed in maintenance diet than one fed for rapid growth.
3. Protein quality: protein that is deficient in one or more of the 10 essential amino acids will produce less growth than a protein that is balanced in essential amino acids.

4. Nonprotein energy in the diet: If the diet is deficient in energy the fish will use part of the protein to meet energy needs thus reducing the amount of dietary protein available for growth. Protein: energy (P: E) ratio between 95–113 mg protein/kcal and 130-158 mg protein/kcal yielded the highest weight gain of carps species and freshwater prawn, respectively. For brood stock of freshwater prawn P: E ratio should be 92-99 mg protein/Kcal. The use of protein as an energy source by carps and prawn can be minimized at a 1:4 ratio of lipid to carbohydrate and growth and survival to be highest at a dietary protein: starch ratio of 1: or 1:1.5.
5. Feeding rate: Fish fed to less than satiation, as frequently occurs in intensive pond culture of food fish benefited from diets containing higher% of protein than fish fed at or near the satiation rate.
6. Natural foods: if natural aquatic organisms contribute significantly to the daily food intake of the fish the protein level in the prepared diet may be reduced. For example aquatic fauna that is consumed by various fish contain 60–80% protein, thus if these are in abundance the supplemental diet would need only a low level of protein.
7. Economics: The cost and availability of protein sources is a major factor in determining how much protein to be used in commercial diet. Protein levels of 30–36% and 40–43% may probably be adequate for most warm water and cold water fish diet, respectively.
8. Sources of protein: High levels of protein are required for maximum growth rate in all plant diets than in diet containing some fish meal. Additions of fish meal which is rich in methionine, to all plant diets which are low in methionine, increased gain per unit of protein fed and reduce the amount of protein required for maximum growth. Among plant protein sources sesame oil cake and palm kernel are rich in sulphur containing amino acid. When sesame oil cake is used with soybean meal, it would help achieve the proper balance of sulphur containing amino acid and lysine in the diet.
9. Digestibility: Another factor affecting protein quality is digestibility. Fish digest protein in natural aquatic fauna quite well and phytoplankton relatively well. Protein in commercial feedstuff such as fish meal, soybean meal is highly available to fish. Cooking improves the protein digestibility in corn and other grain. The level of starch in the diet has been found to have an inverse effect on protein digestibility, as starch increases above 50% of diet reduced protein digestibility significantly.

Energy requirement

Like other animals, fish cannot directly utilize the radiant energy from the sun but get it through oxidation of the ingested complex molecules, which are broken down by digestion into simpler molecules. Dietary lipid and carbohydrates act as a source of energy. The energetic value of protein, lipid and carbohydrate for fish are 5.6 kcal/g, 9.4 kcal/g and 4.1 kcal/g, respectively. The Energy level in fish feed has been treated casually because a deficiency or excess of energy will not affect the health of fish appreciably and practical feeds made with commonly available ingredients are not likely to be extremely high and low in energy. There is a positive correlation between the energy and protein level of ration as the energy plane of ration increases the percentage of protein increases proportionately. The Energy needs of fish are less than those of warm blooded animals because (i) fish do not have to maintain a constant body temperature (ii) fish requires less energy for muscle activity to maintain their position in the water than do animals on land, (iii) fish requires less energy to excrete nitrogen waste product than warm blooded animals. Digestible energy requirements for maximum growth of fish range between 2800–4063 kcal/kg feed, while the gross energy ranges between 4000-4800 kcal/kg diets.

Protein to energy ratio (P:E)

Fish eat to satisfy their ME requirement and consequently cease feeding when their calorie needs are satisfied. Because of this phenomenon fish eat less of high-energy diet than a low-energy diet. Therefore, too much energy to percentage of protein in the ration can prevent fish from consuming enough protein to meet their dietary need for optimum growth rate, even though the fishes are allowed to eat as much as they will consume. For fish ration 6-10 kcal ME/g of protein is adequate. Variations in energy protein ratios are due to variations in energy source and fish size.

High energy diet especially when a high percentage of calories is from fat, produces fatty fish which have a lower dressing percentage than fish fed a low-energy diet. In general 10–20% lipid in fish diet gives optimal growth without excessive fat. When the non protein calories in the ration are primarily from carbohydrates body fat content is affected in only extremely high energy diet. On the other hand, less non-protein energy relative to protein content in the diet may result in utilization of protein for energy supply rather than muscle growth. In this condition metabolic nitrogenous waste in the form of ammonia is excreted through gills and pollutes water where fish inhabits. Thus, excess protein is not only wasteful and uneconomical but also causes aquatic pollution leading to the stress of fish.

Factors affecting energy requirement

There are several factors, which can alter the energy requirements of fish. Feeding rates should be adjusted to compensate for these factors to avoid over feeding, but still provide sufficient energy for optimum growth.

1. Temperature: As environmental temperature declines, homeotherms must increase their metabolic rate to compensate for the additional heat loss if they are to maintain a constant body temperature. Most freshwater fish do not attempt to maintain a body temperature, which is different from the environment. As water temperature declines, the body temperature of the fish declines and metabolic rate is reduced. The low metabolic rate at low temperatures enables fish to survive for long periods under the ice where little food is available. There is a considerable special difference in metabolic adoptions to environmental temperature changes. Each species seems to have a preferred temperature at which it functions most efficiently. If temperature gradients exist, the fish will seek the most favourable

temperature. Usually, this is the temperature at which the difference between the maintenance requirement and voluntary food intake is greatest and at which optimum efficiency growth occurs.

2. Water flow: Energy, which is used for physical activity, is not available for growth. Fish, which are forced to swim against a strong current, are expending energy, which would otherwise be used for growth. However, still, water allows stratification and to accumulation of waste products. Fish rearing facilities should be designed to obtain maximum use of water without undue stress on the fish.
3. Body size: Small animals produces more heat per unit weight than do large animals. Small fish should be fed a higher percentage of body weight than large fish. In mammals the metabolic rate is proportional to the three-fourths of power of body weight ($W^{0.75}$). The exponent applicable to fish has been reported from 0.34–1. The factor $W^{0.8}$ is usually used. Obviously, more work is needed in this area. Work of the Tunison Laboratory of Fish Nutrition (Idaho, USA) has indicated that rainbow trout from 1.0–4.0 g in weight have a metabolic rate proportional to $W^{1.0}$. Fish from 4.0–50.0 g in weight have metabolic rates proportional to $W^{0.63}$.
4. Level of feeding: The level of feeding also affects the energy expenditure of fish. This becomes important in the design of fish rearing facilities. Dissolved oxygen is usually the first limiting factor in fish rearing. The oxygen consumption increases shortly after feeding due to the physical activity of feed and the heat of nutrient metabolism. Facilities must be designed with adequate safety margins. The oxygen required per unit weight of feed also varies with feed level, being higher at maintenance level when all the food is oxidized than at high feeding levels when much of the energy is stored as growth.
5. Other factors: Several other factors can contribute to high energy requirements. Anything, which makes the fish uncomfortable increases physical activity, reduces growth. Crowding, low oxygen and waste accumulation are some of the important factors.

Carbohydrate requirement

No dietary requirement of carbohydrates has been demonstrated in fish and shellfish, however, if carbohydrates are not provided in the diet, other compounds such as protein and lipids are catabolized for energy. Thus for protein-sparing action it is important to provide the appropriate concentration of carbohydrates in the diet of fish and shellfish species being cultured. Generally fish has a limited capacity to utilize dietary carbohydrates. However, carbohydrate utilization is more in herbivores and omnivores than the carnivores. In general, carnivores cannot utilize more than 20% of dietary carbohydrates, whereas, herbivores and omnivores can utilize about 40-50%. Gelatinization of carbohydrates still improves its utilization. Carps and prawns utilize complex polysaccharides like starch more efficiently than simple sugars like glucose. The crude fibre in the carp diet should not be more than 4-8%, which can not be digested but provides the bulk for proper digestion and excretion of faeces. For both fish and prawns less than 4% CF is desirable.

Lipid and essential fatty acids requirements

Next to protein-lipid forms the major dietary component of finfish and shellfish. Lipid is a complex mixture of simple fat, phospholipids, steroids, free fatty acids and other fat-soluble substances such as carotenoids, vitamin A, D, E & K. Lipid is the most energy rich of all classes of nutrients and thus being the important energy source for fish and prawn. It is the source of various fatty acids some of which are essential for maintenance and integrity of cell membrane, carrier of fat-soluble vitamins *etc.* Carps and prawn have no fixed dietary lipid requirement. The required amount is essentially based upon satisfaction of the requirements for essential fatty acids, in combination with its supply as a good source of energy to spare dietary protein requirements. Depending on the quality and quantity of dietary protein, requirement of dietary lipid, which contain the appropriate levels of essential fatty acids should range from 5-9% and 2-10% for carps and freshwater prawn, respectively. Lipid requirement for carnivores may range from 10-15% in the diet. Phospholipids are dietary essential for larvae of fish and prawns for their better growth and survival. 2-4% dietary supplementation of phospholipids (lecithin/cephalin) is necessary for carps and freshwater prawn only at young stages but supplementation of phospholipid to broodstock diet has no beneficial effect on larval quality. Cholesterol is used as a precursor of important steroids, brain, molting hormones and vitamin D. In carps cholesterol can be synthesized via a complex process, which utilizes acetate as a substrate but freshwater prawn like other crustaceans unable to synthesize sterol de novo. The requirement of the freshwater prawn for dietary cholesterol is approximately 0.5-0.6%.

Essential fatty acids

Carps and prawn appear to require a mixture of polyunsaturated fatty acids (PUFA) like linoleic acid (18:3, ω 6) and linolenic (18:2, ω 3) at 1-2% of the dry matter of diet, which can be reduced by feeding ω 3 and ω 6 highly unsaturated fatty acids (HUFA) like 22:6, ω 3, 20:5, ω 3 and 20:4, ω 6 at a dietary level of 0.1–0.5% because PUFAs can be synthesized from HUFAs but bioconversion in opposite direction is found to be lacking. The requirements for essential fatty acids (mainly ω 3 PUFAs and HUFAs) are greater in larvae and broodstock than juvenile and grow-out stage for better hatchability and survivorship of larvae, which is more tolerant to stress. EFA gives better hatchability of fertilized eggs. Adding vegetable oil (sunflower oil, soyabean oil, linseed oil *etc.*) or fish oil (cod liver oil, sardine oil, herring oil *etc.*) at the optimum level either alone or in combination in the diet can supply EFA to the fish at the required level.

Vitamins requirements

Vitamins are organic compounds, which are essential for transformation of energy but they themselves cannot supply energy to the body and a trace amount of it is required from an exogenous source for normal growth, reproduction and health. One of the first symptoms of deficiency of any of the 15 vitamins of warm water fish is depressed appetite and reduced growth rate. Other common symptoms are abnormal colour, lack of co-ordination, sway back syndrome, nervousness, haemorrhage, fatty liver and increase susceptibility to bacterial infection. All fishes do not require all 15 of the vitamins. Coldwater fishes require all 15 vitamins. Vitamin $B_{12}$is synthesized by the intestinal bacteria in warm water fish like catfish, carp and dietary needs are marginal or nil. Supplementation of vitamin C and E in brood stock diet increased viable egg production. Larval diet should be over fortified with vitamins particularly vitamin C, which protect larvae from stress. Brine shrimp naupli is deficient in vitamin C but rich in other vitamins should be enriched with vitamin C. But for larvae and brood stock other kinds of vitamins that should also be supplemented. In indoor conditions larvae and brood stock require complete diet but in pond conditions it requires only supplementary feed with optimum fertilization. The requirements of vitamins for carps and prawns are as follows (Table 4):

Table 4. Dietary vitamins requirement of fishes and prawns

Vitamins	Warm water fish	Cold water fish	Prawns
Thiamin (mg/kg)	20–30	10	50–100
Riboflavin (mg/kg)	20–30	10	30–58
Pyridoxine (mg/kg)	20–30	10	30–50
Pantothenate (mg/kg)	30–40	80	50–100
Niacin (mg/kg)	150	150	100–150
Folacin (mg/kg)	15	3	5–10
Cyanocobalamin (mg/kg)	Nil	0.02	0.02–0.1
Myo-Inositol (mg/kg)	Nil	400	200–300
Choline (mg/kg)	500–600	800	400–2000
Biotin (mg/kg)	0.6–1.0	1.0	1.0
Ascorbate (mg/kg)	30–50	100	50–100
Vitamin A (I.U./kg)	1000–2000	4000	5000–10000
Vitamin E (I.U./kg)	80–100	400	100–200
Vitamin K (mg/kg)	10–20	40	5–20
Vitamin D_3 (I.U./kg)	500	–	1000–2000

Commercial grade vitamin premix as shown in Table 5 can be supplemented in the fish diet @ 1–2% level to supply each vitamin at required level. As vitamin C is heat labile and prone to leaching loss, in general, fish diet should be supplemented with vitamin C extra @ 100–300 mg/kg diet. Extra supplementation of vitamin C @300-600 mg/kg in freshwater fish and @ 1500–2000 mg/g in brackish water or marine fish) and E (@ 50–250 mg/kg for freshwater fish and @ 1800–2000 mg/g for brackish water or marine fish) in brood stock diet increased viable egg production. Larval diet should be over fortified with vitamins particularly with extra vitamin C (@ 300–600 mg/kg), which protect larvae from stress. Brine shrimp naupli is deficient in vitamin C but rich in other vitamins should be enriched with vitamin C.

Table 5. Composition vitamin premix for carp and prawn diet

Vitamin	Quantity/kg diet
A	5000–10000 IU
D_3	100–200 IU
E	100–200 IU
K	200–400 mg
C	50–100 mg
Thiamine	30–50 mg
Riboflavin	30–50 mg
Pyridoxine	0.02–1 mg
B_{12}	0.5–1 mg
Biotin	400–2000 mg
Choline	5–10 mg
Folic acid	200–300 mg
Inositol	100–150 mg
Niacin	50–100 mg

Minerals requirements

Minerals or inorganic elements are required to maintain many metabolic processes including the formation of skeletal tissue, respiration, digestion and osmoregulation. Finfish and shellfish unlike most terrestrial animals can absorb some minerals from the aquatic environment in which they inhabit. Not all elements that are used in metabolism are required in the animal's diet. Fish, particularly marine fish, have an advantage in that their ambient medium contains many of the elements that they need for growth and survival.

The minerals required for normal metabolism can be divided into two groups. Major and trace minerals. Major minerals are required in large quantities and include calcium, phosphorus, magnesium, sodium, potassium, chlorine and sulphur. Trace minerals are those required in trace amounts and include iron, iodine, manganese, copper, cobalt, zinc, selenium, molybdenum, fluorine, aluminium, nickel, vanadium, silicon, tin and chromium. Mineral requirement of fin fish and shell fish are given in Table 6.

Table 6. Mineral requirement of fin fish and shell fish

Mineral Elements	Carps	Channel catfish	Rainbow trout	Tilapia	Eel	Prawn
Calcium (%)	0.1–0.5, 0.19(IMC)	< 0.1	< 0.1	–	0.27	0.1–0.5
Phosphorus (%)	0.6–0.7, 75 (IMC)	0.45	0.6	0.9	0.3	0.6–0.7
Magnesium (%)	0.05	0.04	0.05	0.06	0.04	0.05
Sodium (%)	0.1–0.3	–	–	–	–	0.1–0.3

Mineral Elements	Carps	Channel catfish	Rainbow trout	Tilapia	Eel	Prawn
Potassium (%)	0.1–0.3	Trace	Trace	Trace	Trace	0.1–0.3
Sulphur (%)	0.3–0.5	–	–	–	–	0.3–0.5
Chlorine (%)	0.1–0.5	–	–	–	–	0.1–0.5
Iron (mg/kg)	50–150	30	Trace	Trace	170	50–150
Copper (mg/kg)	1–4	5	3	3.5	Trace	1–4
Manganese (mg/kg)	13	2.4	13	12	Trace	13
Cobalt (mg/kg)	5–10	–	–	–	–	5–10
Zinc (mg/kg)	15–30	20	15–30	20	Trace	15–30
Iodine (mg/kg)	100–300 mg	1.1	1.1	Trace	Trace	100–300 mg
Molybdenum	(trace)	–	–	–	–	(trace)
Chromium	(trace)	–	–	–	–	(trace)
Fluorine	(trace)	–	–	–	–	(trace)
Selenium	(trace)	0.25	0.15–0.3	Trace	Trace	(trace)

Commercial grade mineral premix (Table 7) can be supplemented at 2-4% level to supply the minerals at required level.

Table 7. Composition mineral premix for carp and prawn diet

Minerals	Quantity/kg diet
Ca	10–18 g
P	18 g
Mg	0.8–1 g
Na	6g
K	9g
S	0.2 g
Mn	20 mg
Zn	50–100 mg
Fe	5–20 mg
Co	10 mg
Se	1 mg
Cl	Traces
Mo	Traces
Cr	Traces
Fl	Traces
Cu	25 mg

Feed supplements and feed additives

Feed based intensified aquaculture has been aimed at increased nutrient utilization, growth and survival of fish to maximize production with minimizing feed borne aquatic pollution. For this purpose different feed supplements and feed additives should be added in formulated feed. Critical nutrients such as limiting amino acids, EFAs, vitamins, minerals *etc.*, which have the chances of deficiency need to be supplemented to overcome deficiency in the diet are generally termed as feed supplements. Feed additives are non-nutritive, natural or synthetic substances supplemented in the animal's diet usually in very small quantity for fortifying the diet to improve feed intake and nutrient utilization, enhance growth and increase immunity and survival of animals including fish. The recently used term for feed supplements and feed additives is nutraceuticals. Nutraceutical, a portmanteau of the words "nutrition" and "pharmaceutical", is a food or food product that provides health and medical benefits, including the prevention and treatment of disease.

Limiting amino acids

In formulated diet there is often deficiency of limiting amino acids such as lysine and methionine because most of the feed ingredients are deficient in these amino acids. Thus these amino acids need to be supplemented in formulated diet to overcome the deficiency. Synthetic forms such as L-lysine and DL-methionine and naturally purified herbomethionine are commercially available in the market. L-lysine is supplemented @ 0.25-0.5% and DL-methionine or herbomethionine is supplemented @ 0.5-1% in the diet.

Vitamins

Individual vitamins or vitamin premix are commercially available in the market. Vitamin premix can also be formulated and prepared at the laboratory level. Vitamin premix is a concentrate in which stable forms of essential vitamins are mixed with a carrier usually a basal feed such as wheat flour. Mixing and storage of vitamins need special care and facilities. Thus farmers should not attempt to make vitamin premix and also not add individual vitamins in the farm made feed. Vitamin premix is supplemented in formulated compound feed to overcome the deficiency. Depending on the formulation, vitamin premix can be supplemented in formulated diet @ 0.4-1%. Vitamin C is water soluble anti-oxidant/antistress vitamin which also acts as a nutraceutical in aquaculture. But it is heat labile, thus it is lost during feed processing and storage and it is also prone to leaching loss. Therefore, often separate supplementation of vitamin C @ 100 to 300 mg/kg is required. Extra supplementation of vitamin C @ 300-600 mg/kg in freshwater fish and @ 1500-2000 mg/g in brackish water or marine fish) and E (@ 50-250 mg/kg for freshwater fish and @ 1800-2000 mg/g for brackish water or marine fish) in brood stock diet increased viable egg production. Larval diet should be over fortified with vitamins particularly with extra vitamin C (@ 300-600 mg/kg), which protect larvae from stress. Both Vitamin C and E play a significant role in boosting the immunity of fish due to their free radical scavenging activity, which increases during stress, thus giving the disease resistance. Supplemental level of 3000 mg ascorbic acid /kg diet significantly enhances immunity and disease resistance. Similarly Vit E (Tocopherol) at a higher dietary supplemental level increases immunity and disease resistance in fish.

Minerals

Minerals are of essential elements added to the diet. Fish get most of the macro elements from their aquatic habitat except phosphorus (P). Thus P needs to be supplemented in formulated diet. Some feed ingredients such as fish meal are the good source of P. In oilseed cake and grains/grain by-products about 70-80% remains as phytic acid (phytate) form. Thus fish cannot utilize P from plant-based diet as it is lacking phytase enzyme required for breaking the phytate to make the P available to the animal. Thus formulated diet of fish with plant based ingredients needs to be supplemented with dicalcium phosphate (DCP) @ 0.5% as a P to overcome the deficiency. Trace minerals are less available from water body. Thus, plant based diet, which is often deficient of trace minerals is supplemented with trace element premix @ 0.2-0.4%. Complete mineral premix containing both macro and trace minerals are commercially available and can be added in the formulated diet @ 1-2% level. Sometimes salt (NaCl) can be added separately at 1-2% level in formulated diet. Vitamin-mineral mixture is also available in the market, can be supplemented @ 1-2% level.

Essential fatty acids (EFA)

For freshwater fish, linolic acid (18:2w6) and linolenic acid (18:3w3) are essential fatty acids, whereas arachidonic acid, eicosapentaenoic acid (EPA), 20:5w3 and docosahexaenoic acid (DHA), 22:6w3 are essential for marine fish. Depending on the species, EFA is supplemented @ 0.5-1% level in the formulated diet, especially in brood stock diet to increase viable egg and in larval diet to increase survivability. PUFAs of n3 family act as nutraceutical in the fish diet. It serves as precursors of biologically active eicosanoids, which are in turn important mediators in inflammatory reactions and partly also in the regulation of immune response. Increasing the level of n-3 PUFAs in the diet with fish oils influences the immune response and hence shows disease resistance in cultured fish. It has been shown in fish that HUFAs enriched diet increased the resistance of larvae to different stresses such as handling and variations in temperature and salinity. Non-gelatinized carbohydrate supplemented with 1% n-3 PUFA is found to be optimum to enhance the immunity in *Labeo rohita* juveniles. It is also observed that higher supplementation of ω-3 fatty acid (3%) in the diet causes immunosuppression in *C. catla* juveniles.

Phospholipid

Phospholipid (Lecithin) is commonly supplemented @ 2-4% in fish diet for optimum growth and survival whereas in the formulated feed of marine shrimp supplemental level is 0.2-2%. Soya lecithin is preferable phospholipid for fish diet.

Cholesterol

Shellfish cannot synthesize cholesterol need dietary addition @0.5%. The main function of cholesterol in crustacean is the synthesis of moulting steroid hormone.

Binders

Binders are used in the formulated diet of finfish and shellfish to improve palatability, to enhance pellet durability for preserving physical form during storage, to prevent disintegration during handling and shipping, to enhance their water stability. Binders used in formulated feed are mainly complex polysaccharides. Sometimes some protein sources are also used in fish feed as binder. Though a wide range of binders are available in the market, most commonly used binders in formulated feed are (i) Carboxymethyl cellulose (CMC): 2-4% (ii) Gnm acacia: 2-5% (iii) Na or K bentonite: not > 2%

(iv) Agar agar: 2-5% (v) Gnar gnar: 1-2% (vi) Wheat gluten: 10-12% (vii) Starch powder 2-5% (viii) Heat treatment during diet preparation results in gelatinization of starch that along with energy supply also acts as binder.

Antioxidants

Antioxidants are substrates that can be easily oxidized and thus they protect other compounds which are sensitive to oxidation. Thus antioxidants are broken themselves and slow down the chain reaction involved in peroxidation. In formulated diet antioxidants are added to vitamin premix or to the lipid to delay the onset of the rancidity of these substances. Rancidity makes the feed unpalatable and generates toxic substances such as aldehyde or ketone. Lipids rich in PUFA and vitamin A, E, riboflavin, folic acid is more prone to oxidation. This phenomenon occurs during storage of feed. Thus diet containing PUFA rich lipid and vitamins needs to be supplemented with antioxidants. Natural antioxidants are vitamin C and E and synthetic antioxidants are butylated hydroxyl anisol (BHA) and butylated hydroxyl toluene (BHT) and ethoxyquin. The supplemental doses are i) Vitamin C: 100-300 mg/kg ii) Vitamin E: 300-390 mg/kg iii) BHA: 0.1% iv) BHT: 0.1% v) Ethoxyquin: 0.015%. A better approach is the supplementation of vitamin C and E along with any one of synthetic antioxidants.

Feeding Stimulants or Chemo-attractants

The compounds which stimulate gustatory receptors cells which result in enhanced feed intake called feeding stimulants. Feeding stimulants also enhance flavor. Fish reject unpalatable feed resulting in less feed intake. Thus plant based formulated feed should be supplemented with feeding stimulants which increases palatability of feed, thus increasing feed intake. Feeding stimulants are also called gustatory stimulants or palatability enhancers or flavouring attractants. Medicated feed also needs to be supplemented with feeding stimulants. It is also effective to train young fish or larvae to accept formulated diet after weaning from live foods. Chemicals identified as feeding stimulants are amino acids, betaine, quaternary ammonium bases, nucleoside (inosin) and nucleotide (IMP, AMP, UMP etc), organic acids (propionic acid), bile salts *etc.* Effectiveness of different compounds differs among different species. L forms of amino acids are more effective than their D-isomer. Mixtures of several amino acids are more effective than individual amino acids. Mixtures of amino acids and other stimulants are more effective, e.g betaine plus amino acid mixture. There are species specific sensitivities to different classes of taste stimuli. Feeding stimulants of common carp is a mixture containing betaine and L form of amino acid mixture such as proline, alanine, cysteine, glutamic acid and glycine. A mixture of proline, alanine, cysteine, glutamic acid and glycine at 0.1-0.5% acts as feeding stimulant. Addition of betaine to this mixture @ 0.25% and nucleotide rich spirulina or yeast @ 1% gives better result and also improve immunity.

Preservatives (Acidifiers) & enzymes

In tropical country increasing humidity makes the feed moist during storage. Storage conditions like temperature >25°C, relative humidity >65% and moisture 12% facilitate the mould and bacterial growth that deteriorate the feed quality during storage. Mould like *Aspergillus flavus* contaminate the feed with aflatoxins that produce ill effect on fish. Thus to prevent mould growth antifungal agents are used. Use of antifungal agents in feed to prevent mould growth during storage is called preservatives. Application of feed acidifiers in the species of livestock such as poultry and cattle is currently in the experimental stage and is likely to emerge into an important feed additives for all classes of animal species, given the market's shift from pharmaceutical products to natural feed and hygiene management as nutraceuticals. The addition of phytase (@ 500 FTU) to plant-based diets increased the bioavailability of P and other minerals, thereby increasing bone mineralization in *L. rohita* fingerlings. The effect of phytase was increased because of addition of citric acid (3%) which is an acidifier. Commonly used preservatives and their dose in fish feed are i) Na or Ca propionate: not > 1% ii) K propionate: not > 1% iii) Na benzoate: not > 1% iv) Na or Ca sorbate: not > 1% and v) Methyl paraben: not > 0.1%.

Carotenoids

Carotenoids are a family of pigments the fish can't synthesize and are obtained as part of the diet. These pigments result in red, yellow and orange colors. Fish use oxygenated carotenoids, one of the most important groups of natural pigments, for pigmentation of skin and flesh. Carotenoids commonly occurring in freshwater include beta carotene, lutein, taraxanthin, astaxanthin, tunaxanthin, alpha-, beta-doradexanthins, and zeaxanthin. As fish cannot synthesize these pigments, they rely on dietary supply of carotenoids to achieve their natural skin pigmentation, one of the most important quality criteria informing the market value of ornamental high-value species such as Koi carp (*Cyprinus carpio*) and goldfish (*Carassius auratus*). Fish have cells called chromatophores. Those cells convert yellow pigment zeaxanthin into astaxanthin which is the red pigment and thus gives red colouration in goldfish and common carp. Goldfish metabolized very little beta-carotene and no lutein to astaxanthin. Success at shows and exhibitions of ornamental fishes is very much dependent on achieving vibrant colour. Under certain well-defined culture conditions (nitrogen depletion, high salinity and light intensity) the algae *Chlorella vulgaris*, *Haematococcus pluvialis* and *Arthrospira maxima* (*Spirulina*) will accumulate secondary carotenoids and might be used to replace costly synthetic colouring materials in ornamental fish feed. Supplementation of spirulina @ 4 mg/kg diet is effective in skin pigmentation of blue gouramis (*Trichogaster trichopterus* Pallas) and withdrawal of supplementation diminishes the colour intensity. Besides various plants such as marigold flowers, tomatoes, sweet red peppers, yellow maize, carrots, yam, pumpkin, paprika, beetroot and mushrooms, alfalfa meal, grass meal, chlorella; aquatic animals like mollusks, crustaceans, shrimp, prawns, krill and terrestrial animals and animal products such as bird plumage, insects, butter, egg yolk and cheese are the good natural source of carotenoids, which shows better results than synthetic carotenoids (roche carophyll pink). Diets of ornamental fishes should not only contain adequate levels of protein, energy, oils, vitamins and minerals but also a constant supply of carotenoids with correct balance of ingredients. Supplementation of artificial feeds with a balanced mixture of natural carotenoids can enhance the pigmentation in ornamental fishes. It is reported that supplementation of China rose (*Hibiscus rosasinensis*) petals in the diet of gold fish @ 5 mg/kg increased both skin colouration and gonadal maturation.

Probiotics

Feed supplements with live microbials are called probiotics. Different bacterial species such as Bacillus sp., Bifidobacterium sp. and many others are used as probiotics in formulated fish feed. Thus, Probiotics are single or mixture of live microorganisms like *Lactobacillus*, *Streptococcus*, *Bifidobacterium* species *etc.* which offer new dietary alternatives of immunotherapy to counteract local immunological dysfunctions and to stabilize the natural gut mucosal barrier mechanisms. Probiotics prevent the colonization of harmful bacteria in fish gut, they may be the source of various nutrients such as Vitamin B_{12} and it enhances immunity in the host animal. *Lactobacillus* sp. when administered orally stimulated the immune system of non-specific way. Dry feed containing lactic acid bacteria (*Carnobacterium divergens*) isolated from Atlantic cod (*Gadus morhua*) intestines improved disease resistance of cod fry exposed to a virulent strain of *Vibrio anguillarium*. The Addition of probiotics in the diet (2-3%) improves the growth performance of *Macrobrachium rosenbergii* larvae. Probiotic feeding has a significant role in larvae as the survival rate of larvae is poor as they lack a well-developed immune system. Hence mode of delivery of probiotics to larvae is a challenging task. It was reported that higher survival of *Macrobrachium rosenbergii* when *Lactobacillus* was fed bioencapsulated with Artemisia.

Prebiotics

Prebiotics are non-digestible oligosaccharides (NDO) that are utilized by probiotic bacteria. Some important prebiotics are Mannanoligosaccharides (MOS), fructooligosaccharides (FOS), galactooligosaccharides (GOS) *etc.* Prebiotics improve gut health, proliferate probiotic bacteria, suppress harmful bacteria, improve growth of host animal, increase feed intake, digestibility of nutrients and enhance non-specific immunity. Thus use of prebiotics along with probiotics in diet gives better benefits. Prebiotics can be added in the diet @ 1-2%. When probiotics and prebiotics work together, it is termed synbiotics.

Phytobiotics

After dietary supplementation when extracts of different medicinal herbs such as *C. dactylon*, *A. marmelos*, *T. cordifolia*, *P. kurooa*, *E. alba*, *Ricinus communis* and many others increases immunity and gives disease resistance to the animals including fish, it is termed as phytobiotics. Methanolic extract of various medicinal herbs if supplemented @0.5-1% in the larval diet increases immunity and larval survivability. It was observed that the bacterial (*Vibrio parahaemolyticus*) load of shrimp *P. indicus* juveniles fed with seaweed and herbal extracts was reduced significantly.

Immunostimulants

Immunostimulants like beta-glucans, EF203, lactoferrin, levamisole and chitosan are used as immunostimulants or nutraceuticals in aquaculture. It was showed that peptidoglycan fed black tiger shrimp exhibited higher tolerance to dissolved oxygen, salinity and stress than that fed a control diet. Feeding carp with levamisole (5 mg/kg body weight) resulted in enhanced phagocytic activity of blood leucocytes. Dietary supplementation of immunostimulants at 1% level promotes growth and survival in *L. rohita* fingerlings. In contrast, higher inclusion levels of immunostimulants led to an immunosuppressive effect in *L. rohita* fingerlings. The immunostimulants mainly enhances bactericidal activities of phagocytes. Several immunostimulants also stimulate the natural killer cells, complement, lysozyme and antibody responses of fish. The activation of these immunological functions is associated with increased protection against infectious disease. Dietary yeast RNA supplementation reduces mortality by *Aeromonas hydrophila* in Rohu (*Labeo rohita* L.) juveniles. The inclusion of 0.8% nucleotide in the diet would enhance the immune responses in *Catla catla* fingerlings. Some researchers reported that *Labeo rohita* fed with nucleotide rich ingredients like yeast, yeast extract or spirulina also boosts immunity. Peptides are also having nutraceutical activity e.g. lactoferrin which is a polypeptide and can activate macrophages *in vitro*. Red seabreams orally administrated bovine lactoferrin showed increased numbers of granulocytes in the blood and elevated secretion of body mucus.

Feeding strategies

To achieve best feed efficiency of a given feed for maximum growth of fish in a culture system, implementation of appropriate feeding strategies in terms of types of feed, feeding rate, feeding frequency and feeding methods are extremely important.

Feeding rate

The amount of feed offered should be regulated with reference to the biomass of the fish or prawns being cultured as well as an observation on their daily feed intake. Daily observations on feed intake in lift nets or check trays for prawns are very important to decide on the amount of feed to be offered on subsequent days. Factors that may affect feed intake are: Poor quality, low oxygen level, high temperature, high ammonia, nitrite and hydrogen sulphide levels. Increasing temperature and salinity enhance the energy requirements of fish and prawn. Fish fry and fingerlings and prawn post

larvae and juveniles require more food to meet the demand for best growth. Both over feeding and under feeding affect growth, Production and FCR. The daily feeding rate for prawn (% of biomass) varies from 25 to 2% during crop period, maximum during post- larval stage (PL20) to the maximum when the animal reaches marketable size. Feeding at the constant rate should be avoided. Feeding rates for fish also vary according to water temperature and size. The amount of feed to be given daily can be calculated as follows:

$$\text{Feed to be given (kg/day)} = \frac{\text{Nos. of animals} \times \text{average weight} \times \text{Feeding (\% biomass)}}{100}$$

Feeding frequency

The number of meals offered daily and time feeding is also factors that affect growth and feed efficiency. Frequent feeding reduces starvation and stunting, enables uniform growth and result in minimum feed wastage. In the case of fish daily ration of feed is offered in several meals often 4 to 6 times a day. Feeding in finfish is mostly done during the day, between 6 A.M to 6 P.M but during fry stage a continuous feed supply is maintained. In the case of prawns the number of meals offered per day range from 4 to 6 for post larvae and juveniles, to 3 to 6 times day for sub adults and adults. The total amount of feed to be offered each day is divided into small quantities and fed. In case of burrowing prawn species like *Penaeus semisulcutus* and *P. japonicas* late afternoon, evenong and night feeding is preferred. In the case of *P. monodon* and *P. indicus* about 40 to 45% of the daily is offered between 6 A.M and 11 A.M and the balance between 2 P.M and 12 midnight.

Feeding methods

Dry pellets, granules for fish and prawns could be broadcasted. Fish in general are fast feeders and good palatable feeds are consumed within 15 to 30 minutes by most species but, prawns being slow feeders, it is necessary to evenly distribute granules and pellets. Broadcasting the feeds from pond bunds is quite adequate for small ponds (<0.5 ha). But in larger ponds (>0.5ha) broadcasting the feeds from bunds should be supplemented by distribution in slightly interior areas using small boats. Moist feeds and meals should not be broadcasted but kept on earthen or plastic trays, placed in the peripheral areas of the pond bottom. The feeding method adopted in semi-intensive carp culture systems is unique in West Bengal. The outline of the method is as follows: feed mixture is kept in perforated fertilizer bags tied to bamboo poles. About 20 to 30 bags are kept per hectare. Fish browse on the feed through the perforations in the bags and within 2 hours most of the feed kept in the bags is consumed.

Feeding practices for carps

In nursery pond

Though plankton is the main food for carp spawn, egg yolk suspension is fed @ 100 gms yolk and 5 gms yeast per lakh spawn twice daily once at morning 8-10 am and another evening 5 pm for the first 5 days. The suspension is uniformly spread in nursery ponds or tanks. Instead of egg yolk suspension, finely powdered mash (50-70 μ) can also be broadcasted during initial period of rearing. Thereafter, finely powdered feed or fine crumbles (>70-400 μ) is broadcasted for spawn rearing in well prepared nursery ponds up to 13th day out of total 15 days rearing period. The larvae are starved on day 14 and on day 15 harvesting of fry is done. Daily allowance of feed in nursery pond is 4 times or 400% of initial body weight of spawn for first week and 8 times or 800% of initial body weight of spawn for second weeks and can be fed to the fish in two equal split doses once at morning 10 AM and another at late afternoon at 5 PM. If possible, per day feeding frequency may be increased to 6-8 times because it is more beneficial for tiny spawn in nursery ponds.

In rearing pond

For feeding fry in well prepared rearing pond for 90 days period initially crumbles of 0.5 mm dia can be used and gradually crumble size can be increased up to 0.8-1 mm dia. Considering the plenty of live food available for larvae, daily allowance of feed in rearing pond is 6-8% of body weight during first month, 5-6% of body weight during second month and 3-4% of body weight during third month and can be fed to the fish in two equal split doses once at morning 10 AM and another at late afternoon at 5 PM, if feed is broadcasted. Feeding frequency 3-4 times per day is always beneficial. However, feeding frequency is depended on feeding method. Tray (plastic or aluminum) system of feeding method is always preferable for controlling the feed loss. Total amount of required feed per day is taken either in a tray, which is then hung from bamboo pole from different places of the pond 8-10 ft away from the pond side. 14-16 trays are required per ha area. This methods of feeding is done once per day and in the next day trays are taken out, washed properly and continued the feeding in the same way.

In grow out pond

During 10-12 months culture period, for feeding fingerlings and growers in grow out pond under composite fish culture system different types of feed such as dry mash, wet ball, cooked paste, cooked ball or dry pellets can be used. Under semi-intensive culture system supplementary artificial feed and intensive culture system complete artificial feed should be provided. Fish are fed 5% of body weight during first two months, 4% of body weight during next two months, 3% of body weight during next two months, 2% of body weight during next two months and 1% of body weight during final 2-4 months. Depending on the feed types either broadcast or tray (plastic or aluminum) or basket (bamboo basket) or bag (cement bag or gunny bag) system of feeding method is employed in grow out pond. A mixture of floating and sinking pellets at 2:1 ration can be broadcasted in the pond twice daily once at morning 10 AM and another in late afternoon at 5 PM. Wind may displace the floating pellets which may congregate at the side of the pond. To prevent this feed may be broadcasted within the plastic ring placed in different places of the pond. Floating pellets are suitable for feeding carps in cages. For other kinds of feeding methods as mentioned earlier, feeding is done once daily. Either wet ball or cooked paste or cooked ball or dry sinking pellets can be offered to the carps through three tier system of tray or basket method in which total amount of required feed per day is distributed in different trays or basket which are tied up in and hanged from bamboo pole that is placed 8-10 ft away from the pond side and trays or basket in are submerged in the water at 1.5 ft, 3.5ft and 5.5ft depth. For easy submersion weighty stone or brick can be tied at the bottom of the tray or baskets. In case of bamboo basket polythene paper can be placed inside bottom of the basket to prevent loss of disintegrated feed. This kind of arrangement should be done at 14-16 places per ha area. Next day morning trays or basket are removed, washed and continued the feeding in the same way. Mash feed and also sinking pellets can be offered to the fish through three tier bag system of feeding method. Perforated nylon or plastic cement or fertilizer bags of 20 kg capacity are generally used for this purpose. After distributing the daily required feed inside the bag, mouth is tied and bags are hung in the same way as tray or basket method. This sort of arrangement is required at 14-16 places per ha area. When fish nibbles near holes, a certain amount of feed mixture or pellets comes out through holes that are consumed by the fish, thus this system acts as the indigenous type of demand feeder (which are generally used in developed country). Such feeding method is common in carp farms of Andhra

Pradesh. In Punjab, farmers use several feed baskets or perforated bags tied up in a row in a floating material which is kept floating across water bodies. Tray/basket and bag systems of feeding methods are useful for controlling the feed loss or waste.

In polyculture of carps and prawn, carps are fed in similar way as described above but prawn feed is given in tray or basket hanged from the bamboo pole 1-1.5 ft away from pond side and submerged the tray 1 ft underneath the water. Prawn feed is offered at 8 PM since prawn is having nocturnal feeding habit. Wet ball or pellet feed can be used for feeding of prawn. Besides snail meat/meat meal/fish meal/meat scraping can also be used at 15 days intervals for feeding of prawn. Prawn juveniles are fed @ 25% of body weight for first 2 months and gradually reducing to 3% of body weight towards the end of the culture period on daily basis or @ 5-3% of body weight on daily basis for the first month and then at the same rate on alternate days from the second month onwards. Under composite fish culture system, for feeding of grass carp separate arrangement is required. Chopped aquatic weeds, fooder grasses (napier etc), lawn grass, vegetable waste *etc.* can be placed on rectangular bamboo platform fixed at corner of ponds at certain depth for feeding of grass carp. The grass carp should be fed until they stop eating. Usually they consume aquatic weeds about 50% of their body weight daily. Hence it is advisable to feed them at least 1 hour before the application of supplementary feed to other fish. Sometimes, mixed feeding schedule such as 1-2 days feeding with low protein diet followed by 3 days feeding with high protein diet can also be practiced. Through proper feeding management, FCR in carp culture is possible to maintain as 2:1. Trash fish and floating pellets are used for feeding fish in cages where fish production of 35-65 kg/m3 is achieved after 8-12 months.

Feeding practices for magur

For magur Larvae in indoor tank

1. Mixed zooplankton, Artemia nauplii, molluscan meat, tubifex or egg custard are considered to be the larval feed during hatchery rearing of *C. batrachus* larvae or spawn
2. These feed items contain 41-65% protein
3. Mixed zooplankton is observed to be well-accepted feed for these catfish larvae, which can be easily collected from a well prepared carp nursery ponds
4. Live plankton is considered to be the well accepted feed for rearing of fish larvae as observed in other fish larvae
5. As the plankton remains in live condition in the rearing tanks, the larvae get opportunity to feed on them as and when required
6. Feed containing 45% protein in the form of small ball is offered along with live plankton from 7-8 days of rearing
7. The supply of live plankton may be withdrawn gradually during the rearing period of 13-14 days.
8. This mixed feeding not only enhances growth, but also ensures higher survival rate.
9. Organisms/particles ranging from 20-30μ are ideal for the initial feeding

10. Size can be increased gradually to 50-60 micrometre for a week old fry
11. Since there may be a differential growth in fry from the beginning, it is wise to proceed with the visual observation for selecting the size of the feed
12. The fry develop gregarious habits within a week and being nocturnal and photonegative, they normally congregate in the corners of the rearing container to avoid light during daytime
13. However, they get fully dispersed all over the container during the night and as soon as they are exposed to light, they move to the corners of the container in groups.

Fry are usually reared in indoor tanks for a few weeks before releasing them into ponds. During this period they are fed with crumbles (0.3-0.5 mm) at an hourly interval. The feeding rate should be adjusted by visual observation.

For magur fingerlings and grower in pond
In a pond with a high density of zooplankton, artificial feed @ 10-5% of body weight is normally dispensed or broadcasted from all sides to provide feeding opportunities to all fish. Feeding should be done twice daily once at very early morning and another in late evening as magur prefers to eat under less light.

Water quality is very much important for feeding of catfish. At low oxygen level feeding activity of magur is reduced. Thus pelleted feed needs to have high degree of water stability. Mash and wet ball is less preferable for catfish. Sometimes molluscan meat, chopped chicken viscera can also be fed to magur under pond condition. These feeds are placed at shallow zone near the side of the pond. Through proper feeding management FCR can be maintained as 3-4:1 under pond condition.

Feeding practices for pangasius
Under pond condition a mixture of rice bran, broken rice and small quantity of trash fish can be fed to the stocked fingerlings for first two months. From third months onward, fish are fed various formulated diets. The feed is broadcasted to fingerlings @ 10% of body weight and gradually reduced to 5% for juvenile, grower and adult stage. Through proper feeding management in ponds, fish can attain an average weight of 1-1.5 kg with FCR of 4-6:1 at the end of 8-12 months culture period.

Feeding practices for freshwater prawn

For freshwater prawn larvae
(i) Freshwater prawn larvae are called zoea (ii) 11 zoeal stages *i.e.*, Z1-Z11 or I-XI are completed between 23 and 32 days depending on the temperature, food and water quality (iii) Larval stages are planktonic in nature (iv) I to XI developing larval stages requires either artificial or natural brackishwater (12-14 ppt) at 28-31°C to attain the post-larval stage (v) The postlarvae settle down at the bottom as crawlers or cling to vegetation or submerged objects.

Stocking in larval rearing tank: (i) Initially small tanks at high density of 700-1,000/L (ii) After 6-10 days, larvae are moved to larger tanks and the density reduced to 50-100/L.

Feeding: (i) In nature newly hatched zoea (1.6 to 2.40 mm) feed on minute zooplankton, diatoms and detritus. (ii) However, in hatchery they prefer to feed on minute zooplankton especially Cladocerans and Copepods. (iii) In hatchery they prefer to feed on minute zooplankton especially Rotifers, Brine shrimp naupli, Flesh of prawn and fish, Molluscan meat, Chopped earthworm, Chopped tubificid worm, Egg custard *etc.* (iv) From stage I to V (up to 6 days), larvae prefer to take *Branchionus plicatilis,* Brine shrimp nauplii *etc.* (v) Whereas from stage VI onwards (up to 30–32 days), the supplementary feeding with egg custard, animal meat *etc.* can be done.

Strategy: A gradual replacement of up to 50% of the Artemia nauplii ration with wet and dry diets (egg custard *etc.*) show similar results compared to a 100% Artemia control in terms of larval development, survival and larval quality.

Feeding Schedule-I

1. The larvae are fed with egg custard, *Moina micrura* and *Artemia nauplii.*
2. The feed is given five times a day at 0600, 1000, 1400, 1800 and 2200 hours.
3. The amount of egg custard varied from 0.1 to 1.0 g per 1000 larvae per time, Artemia nauplii 5 to 10 per larva per feed and Moina 2 to 6 per larva per feed.
4. One day's feed consisted of 2 times Moina, 2 times egg custard and 1 time Artemia nauplii or 2 times Moina, 2 times Artemia nauplii and 1 time egg custard.

Feeding Schedule-II

Age of Larvae in days	Stage	Feed constituents and amount					
		Artemia nauplii		Moina		Egg custard	
		No./ml	Times/day	No./ml	Times/day	g/1000 larvae	Times/day
2–3	I–II	2	–2	4–	–	–	–
4–6	III–IV	4–5	3	–	–	–	–
7–15	IV–VI	5–6	2	2	1	0.10–0.25	1
16–25	VI–IX	5–6	1	3	2	0.40–0.60	2
26–35	IX–XI &PL	6–7	1	3	2	0.75–1.25	2
36–45	X–PL	6–7	1	3	2	1.50–2.00	2

For juveniles and growers in pond

To enhance the growth and as a precaution against cannibalism, the prawn juveniles are given feed mix (rice bran: oil cake in a ratio of 1: 1) @ 25% of body weight for first 2 months and gradually reducing to 3% of body weight towards the end of the culture period on daily basis (following table) or @ 3-5% of body weight on daily basis for the first month and then at the same rate on alternate days from the second month onwards. However, quantity of feed should be adjusted through trial and error after verifying the consumption on the following morning. To avoid cannibalism, prawn should not be hungry. Wet ball may be prepared using these ingredients and provided through plastic or aluminium tray or bamboo basket hanging from bamboo pole fixed 1-1.5 ft away from the pond dike and submerged 1-1.5 ft underneath the water. Per hectare area at 14- 16 places this sort of arrangement should be made. Ball can also be prepared with more ingredients (different oil cakes especially ground nut oil cake, fish meal, shrimp meal, silkworm pupae, beef liver meal, meat meal, squid waste, dry fish, dry acetes, broken rice, rice bran, tapioca root powder, yeast, *etc.*) along with vitamin-mineral mixture following improved formula. Farm made or commercial sinking pelleted feed may also be used and given through same tray/ basket method. Mash feed or sinking pellets can also be given through holed bag method in which bags are arranged in a similar way to tray method. Feed can also be spread around the periphery of the pond in the shallow areas. Check trays kept in the different areas of the pond will help in deciding the quantum of the feed per day. In general prawns require 28-30% protein and 8-10% fat in their diet. As prawn is having nocturnal feeding habit, the feed should be given at 8 pm. Besides, special diets like boiled tilapia flesh, chopped raw meat of gastropods or trash fish, cooked chicken entrails @ 10% of the bodyweight are also administered on fortnightly basis. Sometimes compound chicken feed mixed with trash fish and prawn meal in mincer and formulated shrimp feed may be used. In monoculture the feed conversion ratio (FCR) is 7-9:1 for wet feed and 2-3:1 for compound dry feed. FCR is reduced when culture period is extended beyond 8 months. Prawn should be sampled using cast net on monthly basis and based on the average body weight new feeding rate may be calculated.

Weight dependent feeding rates for giant freshwater prawn

Prawn Weight (g)	Percentage of body weight fed daily
< 1	≥ 25
1–2	20
2–5	12
5–10	10
10–15	8
15–20	6
20–25	5
25–30	4
30	3

In polyculture pond, for carp either wet ball or mash feed or sinking pellet can be used. Wet ball or mash feed can be prepared using ingredients following either traditional formula or improved formula. Pellet feed may be either farm made or commercially manufactured. Mash feed may be given by three tier bag method in which bags with small holes and filled with feed are hanged from bamboo pole 10 ft away from pond dike and submerged at 1.5 ft, 3.5 ft and 5.5ft underneath the water. Wet ball can be given through plastic or aluminium tray or bamboo basket arranged in the same way of bag method. Sinking pellets can be given either through bag method or tray method. Per hectare area at 14-16 places this sort of arrangement should be made and feed should be given at 5% of body weight for first 2 months, 4% of body weight in second two months, 3% of body weight in third two months, 2% of body weight in fourth 2 months and 1% of body weight in last 2-4 months on daily basis at morning 10 am.

A mixture of floating and sinking pellets (2:1) can also be broadcasted for feeding of carps. To avoid wind mediated aggregation of floating pellets at the side of pond, broadcasting may be done within the rings made by plastic pipe and fixed different places of pond. Prawn should be given feed in the same way with the same amount and the same time as described earlier. In polyculture the feed conversion ratio (FCR) is 8:1 for wet feed and 1-2:1 for compound dry feed. Both carps and prawn should be sampled using cast net on monthly basis and based on the average body weight new feeding rate may be calculated.

Conclusion

With the target of fulfilling future demand of fish, intensified feed based aquaculture can only be successful by using proper feed which can be efficiently utilized for fulfilling the nutrient requirement and through the implementation of appropriate feeding strategy in terms of feed type, feeding level, feeding frequency and feeding methods. Feed should be formulated according to food and feeding habits and nutrient requirements of fish.

References

Ayyappan S, Ali SA (2007) Analysis of feeds and fertilizers for sustainable aquaculture development in India. *In*: M.R. Hasan, T. Hecht, S.S. De Silva and A.G.J. Tacon (eds), Study and analysis of feeds and fertilizers for sustainable aquaculture development, *FAO* Fisheries Technical Paper, No. 497. Rome, FAO. pp. 191–219.

Ayyappan S, Jena JK (1998) Grow-Out Production of Carps in India. Journal of Applied Aquaculture, 13(3/4): 251-282.

Ayyappan S, Moza U, Gopalkrishan A, Meenakumari B, Jena JK, Pandey AK (eds.) (2013) Hanbook of Fisheries and Aquaculture, ICAR, New Delhi, 1116p.

Chandrapal GD (2005) Status of trash fish utilization and fish feed requirements in aquaculture India. Paper presented at the "Regional Workshop On Low Value And "Trash Fish" In The Asia-Pacific Region" Hanoi, Vietman, 7-9 June 2005.

DAHD (2009) Annual Report 2008-09. Department of Animal Husbandry, Dairying and Fisheries, Ministry of Agriculture, Government of India, New Delhi, pp. 60-61. De Silva SS, Hasan MR (2007) Feeds and fertilizers: the key to long-term sustainability of Asian aquaculture. In MR Hasan, T Hecht SS, De Silva, AGJ Tacon (eds). Study and analysis of feeds and fertilizers for sustainable aquaculture development. FAO Fisheries Technical Paper. No. 497. Rome, FAO. pp. 19–47.

De Silva SS, Turchini GM (2009) Use of wild fish and other aquatic organisms as feed in aquaculture–a review of practices and implications in the Asia-Pacific. *In* MR Hasan, M Halwart (eds). Fish as feed inputs for aquaculture: practices, sustainability and implications. FAO Fisheries and Aquaculture Technical Paper. No. 518. Rome, FAO. pp. 63–127.

Dhawan A, Kaur VI, Virk P (2004) Non-conventional fish feed resources: an overview. Fishing Chimes, 23 (10 and 11): 66–72.

FAO (2002) Use of fishmeal and fish oil in aquafeeds: further thoughts on the fishmeal trap, by MB New, UN Wijkström. FAO Fisheries Circular No. 975. Rome. 61 pp.

FAO (2014) State of World Fisheries and Aquaculture, Food and Agriculture Organization of the United Nations, Rome (Italy), Fisheries and Aquaculture Dept, 2014.

Hasan MR (2001) Nutrition and feeding for sustainable aquaculture development in the third millennium. *In* RP Subasinghe, P Bueno, MJ Phillips, C Hough, SE McGladdery, JR Arthur, eds. Aquaculture in the third millennium, 193–219 pp. Technical proceedings of the conference on aquaculture in the third millennium, Bangkok, Thailand, 20-25 February 2000, Bangkok, NACA and Rome, FAO.

Hasan MR, Hecht T, De Silva SS, Tacon AGJ (eds) (2007) Study and analysis of feeds and fertilizers for sustainable aquaculture development. FAO Fisheries Technical Paper. No. 497. Rome, FAO. 2007. 510p.

NRC (National Research Council), (1993) Nutrient requirements of fish. Committee on Animal Nutrition, Board on Agriculture. National Research Council, National Academy Press, Washington DC., USA, 114p.

Rana KJ, Siriwardena S, Hasan MR (2009) Impact of rising feed ingredient prices on aquafeeds and aquaculture production, FAO Fisheries and Aquaculture Technical Paper, No. 541, Rome, FAO, 2009. 63p.

11

Defining The Role of Occupational Physiology and Ergonomics for Improvement of Health and Productivity of Indian Inland Fishermen

Rajib Biswas

Project Coordinator–Foundation for Occupational Health Reform and Developmental Research, Kolkata-700030, West Bengal
Associate Professor of Physiology, Himachal Dental College Sundernagar, Mandi –175002, Himachal Pradesh

Alok Ghosh Chaudhuri

Associate Professor, Department of Physiology
Vidyasagar College, 39 Shankar Ghosh Lane, Kolkata-700006, West Bengal

Introduction

Any work condition revolves around three main components - the man, machine and environment. 'Man'-is represented by the worker who is either the controller or the executor of an action. Therefore the work output depends on how efficiently the workers are performing. In this context, the health of the worker is of utmost importance. It is one of the prime supporting pillars of productivity. If the health condition declines, efficiency is reduced and productivity suffers. Work involves a variety of physical and cognitive activities performed to achieve a desired or specified productivity. It may include a single individual or a small or large group of people as the worker. It is characterized by a specified duration, specific speed or work pace and a required amount of effort. The performance and efficiency expected from the workers have a direct bearing on the work process or work tool and the work environment. All these stress the bodily systems and affect the health of the worker. The stress could be classified as physiological stress and psychological stress Occupational health deals with the study and maintenance of physical, mental and social well-being of workers in the workplace (WHO, 1957). Occupational Physiology and Ergonomics are related branches of Occupational health that are in particular concerned with the study and maintenance of health and well-being during work.

The principles and methods of occupational physiology are concerned with the assessment of physiological capabilities and limitations of an individual for performing a particular task. It can be well- understood from a physiological perspective as the work demands physiological energy expenditure. In accordance the muscular power, efficiency of cardiovascular system, amount of maximum oxygen intake and its utilization, level of fatigability, speed of recovery after the work is over and efficiency of body temperature regulation- all these determine the working capacity of an individual. The methods of occupational physiology are also concerned with measuring the physiological reactions arising from work mainly in terms of cardiorespiratory and musculoskeletal and biomechanical parameters. This enables for a physiological classification of physical workload. Therefore by comparing the physiological working capacity of the individual with the physiological demand expected from physical work, it is possible to determine what an individual can do safely, without stretching his physiological capabilities (Brouha 1960). These evaluations come under the purview of occupational physiology.

The principles of occupational physiology are well-knitted with Ergonomics. The word 'Ergonomics' is derived from the Greek words *ergon* (work) and *nomos* (law). In essence, this scientific discipline is the 'science and art of man at work'. It is concerned with scientific studies that help us to understand the interactions between man, machine and environment in a working system. It applies theory, principles, and methods for designing the work to optimize the interaction between the worker with work processes and work environment to solve any problem arising out of unsafe, unhealthy, uncomfortable or inefficient situations which may affect the health of workers. Therefore the main focus of ergonomics relies upon the worker. Its main objective is to maintain health and well-being at work and at the same time to increase overall performance in terms of efficiency and productivity. Knowledge of occupational physiology is a prerequisite in ergonomic studies to evaluate the physiological capabilities and limitations of humans.

In many work situations the manual labour is inevitable and often arduous. From the viewpoint of an individual's capacity and limitations, a job that requires physical labour may not always be suitable for a group of workers particularly the older or female workers or workers with some sort of disabilities or illness. In such a situation, applying the methods of occupational physiology will help in assessing the physiological stress of work and to derive the rationale of the suitability of such workload for workers of varying physical and physiological characteristics. Once a job is found physiologically unsuitable for a group of workers, the principles of ergonomics can be applied for reduction of workload for the vulnerable group and at the same time taking care of productivity.

Nevertheless, the physical stress of work is an occupational health hazard arising out of ergonomic and work physiological problems. Therefore it needs to be controlled to prevent work related illnesses. A classical approach of solving such problems usually involves identifying the job or task at risk, analyzing the problem, developing alternative solutions and selecting the best one, implementing the preferred solution and doing a follow up study to ensure that the problem has been solved.

Ergonomic interventions include formulating control measures to reduce job stress. In particular, it involves developing alternative solutions and selecting and implementing the best one by the classical six step method of Ergonomic intervention. Control measures are often successfully applied in industrial settings to improve working conditions and to reduce physical stress as well as to prevent work related illnesses(Eklöfand Hagberg, 2006).

Different kinds of control measures can be implemented during intervention. The initial control measure includes engineering control where the objective aims to redesign the job. However, this is not always possible and so the intervention focuses on the next control procedures which are called organizational measures. Such interventions are to be implemented by the discretions of the organization and guided by its policy.

The organizational measure is one of the widely used control measures taken in ergonomic intervention in industrial or office settings. Organizational measures include providing suitable rest breaks to the workers during work and implementing job rotation during work. Usually, the method of job rotation increases the possibility of providing rest pauses between work periods. In simple terms, the job rotation refers to the rotation from one job to another. It can be defined as "regular, alternating between jobs within an organization on basis of a scheme or spontaneously on basis of personal appointment" (Kuijer 1999). It is one of the most practiced organizational interventions that has been widely implemented in various industrial situations. Claimed benefits of job rotation include morale building, productivity improvement and improved worker retention. (Farrant, 1987; Cheraskin and Campion, 1996; Comper and Padula, 2014).

Job rotation can also be implemented in work situations where the work involves physical exertion due to predominance of manual labour. In many of these work conditions the workload or exposure of the individual to physical exertion cannot be lowered due to the characteristics of the tasks. In these conditions the application of job rotation would aim at reducing the physical workload by a reduction in physical work demands (Mathiassen. 2006; Sato and Coury, 2009). Objectively in such situations, the job rotation is used as a means to alternate between jobs with different grades of mechanical or energetic loads. It has been reported that workers engaged in jobs involving a dynamic type of activity with more muscular exertion and energetic load could be able to benefit from this intervention principle (Jonsson, 1998). Job rotation reduces the cumulative work stress with reduction in physical, energetic and musculoskeletal overloads (Keir, *et al.*, 2011) and therefore acts as an important intervention tool of health promotion.

In the last two decades our country has witnessed a paradigm shift in terms of globalization, urbanization and industrialization parallely with economic transition. Today technology has become the single and paramount driving force of civilization attempting to ease out our difficulties by increasing the luxuries of daily living conditions. However, despite all these transitions most of the Indians still live in villages. Agriculture and fishery are still the sunshine sector of Indian economy and widely practiced in the nook and corner of the subcontinent. They provide livelihood to the majority of the country's population including the economically backward classes. But unlike different industrial scenarios, where the introduction of automation has reduced the manual labour to a great extent, various areas of agriculture and fisheries sectors are yet to taste its full fervor. These jobs are labor intensive. Manual work is indispensable and the nature of the job often calls for exaggerated physical and physiological stresses.

The occupation of inland fishing forms the rural economic backbone for many states of India. The state of West Bengal holds a key position in fish production of our country. Fishermen engaged in inland fishing represent an important unorganized sector of the state. In the last few years a significant contribution has been made by the government for betterment of standard of living and working conditions of the unorganized sector workforce. It appears that such approaches should be complemented with the integration of various occupational health programs for betterment of working health to enhance the overall well-being and quality of life of the workers. Therefore it would not be irrelevant to state that occupational health studies on the inland fishing community are essential to utilize the potential of the fishermen more effectively. However, occupational health studies among Indian fishermen are scanty and this still remains an almost answer area that needs to be explored. A few systematic work-physiological attempts were conducted by the author among inland fishermen. These studies were aimed at evaluating the physical work stress associated with inland fishing that involved individual effort using special fishing appliances (Biswas *et al.*, 2001; Biswas and Samnta, 2006), and group effort conducted in pond (Biswas and Samanta, 2005), river (Biswas and Samanta, 2005a) and large reservoirs (Biswas and Samanta 2009). The state of west Bengal has a long history of traditional practice of Brackish water aquaculture which is performed in water bodies called '*bheries*' of '*bhasabadha*' in local parlance. A previous study by the author on fishermen engaged in Bheri fishing revealed that physical stress in Bheri fishing ranged from very heavy to heavy. This type of work was deemed unsuitable for older workers who often fail to cope with the work pace and the dynamic workload involved in the different tasks. In this context, the present study was planned. The study involved a physiological assessment of workload to evaluate the physical and metabolic demand of different *Bheri* fishing tasks as encountered by the fishermen during actual conditions of work about their maximal functional capabilities. The study also intends to define the heaviness of different activities in terms of physiological parameters.

The main objectives of the study can be summarized as follows:

- To collect baseline physical and physiological data of fishermen including maximum functional capabilities
- To identify and report the pattern of work followed during actual situation of work
- To compare the magnitude of physiological stress involved in various fishing tasks with a physiological classification of workload
- To formulate a new job rotation schedule
- To compare the magnitude of physiological stress before and after job rotation.

Method

Subjects

A group of seventeen professional whole timer fishermen was selected for the study. As the study involved multiple days of follow up, interactions were carried out with fishermen before the study. During these interactions fishermen were explained about the study and the extent of their involvement as required by the design of the study. They were explained and motivated to cooperate for both laboratory and field investigations. A minimum work experience of five years, no reported symptoms of illness and regular involvement of two weeks before the study were selected as inclusion criteria. Among the twenty one subjects selected initially, three declined for laboratory investigations and one subject was not available for follow up. The finally selected subjects were divided into two age groups; the young group with age below 40 years (N=8) and an older group with age above 40 years (n=9)

Study Design

This study was conducted in different phases. The scheme of the study is presented in Box 1. After the initial process of site selection and data collection, a laboratory investigation was conducted to collect the baseline physical and physiological data and maximal functional capabilities of fishermen. In the next phase, field investigations were conducted. Field methods comprised work study to explore the nature of the work practiced and assessment of physiological workload connected with different activities.

Evaluating the data obtained in field studies in terms of physiological characteristics of the fishermen as obtained in laboratory findings, the physiological characterization of work was made to identify the activities and work patterns that were most demanding. In the next phase, a well-planned job rotation scheme was administered to the entire work process. This was done by following a simple guideline that no back- to back high stress jobs was to be performed. The entire work was re-evaluated in terms of physiological workload.

Box 1. Schematic presentation of the study design

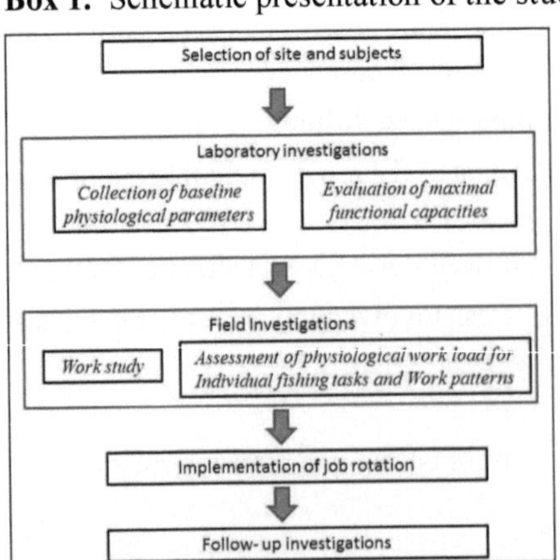

Laboratory investigations

A semi-structured questionnaire was administered to gather information on self reported age, work experience and duration of work shift and other working periods. Height and weight were obtained by standard anthropometric methods and body mass index (BMI) was calculated as an indicator of nutritional standard (Key *et al.*, 1972). Resting heart rate was measured by taking the radial pulse for one minute period while the subjects were allowed to sit comfortably in a reclining position. Maximal functional capacity of the subjects was assessed by a standard bicycle ergometry test protocol at graded workloads (Aminoff *et al.*, 1999). During the test, heart rate (HR) and oxygen consumption (VO_2) were continuously monitored. The test was discontinued when the subjects felt maximal exertion. The heart rate and oxygen consumption obtained at the endpoint of the test were considered to be the maximal heart rate and maximal oxygen consumption.

Field investigations

The work-study was performed by observing and identifying the work patterns and measuring the duration of different activities performed during the habitual work shift. Assessment of workload was done by two approaches- evaluation of the workload connected with individual fishing tasks and evaluation of workload entailed in the whole shift.

To obtain the cardiovascular reactions of work, the pulse rate was measured from radial pulse during work at multiple times. Netcardiac cost (NCC) and relative cardiac cost (RCC) were used as indicators of the cardiac strain. The methods of calculations are summarized in Box 2.

Box 2. Description of the cardiac indices

Heart rate reserve (HRR) = Maximum heart rate–Resting heart rate (RPR) Net cardiac cost (NCC) = Working pulse rate (WPR)–Resting pulse rate (RPR) Relative cardiac cost (RCC) = NCC* 100/HRR

The subjects also measured their perceived level of exertion (RPE) by following a 10-point rating scale. Measurements were taken as quickly as possible in order not to disturb the normal work pace of the subjects. No instructions were given to the fishermen to control their work method as it might interfere with the primary exploratory objective of the study. The fishermen maintained their habitual pattern for work, work–rest regimen and normal work pace.

Description of the tasks examined

The total daily fishing period consisted of multiple work cycles. In each cycle the fishing started with two activities that were performed simultaneously. While a group of fishermen pulled a long drag net (net pulling) to form a barricade across the coastline in a semicircular way, another group of fishermen waded in knee deep (wading) to a distance of about 200 meters from the coast line and then approached towards the net by running and simultaneously beating the water with a stick (Striking). This striking made the fishes to converge in the barricade. The net was then gradually closed by bringing its both ends together to entrap the fishes. The entrapped fishes have finally sorted out size-wise as well as species - wise (Catch Handling). The same activities were repeated in the next cycle of fishing.

Analysis of work activities

The entire fishing process involved multiple work cycles. A number of cycles ranged between 4 and 7 (mean 5.4 ± 1.1). In each cycle, fishermen performed three activities, viz, pulling the net, striking the water and handling the catch.

The fishermen worked in two groups and each group maintained a fixed task assignment throughout the work shift. One group was involved in striking followed by net pulling and finally catch handling (SNC), while the other group performed net spreading and catch handling (NC). These task assignments were repeated in each cycle of work. Therefore, these types of activities were found to be non-rotating types. The mean duration of total work shift was obtained to be 264 ± 28 (range 238-301) min and average cycle time was 46 ± 5.6 (range 33-54) min. The number of work cycles varied between 5 and 7.

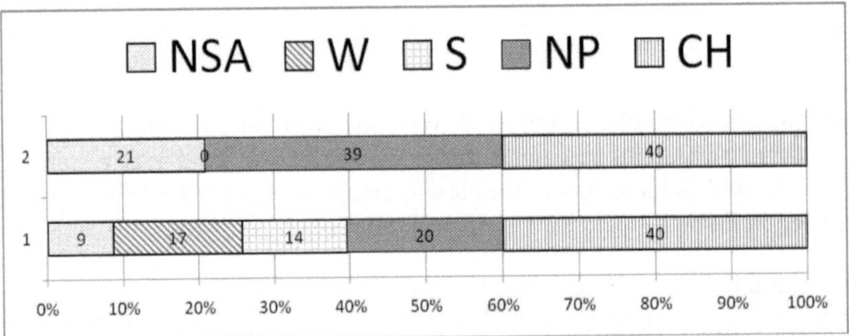

Fig. 1. Duration of different activities expressed as percentage of the total work shift (NSA–Nn–specific activity, W- wading, S-Striking, NP- Net puling, CH- Catch handling)

Duration of different activities expressed as percentage of the total work shift is presented in figure 1. The duration of total work shift, work cycle and catch-handling task was similar for both the groups. The fishermen spent 40 percent of the total activity period in catch handling. However, the duration of net pulling and non-specific period varied significantly among the groups. Net pulling time was more for NC group (39% of the total period) as compared to SNC group (20% of total period). Periods of non–specific activities were also higher in NC group (21% of total time) as compared to SNC group (9% of total period). . A considerable time was spent by the SNC group in wading.

Workload in individual fishing activities

Descriptive statistics comprising mean, standard deviation and range of the physiological responses obtained for different activities are presented in Table 1. The maximum workload was involved in 'striking' where 82% of VO_2max was used. Mean heart rate attained for this task was 159 ± 9.9 beats/min. 'Net spreading' appeared comparatively lighter than striking with a mean heart rate of 127 beats/min and required 50% of VO_2max on average. The least physiological strain was encountered in 'catch handling' with a mean heart rate of 108 ± 8.3 beats/min. Other physiological responses demonstrated similar gradation.

Table 1. Physiological workload in different fishing activities.

Variables	Striking (n = 10)	Netting (n = 16)	Catch Handling (n =16)
WPR (beats/min)	159 ± 9.9* (142 - 173)	127 ± 8.2 (110-138)	108 ± 8.3 (92-121)
NCC (beats/min)	88 ± 12.3 (67–107)	56 ± 7.0 (43-67)	37 ± 8.1 (21-50)
RCC (%)	83 ± 7.2 (66-91)	54 ± 6.4 (42-65)	36 ± 6.7 (24- 46)

Workload in two patterns of work

The descriptive statistics of the different physiological parameters obtained from the fishermen engaged in two non- rotating work patterns namely, SNC and NC are presented in Table 2. The magnitude of all the physiological parameters was conspicuously higher for the SNC group as compared to the NC group.

Table 2. Physiological workload in different patterns of fishing activities

Variables	SNC (n = 8)	NC (n = 9)
WPR (beats/min)	130 ± 11.9 (104-150)	112 ± 8.7 (92-130)
NCC (beats/min)	56.3 ± 12 (30-76)	43.1 ± 9.4 (22-64)
RCC (%)	61 ± 13.6 (35-84)	45.8 ± 12.9 (19-71)
RPE (Rating of Perceived exertion)	7.6 ± 0.99 (6-8.9)	6.6 ± 1.05 (5.4-8.4)

Job rotation

The habitual pattern of work observed in fishing was performed in a non-rotating manner. The fishermen divided them into two groups and each group performed a non-rotating pattern of fixed activities throughout the work shift. The job rotation was implemented in the following manner. The fishermen were grouped and each group was allowed to perform both the patterns of work in different work cycles alternatively. For all the groups, a single cycle of SNC pattern of work was followed by two cycles with NC pattern. Thus, the non–rotating patterns were transformed into a rotating pattern, all the seventeen fishermen performed the job rotation scheme. Fishermen were studied for six work cycles after the introduction of job rotation. Therefore all the groups performed two spells of SNC work and four spells of NC work pattern. The group and task allocation patterns are summarized in Table 3.

Table 3. Group composition and task allocation pattern during job rotation

Group Name	Group composition (Young + Old subjects)	Total subjects	Allocated Task pattern in different cycles (C1-C6)					
			C1	C2	C3	C4	C5	C6
A	3 +3	6	SNC	NC	NC	SNC	NC	NC
B	3 + 3	6	NC	SNC	NC	NC	SNC	NC
C	2 +3	5	NC	NC	SNC	NC	NC	SNC
Total	8+9	17						

Comparative analysis of physiological strain among non-rotating and rotating work pattern.

Descriptive statistics of different physical characteristics of three groups of fishermen involved in non- rotating and rotating work patterns and their physiological reactions are presented in table 3. A one-way ANOVA was performed to test statistically significant differences among various parameters. The test revealed that the groups did not vary in terms of all the baseline physiological and physical parameters. The mean age of the three groups varied between 40 and 42 years and body mass index was almost equal for both the groups and obtained to be 20 kg / m^2.

Descriptive statistics of physiological reactions of three groups of fishermen involved in non-rotating and rotating work patterns are presented in table 4. A statistically significant difference was obtained for working pulse rate values between the groups as determined by one-way ANOVA ($F(2,31) = 86.4$, $p < 0.001$). Statistically significant differences were also obtained for net cardiac cost ($F(2,31) = 25.4$, $p < 0.001$), Relative cardiac cost ($F(2,31) = 8.20$, $p < 0.001$) and rating of perceived exertion ($F(2,31) = 8.20$, $p = 0.001$).

A post hoc Tukey test revealed that WPR was significantly lower after taking NC (113 ± 4.0, p = 0.0001) and SNC-NC-NC (114 ± 3.1, p= 0.0001) as compared to SNC (133 ± 4.1). Similar findings were also obtained for all other parameters when NC and SNC-NC-NC are compared to SNC.

Table 4. Comparison of physical characteristics and workload for three different groups

Variables	SNC	NC	SNC-NC-NC
Age (years)	42.0 ± 9.6	40.4± 17.2	41.1 ± 13.7
Body mass index (kg / m^2)	20.3 ± 1.1	20.9 ± 1.6	20.6 ± 1.4
Resting pulse rate (beats/min)	74.0 ± 3.7	69.0 ± 3.9	71 ± 4.4
Maximal Heart rate (beats/ min)	167 ± 7.8	166 ± 15.4	166 ± 12.1
Heart rate reserve (beats /min)	91 ± 10.1	97± 16.1	95 ± 13.3

Table 5. Comparison of physiological workload for three groups of fishermen in rotating and non-rotating work pattern

Variables	SNC	NC	SNC-NC-NC
Working pulse rate (beats / min)	133 ± 4.1	113 ± 4.0	114 ± 3.1
Net cardiac cost (beats / min)	59 ± 4.2	44 ± 5.9	46 ± 4.8
Relative cardiac cost (%)	64 ±6.7	47 ± 11.1	49 ± 7.2
Perceived exertion	7.8 ± 0.96	6.5 ± 1.0	6.4 ± 0.63

Physiological strain in relation to work pattern and age

Figure 2 demonstrates different physiological parameters in three work patterns in relation to the age of the fishermen. It can be observed from the figure that all the parameters were higher among the SNC group as compared to the other two groups. Moreover, in all the three groups, the values of all parameters for the older fishermen are on a higher side as compared to the younger counterparts.

Attempts were made to compare the stress in all three groups among the older fishermen. A one way ANOVA revealed a statistically significant difference among the groups for working pulse rate ($F(2,15) = 75.6, p < 0.001$), net cardiac cost ($F(2,15) = 21.7, P < 0.0001$), relative cardiac cost ($F(2,15) = 31.2, P < 0.0001$) and rating of perceived exertion ($F(2,15)=6.34, P = 0.01$). Multiple comparisons between groups were done by Tukey post hoc test. Mean working pulse rate was significantly lower after taking NC (116 ± 1.9, $p < 0.001$) and SNC-NC-NC (115 ± 3.41, $p < 0.01$) as compared to SC (136 ± 2.8) group. Group comparison for net cardiac cost yielded exactly similar results. Relative cardiac cost values were found to be significantly higher in NC (54.6 ± 7.1, p= 0.045) and SC (70 ± 2.7, $p < 0.001$) as compared to SNC NC-NC (47.6 ± 3.7).For the perceived exertion, the only statistically significant lower value was obtained in the SNC-NC-NC group (6.5 ± 0.50, p= 0.008) as compared to the SC (8.1 ± 0.87). Other group comparisons for this parameter appeared insignificant.

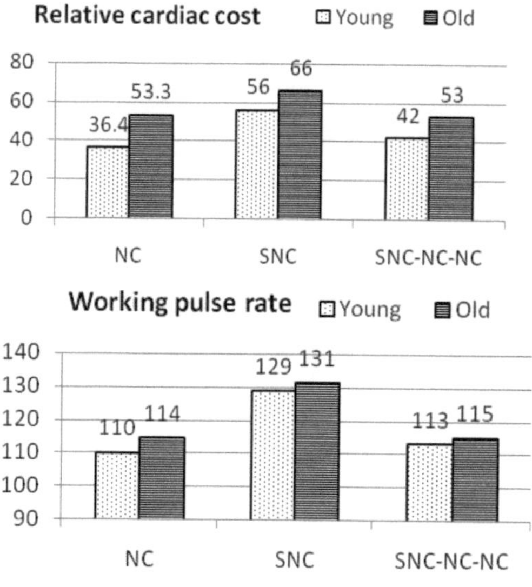

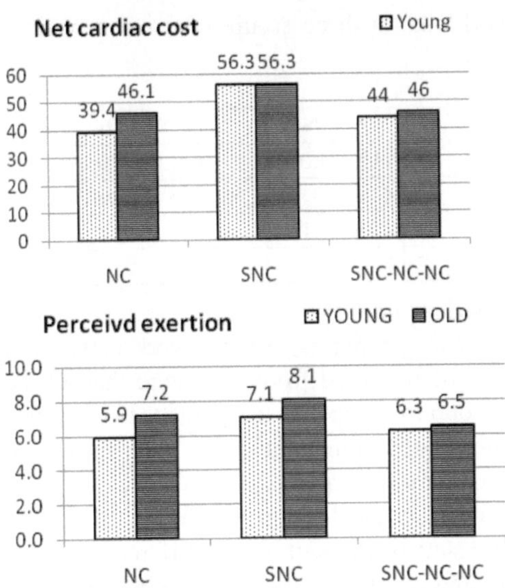

Fig. 2. Physiological parameters in three work patterns in relation to the age of the fishermen

The mean heart rate values obtained in different cycles of work were plotted against the number of cycles, to demonstrate the trend of heart rate in different job patterns. This is presented in figure 3. The figure depicts that except for SNC-NC-NC the trends of heart rate were increasing. This points towards an indication of cumulative stress and non-steady physiological state of the subjects engaged in these patterns of work. Furthermore, the mean working pulse rates for the young and older fishermen in different cycles of work in the SNC-NC-NC pattern were obtained to be lowest, lying between 110 and 120 beats/min. For other categories of work patterns the working pulse rates demonstrated higher values.

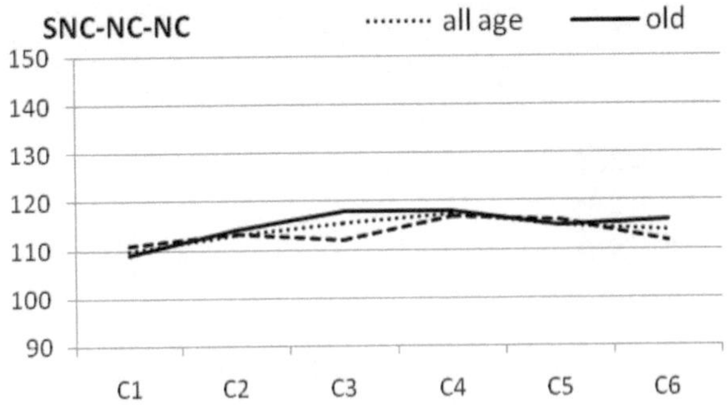

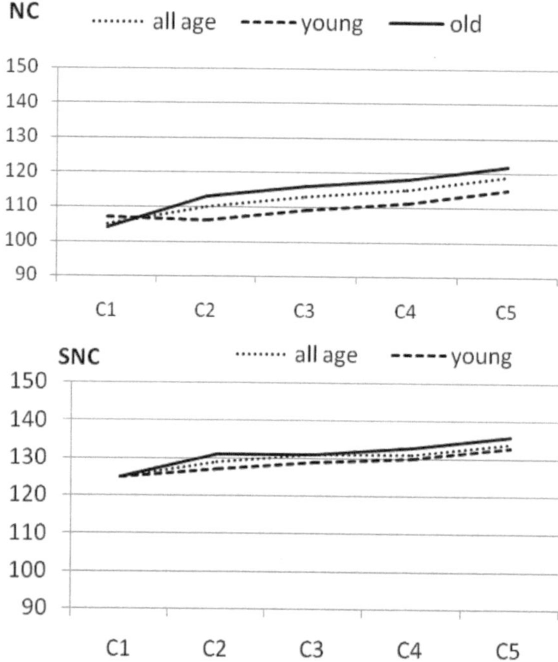

Fig. 3. Trend of working pulse rates in different patterns of work

Rationale of the methodology adopted in the study

Measuring the physiological demand of the work and estimating the functional capabilities of a worker is the key approach in occupational physiology to determine what a man can do safely without stressing his physiological system. In the present study a similar method had been adopted adhering to the standard protocol. The maximal functional capacities of the fishermen were determined and the physiological demands of the different tasks were then evaluated. Muscular exertion in physical activity imparts load on metabolic, musculoskeletal and cardiorespiratory systems. This is reflected by a change in a wide variety of physiological parameters. Measuring one or more of these parameters helps to determine to what degree the 'working level' differs from the 'resting level' and gives an estimate of the physiological workload. In this study, we have chosen heart rate as the principal physiological parameter along with some cardiac strain indices to evaluate the strain of the workers. Studies have indicated the heart rate as the most fundamental index of physical strain due to its close relationship with various physiological functions like cardiac output, oxygen consumption, sweat rate *etc.* (Durnin and Edwards, 1955; Ford and Hellerstein, 1959). It not only permits the evaluation of circulatory strain imposed by the workloads of varying intensities (Brouha 1960) but also provides an integrated response to energy requirements and both thermal and postural demand (Nielsen and Meyer, 1987). It is also suitable for field studies several recordings can be obtained with minimal interference with the subject's freedom of motion.

In the present study the heart rate was therefore chosen as the principal parameter to evaluate the physiological strain. Functional capacities are determined in terms of maximal heart rate and heart rate reserve of the individual fishermen. The workload was also judged in terms of some derived indices of cardiac strain like net cardiac cost and relative cardiac cost. These indices were chosen as they are sensitive to many inter- and intraindividual influences (Gertner *et al.*,1984; Green *et al.*,1986). Net cardiac cost is directly related to resting heart rate and so it evaluates the workload strictly connected with the job; while the relative cardiac cost considers both the resting and maximal heart rate of the subjects and it therefore gives the best expression of the individual circulatory strain (Åstrand and RodhalI, 1986, Costa *et al*, 1989).

Optimization of workload

The concept of physiological safety for men at work is often a most appreciated but commonly ignored concept in the majority of industrial and non - industrial work settings. Too often a task is demanded from a worker without the knowledge of his physical and physiological capabilities for performing it. Industries have a regular practice of defining jobs in terms of time, motion, productivity and efficiency but never in terms of physiological demand. Experts in the field of work physiology tend to agree that the workload in certain tasks is often so heavy that they impose undue physiological stress on the workers and result in the development of fatigue. This leads to a gradual decrement in the working capacity. Brody (1945) suggested that in heavy manual work a safety margin is necessary in terms of the physiological demand of work and maximum rate of work should be determined in such a way that it can be carried out day in and day out and the worker remains vigor to an advanced age. The optimal workload thus chosen to ensure this physiological safety has been termed as an acceptable workload.

The acceptable workload is often expressed in terms of relative aerobic stress. This is the oxygen utilization by the worker expressed as the percentage of his maximal oxygen intake capacity. This is well correlated with the relative cardiac cost (Astrand, 1986). As different factors influence the responses at work, recommendations for acceptable workload requires adjustment not only to age, gender and maximal functional capacities of the subjects but also with the amount of active muscle mass involved, static and dynamic muscular exertions and duration of work and rest periods (Aminoff *et al.*, 1999). Various studies, which have attempted to establish an optimal work rate limit, recommended that the work limit should not exceed 50% of the maximal aerobic capacity of the subject. In the present study, the optimal workload encountered by the subjects has been judged in terms of RCC. It was found that the workload of the older fishermen exceeded the limit of 50%, while for the younger workers the workload was found to be within the acceptable limit after implementation of job rotation.

Heaviness of the work

Gradation of the heaviness of different activities is a decade old approach that was proposed by different researchers with respect to the physiological responses at work.

These classifications are either based on parameters like working heart rates, energy cost, sweat rate *etc.* (Astrand, 1986; Ramanathan, 1967; Christensen, 1967). According to such gradations, the heaviness of work in terms of heart rate is designated as light (WHR varying between 70 to <90 beats/min), moderate (WHR between 90- 110 beats/min), heavy (WHR between 110-<130 beats/min), very heavy (WHR between 130-< 150 beats/min) and extremely heavy (WHR above 150 beats / min). The findings from the present study revealed that in terms of working pulse rates the heaviness of different tasks varied between moderate for catch handling, heavy for net pulling and extremely heavy for striking. It was also obtained that the SNC work pattern appeared to be moderate to very heavy for the fishermen involved in this work, while the group of fishermen engaged in NC activity experienced moderate to heavy physiological stress. The magnitude of physical workload experienced by the fishermen was comparable with the work stress in coastal and sea fishing, as obtained in overseas literatures (Schilling, 1966; Astrand *et al.*,1973; Rodahl *et al.*, 1974, Rodahl and Vokac, 1977).

Job rotation as a means to reduce workload

The main objective of the study was to apply principles of occupational physiology and ergonomics to minimize occupational risk with simultaneous preservation of working capacity of the fishermen. The main occupational risk of concern that is examined in the present study was the excessive physiological workload encountered by the fishermen during work. The methodology adopted and the findings thereof have tried to explain the mechanism responsible for the development of physical fatigue of the subjects by various quantitative assessments.

Observations made on the activities performed by the fishermen revealed that the workload and subsequent physiological responses varied according to the task performed. The fishermen worked in two definite patterns of task assignments. The physiological demand of the individual tasks assigned in each pattern and the sequence of activities followed in each pattern were responsible for a wide range of variation in physiological response across the groups. The task of striking was heavier as compared to netting and catch handling. It involved running in shallow waters and simultaneously beating the water with a stick. This activity demanded exaggerated muscular efforts, which is reflected in elevated physiological reactions. The influence of this task resulted in the significantly higher physiological responses among the SNC group as compared to NC counterpart. Moreover, the SNC group has hardly any chance to have rest in between successive cycles because after completion of catch handling they waded away from the coastline to start a new spell of striking. Lack of rest period and wading might have increased muscular exertions and hindered recovery. In contrast, the movement of the subjects engaged in NC pattern was much limited along the coastline. They had more periods of unspecified work and rest in between successive periods of netting activities. This had resulted in a much lower value of physiological reactions in this group. This demonstrated a polarized effect of workload with an exposure inequality. One group was continuously exposed to high workload while the other was exposed to moderate workload. Based on these observations, attempt taken for optimization of working conditions by implementing the best possible adjustment to alleviate the physical fatigue and stress of the fishermen. The job rotation plan was promoted in accordance. It was also observed that the older workers were engaged in striking activities owing to their experience driving the fishes towards the net by striking. So they were indispensable in the striking group. These appeared to be inherent characteristics of the job which could not be controlled. Therefore, while planning the job rotation, care had been taken so that reduction of physical stress could be achieved for the older worker as well. No new work pattern was formulated in the job rotation plan. However, the entire group of fishermen was divided into three groups. In accordance with the basic principle of job rotation that the work should alternate between tasks with high and low physical and energetic demand, each group was allowed to alternate between the two work patterns in successive work cycles with varying demand. The SNC was identified as the high demand job and the NC as the low demand one. So each group performed one cycle of SNC followed by two cycles of NC. The job rotation method followed in this study had some advantages. Firstly, it did not change the habitual pattern of work which otherwise may create confusion among the fishermen. Secondly, it ensured that all fishermen will be available for net pulling. In terms of productivity, this was important, as the process required a considerable amount of maneuvering to entrap the fishes more effectively which would not be possible with a fewer number of fishermen. The third advantage was that adequate numbers of fishermen were available for catch handling which would otherwise increase the cycle time. Implementation of the present plan of job rotation in the fishing tasks results in some positive effects on diminishing the physical strain of the fishermen. The magnitude of the physiological response was recorded from the workers in the new work pattern was slightly higher than the NC pattern but significantly lower than the SNC pattern. Moreover, it prevented the 'exposure inequality' as observed in the habitual work pattern, where the SNC and NC groups were continuously exposed to high and low physical stresses respectively. The new pattern of task was continued for a longer period of time (6 work cycles) and resulted in a significant decrease of physiological strain. A steady pattern of heart rate was observed for all the fishermen in contrast to the non-steady pattern found in habitual work patterns.

It has been suggested that job rotation may decrease 'task aversion' among workers (Kliujer, 1999). Some indications of task aversion were noted, although not systematically investigated, among the fishermen engaged in striking. This aversion might have resulted from fatigue due to the arduous nature of the task and monotony arising out of its repetition throughout the shift. A symmetric distribution of SNC and NC pattern among the different groups might have been effective in reducing fatigue as indicated by a reduction in perceived exertion scores. The job rotation implemented in the study, however, had failed to maintain the physiological responses within the acceptable limit particularly for the older workers. One explanation can be provided for this. Due to the nature of the job and size of the whole fishing team, it was not possible to provide a rest period to the older workers either after striking or net pulling.

Such provisions would reduce the number of fishermen available for net pulling and catch handling tasks and might pose a negative impact on the overall productivity and efficiency of the work process as mentioned earlier. However, it could be stated with a considerable amount of certainty that with any such provision of rest pause, the physiological strain of older fishers could be reduced to a greater extent which might be possible to examine with a larger group of fishermen.

Conclusion

The present study is an example to demonstrate the effect of the application of principles and methodologies of occupational physiology and ergonomics in reducing the overall stress of work by applying a job rotation scheme. However, due to certain limitations, the authors felt that the study is not complete and can be repeated in larger groups to yield more effective results. The result from the present study reflected that the job rotation has become successful in reducing the overall strain of fishermen to a significant amount. It appeared that the scope of this study is enormous and can be successfully implemented in various other fisheries and agriculture sector work where the job is physically demanding to reduce the overall physical strain of the workers. This will increase productivity and will promote the working health of the workers as well.

References

Aminoff T, Smolander J, Korhonen O, Louhevaara V (1999) Physiological strain during kitchen work in relation to maximal and task specific peak values. Ergonomics 42: 584-92.

Åstrand I, Fugelli P, Karlsson C.G, Rodahl K, Vokac Z (1973) Energy output and work stress in coastal fishing.Scandinavian. J Clinical Lab Investig 31: 105-113.

Åstrand P O, Rodahl K (1986) Textbook of work physiology. McGraw Hill. New York.

Biswas R, Samanta A (2009) Cardiac strain and energy expenditure in inland fishing. In the proceedings of 17th Biennial Congress of International Ergonomics Association 9–14th August, Beijing, China: 149-155.

Biswas R, Samanta A, Chatterjee S P (2001) Physiological strain in a traditional inland fishing task of India. Ind J Physiol Allied Sci 55: 161–167.

Biswas R,Samanta A (2006) Assessment of Physiological strain in inland fishing activity. Ind J Occup Environ Med 10: 19–23.

Biswas R, Samanta A (2005) Physiological cost of pond fishing. Ind J Physiol Allied Sci 59: 58–68.

Biswas R, Samanta A (2005) Work stress in river fishing. In the proceedings of the 3rd International conference of Indian society of ergonomics: Humanizing work and work environment (HWWE), Guwahati, Assam, India, 10th - 12th December 55-59.

Brody S (1945) Bioenergetics and growth. New York: Reinhold.

Brouha L (1960) Evaluation of the physiological requirements of Jobs. In: Physiology in Industry Pergamon press; pp: 82-108.

Cheraskin L, Campion MA (1996) Study clarifies job-rotation benefits. Person J 75

Christensen E H (1969) Man at work-outline of work physiology- Issued by the Chief advisor of factories, Ministry of labour and employment, Govt of India, New Delhi. Comper MLC,

Padula RS (2014) The effectiveness of job rotation to prevent work-related musculoskeletal disorders: protocol of a cluster randomized clinical trial. BMC Musculoskel Disord 15:170

Costa G, Berti F, Betta A (1989) Physiological cost of apple farming activities. Ergonomics *20:* 281-86.

Durnin JVGA, Edwards R G (1955) Pulmonary ventilation as an index of energy expenditure. Quar J Exper Physiol 40: 370-77.

Eklöf M, Hagberg M (2006) Are simple feedback interventions involving workplace data associated with better working environment and health? A cluster randomized controlled study among Swedish VDU workers. Appl Ergon 37:201–210.

Farrant AW (1987) Job rotation is important. Supervision 49: 14–16.

Ford AB, Hellerstein HK (1959) Estimation of energy expenditure from pulmonary ventilation. Journal of Applied Physiology 14: 891-93.

Gertner A, Israeli R, Cassuto Y (1984) Effects of work and motivation on the heart rate of the chronic heat exposed workers during their regular work shifts. Ergonomics 27: 135- 40.

Green MS, Luz Y, Jucha E, Cocos M, Rosenberg N (1986) Factors affecting ambulatory heart rate in industrial workers. Ergonomics 29: 1017-27.

Jonsson, B (1988) Electromyographic studies of job rotation. Scandinavian journal of work environment and health 14 (suppl.):108–109.

Keir PJ, Sanei K, Holmes MWR (2011) Task rotation effects on upper extremity and back muscle activity. Appl Ergon 42(6):814–819

Kuijer PP, Visser B, Kemper HC (1999) Job rotation as a factor in reducing physical workload at a refuse collecting department. Ergonomics 42(9):1167–1178.

Mathiassen SE (2006) Diversity and variation in biomechanical exposure: what is it, and why would we like to know? Appl Ergon 37(4):419–427.

Neilsen R, Meyer J P (1987) Evaluation of metabolism from heart rate in industrial work. Ergonomics 30: 565-572.

Ramanathan NL, Dutta SR, Roy BN, Chatterjee A, Mullick LN (1967) Energy cost of different muscular tests performed by Indian subjects. Ind J Occup Hlth 10: 253-61.

Rodahl K, Vokac Z (1979) The work physiology of fishing. Psychother Psychosom 32; 52-61.

Rodahl K and Vokac Z (1977) Work stress in Norwegian trawler fishermen. Ergonomics 20: 633-642.

Rodahl K, Vokac Z, Fugelli O, Vaage O, Maehlum S (1974) Circulatory strain, estimated energy output and Catecholamine excretion in Norwegian coastal fishermen. Ergonomics 7: 585-602.

Rodahl K, Vokac Z (1977) Work stress in long line bank fishing. Scand J Work Environ Hlth 3: 154-159.

Sato TO, Coury HJ (2009) Evaluation of musculoskeletal health outcomes in the context of job rotation and multifunctional jobs. Appl Ergon 40(4):707–712.

Schilling RSF (1966) Trawler fishing: an extreme occupation. Proceedings of the Royal Society of Medicine 59: 405-409.

WHO Joint ILO/ WHO Committee on occupational Health. 3rd report (1957), 135.

12

Freshwater Fish Transgenics Implications and Issues

Hirak Kumar Barman and Kiran D. Rasal

Fish Genetics and Biotechnology Division, ICAR - Central Institute of Freshwater Aquaculture, Kausalyaganga, Bhubaneswar 751002, Odisha

Introduction

The science of Biotechnology has been making every effort to create new opportunities for the welfare of humanity. Modern biotechnological tools are applied in India to boost fish production through aquaculture as well as conservation of the vast aquatic resources of the country for sustainable utilization. Transgenic technology is widely used in biotechnology, from the generation of genetically modified (GM) foods to the production of pharmaceutical proteins. This technology has been successfully used to develop fast growing super-fish stocks for aquaculture. The main reasons for genetic manipulation of species used in aquaculture are to enhance the growth and efficiency of food conservation, to increase tolerance to environmental variables like temperature and salinity, to produce new colour variants of ornamental fishes, to increase the resistance of species to pathogens, *etc.* Though the conventional selective breeding approach has proven to genetically upgrade rohu19, it is a rather time consuming process. Traditional selective breeding approaches in combination with transgenesis can bring about faster improvement of selected traits.

World-wide Implications of transgenic fishes

Transgenic technology is useful for both basic and applied research. The genes which have been considered of interest in transgenic fish production are growth hormone genes, growth hormone releasing factor genes, metallothionein genes, antifreeze protein genes, crystalline genes, esterase genes, disease resistance genes, regulatory gene sequences such as metallothionein gene promoter, heat shock gene promoter and other tissue-specific promoters. The commercial applications have focused on genetically improving fish stocks, with targeted traits of enhanced growth, disease resistance, freeze resistance, *etc.* (Gong and Hew 1995; Yazawa *et al.*, 2005). Fish transgenics have long been used as a tool for increasing our understanding of developmental biology by expressing the reporter gene, green fluorescent protein (GFP), under the control of a tissue-specific promoter.

Transgenic application for value-addition in ornamental fishes scores advantage over food fishes in those directions. For example, stable lines of transgenic zebrafishes

(*Danio rerio*) expressing several living colour proteins such as GFP, red fluorescent protein (RFP), yellow fluorescent protein (YFP), blue fluorescent protein (BFP) and cyan fluorescent protein (CYF) were successfully generated (Gong *et al.*, 2003). Interestingly, massive expression of fluorescent colours in the skeletal muscle was visible under normal light. The feasibility of stable expression of colour genes was made possible by zygotic injection of expressible constructs driven by the zebrafish *D. rerio* muscle-specific promoter from the myosin light polypeptide 2 (*mylz2*) gene, also known as *MLC2*. The *mylz2* is an isoform of a fast skeletal muscle forming gene. Organ-specific expression depends upon particular regulatory elements. The proximal *mylz2* promoter, consisting of seventy seven base pairs (bp), was proven to be sufficient for reporter gene expression in zebrafish (*D. rerio*) muscle (Ju *et al.*, 2003). The zebrafish (*D. rerio*) *mylz2* promoter has also been used successfully to generate fluorescent white skirt tetra (*Gymnocorymbus ternetzi*) and medaka (*Oryzias latipes*) fishes (Pan *et al.*, 2008; Zeng *et al.*, 2005). These value-added aquarium fishes have already been commercialized in some countries as 'GloFish' with six attractive fluorescent colour combinations, namely starfire red, cosmic blue, electric green, galactic purple, sunburst orange and moonrise pink (www.glofish.com). The research was primarily aimed to produce zebrafish that glow different colours when different pollutants, like heavy metals are present or when the pH of the water changes. These transgenic specimens proved to be very sensitive pollution indicators. The colour fishes can be produced by the use of different types of colour proteins. The most successful commercial ornamental transgenic organism to date has been 'GloFishTM', marketed by Yorktown Technologies. The GloFish is a trademarked brand of genetically modified (GM) fluorescent zebrafish with bright red, green, and orange fluorescent color. It is the first genetically modified animal to become publicly available as a pet. The original zebrafish (*Danio rerio*) from which the GloFish was developed is a native of rivers in India and Bangladesh. It measures three centimeters long and has gold and dark blue stripes, and over 200 million have been sold in the last 50 years in the United States ornamental fish market. GloFish has continued to be successfully marketed throughout the United States. Since their introduction in late 2003, there have been no reports of any ecological concerns associated with their sale. In addition to the red fluorescent zebrafish, trademarked as "Starfire Red", Yorktown Technologies released a green fluorescent zebrafish and an orange fluorescent zebrafish in mid-2006. The new lines of fish are trademarked as "Electric Green" and "Sunburst Orange", and incorporate genes from sea coral. Despite the speculation of aquarium enthusiasts that the eggs are pressure treated to make them infertile, it has been found some GloFish are indeed fertile and will reproduce in a captive environment. The application of transgenic technology in developing novel varieties of ornamental fish and bioreactor fish was explored in different fish species, especially zebrafish (*Danio rerio*).

The fluorescent proteins have become an essential tool in the production and analysis of transgenic organisms in basic and applied biology. The fluorescent proteins are expressed under the tissue-specific promoters. Three living colour fluorescent proteins, green fluorescent protein (GFP), yellow fluorescent protein (YFP) and red fluorescent protein (RFP or dsRed) were expressed under a strong muscle-specific *mylz2* promoter in stable lines of transgenic zebrafish. By using different tissue-specific promoters, the coloured proteins could be targeted into different tissues or body parts. Different varieties of colour patterns can be achieved from different combinations of tissue-specific promoters and colour proteins. The strength of the promoter plays an important role in the successful generation of colourful ornamental fish.

Recent advances in freshwater transgenic fish research in India

The use of an endogenous promoter construct, where the promoter-regulatory element is derived from the same species, was demonstrated to be beneficial in driving foreign gene expression (Nam *et al.*, 2001). This essentially requires the isolation of a species specific functional promoter capable of driving either ubiquitous or tissue-specific expression of a gene of interest.

The Indian major carp, *Labeo rohita* (rohu) is an economically important freshwater fish in India as well as other Asian countries (Barman *et al.*, 2010; Barman *et al.*, 2012; Mohapatra *et al.*, 2010). Isolation of the rohu (*L. rohita*) *mylz2* promoter will have potential use in tissue-specific expression of desired genes of interest for generating transgenic rohu *L. rohita.* We cloned the 5'-flanking region (1.2 kb) of a muscle specific gene, encoding myosin light chain 2 polypeptides (*mylz2*) of a farmed carp, *Labeo rohita* (rohu) (Mohanta *et al.*, 2014). Sequence analysis using TRANSFAC database search identified the consensus cis-acting regulatory elements of TATA-box and E (CANNTG)-box, including the MEF2 (monocyte enhancer factor 2) motif, implying that it is likely to be a functional promoter. The proximal promoter (~620 bp) was highly homologous with that of *Danio rerio* (zebrafish) as compared to *Channa striatus* (snakehead murrel) counterparts and showed less identity with *Sparus auratus* (gilthead sea bream), *Xenopus laevis* (African clawed frog) and *Rattus norvegicus* (Norway rat). Direct muscular (skeletal) injection of the construct containing the mylz2 promoter (0.6 kb) fused to a green fluorescent protein (GFP) reporter gene showed efficient expression in *L. rohita*, validating its functional activity. Further, the functional activity was confirmed by the observation that this promoter drove GFP expression in the skeletal muscle of transgenic rohu (Fig. 1). It will be interesting to examine the significance of each of these regulatory elements for a better understanding of organ-specific or developmental stage-related functionalities.

The promoter may have potential applications for value-addition in ornamental fishes and studying gene regulatory functions. The similar works are being extended for indigenous aquarium fish species of *Chanda nama* and *Laubuca laubuca.* We cloned the 5'-flanking region (2728 bp) of a muscle-specific gene encoding myosin light chain 2 polypeptides (*mylz2*) of a potential aquarium fish, *Laubuca laubuca.* The sequence data analysis using TRANSFAC-database search identified the consensus *cis*-acting regulatory elements of TATA-box and E (CANNTG)-box including MEF2 (monocyte enhancer factor 2) motif implying that it is likely to be a functional promoter. The proximal promoter (~800 bp) was highly homologous with that of zebrafish, *Danio rerio* as compared to *Channa striatus* and *Labeo rohita* counterparts showing least identity with *Sparus auratus*, *Xenopus laevis* and *Rattus norvegicus*. Direct muscular injection of the constructs containing the *mylz2* promoter (1.7 kb) fused to a red and green fluorescent reporter gene showed efficient expressions in *L. laubuca* and heterologous species of *L. rohita*, respectively (Fig. 2), and thus validating its functional activity. The promoter will have potential applications for value-addition in ornamental fishes and to study gene regulatory functions.

The cytosolic β-actin is expressed ubiquitously and abundantly in almost all eukaryotic undifferentiated and differentiated cells1. The β -actin promoter of several fish species has been cloned, characterized and subsequently used for generating transgenics (Takagi *et al.*, 1994; Liu *et al.*, 1990). The use of 'autotransgene' construct, where both the promoter/regulatory element and targeted structural gene derived from the same species, was demonstrated to be beneficial in transgenesis (Nam *et al.*, 2001). This requires isolation of species-specific functional promoters capable of driving either ubiquitous or tissue-specific expression of the gene of interest. Isolation of rohu β -actin promoter will have potential use in expressing desired genes of interest for generating transgenic rohu.

The beta-actin gene promoter of rohu (*Labeo rohita*) was isolated and characterized. Expression analysis of beta-actin gene promoter was undertaken by direct injection into the muscle of the same species (Barman *et al.*, 2010). The promoter region contained the consensus cis-acting regulatory elements of TATA box, CAAT box, proximal CC(A/T)6GG box (CArG or serum response element) including MEF2 box. Direct muscular injection of the construct containing beta-actin promoter fused to a GFP reporter gene showed efficient expression at the site of injection as well as in the areas away from the site. One CArG box positioned between the CAAT box and TATA box is capable of activating reporter gene expression (Fig. 3). The entire rohu beta actin promoter/ regulatory region showed the closest similarity with that of catla (*Catla catla*) among the sequences of other species available in GenBank. Our study has potential implications in the basic research, vaccination, gene therapy and transgenics (Barman *et al.*, 2010). Further, transgenic rohu was generated using this construct showing ubiquitous expression of GFP (Fig. 2A of Annexure I). The same construct was used to raise transgenic rohu fish. About 20% of transgenic offspring showed ubiquitous expression of the reporter GFP gene (Barman *et al.*, 2015). Massive epithelial and/or muscular expressions, with visible green color under normal light, were documented in a few transgenic rohus (Fig. 4). The heightened expression of GFP mRNA was documented in the muscle of transgenic fishes as compared to muscle of non-transgenic fishes.

Ethical and ecological concerns

The greatest concerns regarding transgenic food fish are those related to their inadvertent release and escape to the environment, in addition to controversies about food safety issues (Alison and Paul 2006; Muir and Howard 1999). One way of mitigating environmental risks is to develop effective containment strategies (Devlin *et al.*, 2006).

Even though transgenic fishes have some benefits, but the marketing of these transgenic food fish remains a controversial issue due to ecological and food safety concerns. But in comparison to the transgenic food fish, the transgenic ornamental fish do not possess any threat to the environment. The culturing of GM ornamental fish is less concerned about environmental and ecological issues. There is no food safety issue for ornamental fish and marketing of transgenic ornamental fish is a more viable concept. Ornamental fishes form an important commercial component of aquaculture, providing for aesthetic requirements and upkeep of the environment.

The use of 'autotransgene' construct, where the promoter/regulatory element and targeted structural gene derived from the same species, was demonstrated to be beneficial in transgenesis, without having ethical concerns. With phenomenal increase in population and thereby heightened demands in foods vis-à-vis decrease in cultivable lands will essentially require GMOs in future. The effective and regulatory containment facilities for the auto-transgenic fishes will have great potential for supplying protein rich diets.

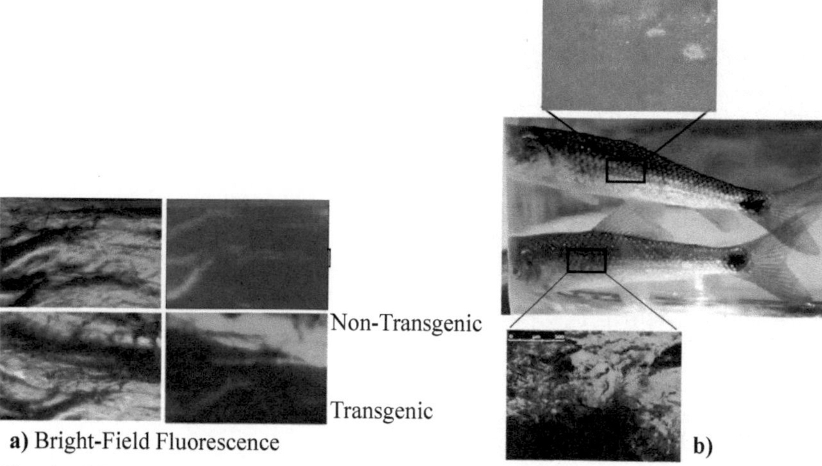

Fig. 1: GFP expressions driven by the mylz 2 promoter in the skeletal muscle of rohu (*L. rohita*): **(a)** Histological slides of skeletal muscle following direct muscular injection of DNA construct; **(b)** Massive GFP expressions in transgenic rohu fishes. *(See colour version on page 255)*

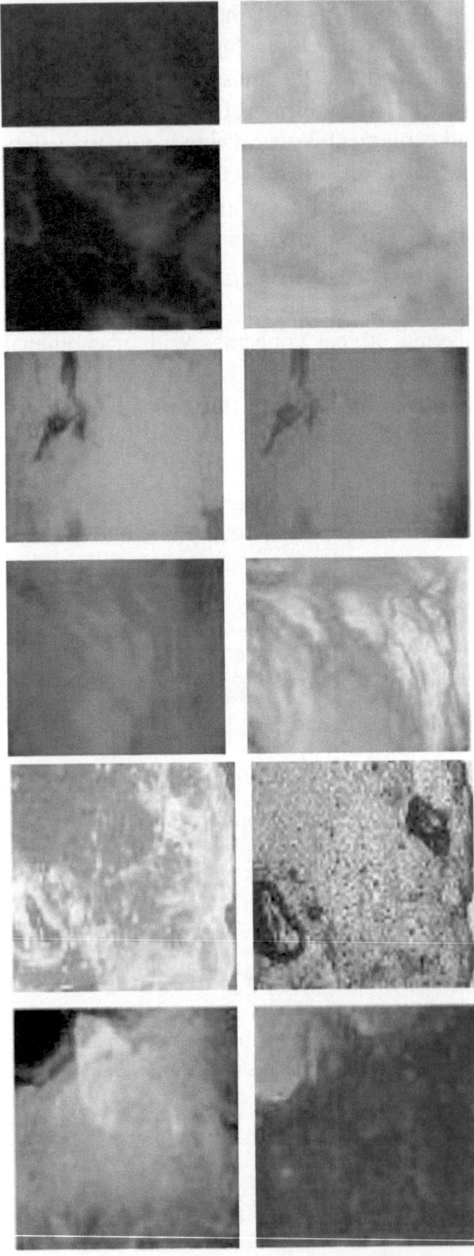

Fig. 2. Fluorescence protein expressions driven by the full-length promoter at the site of injection of the skeletal muscle. Images are taken under fluorescence- (left panel) and bright-field (right panel). RFP expressions driven by the full-length *mylz2* promoter at 15, 30 and 60 days in *L. laubuca* (upper panel). Control is the muscle of non-injected fish. GFP was expressed in the skeletal muscle of *L. rohita* at 15 days of examination (lower panel). *(See colour version on page 256)*

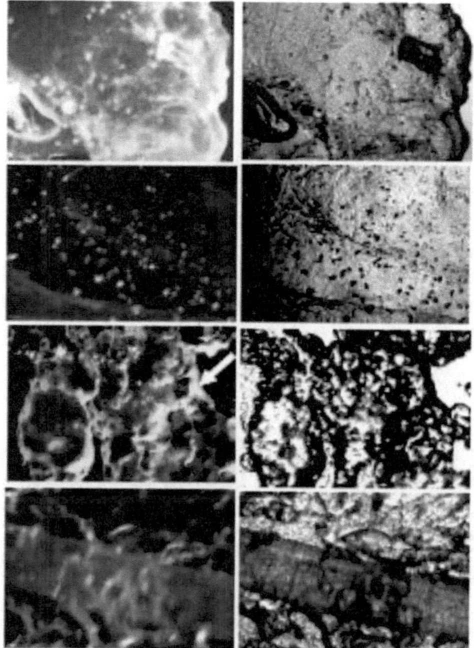

Fig. 3. Green fluorescence protein expression in muscle at the site of injection at 15, 30 and 55 days. Control is the muscle of non-injected fish. Images are taken under fluorescence (left) and bright-field (right). Arrow indicates autofluorescence. (Reproduced from our publication, *Current Science*, 99: 1030-1032) *(See colour version on page 257)*

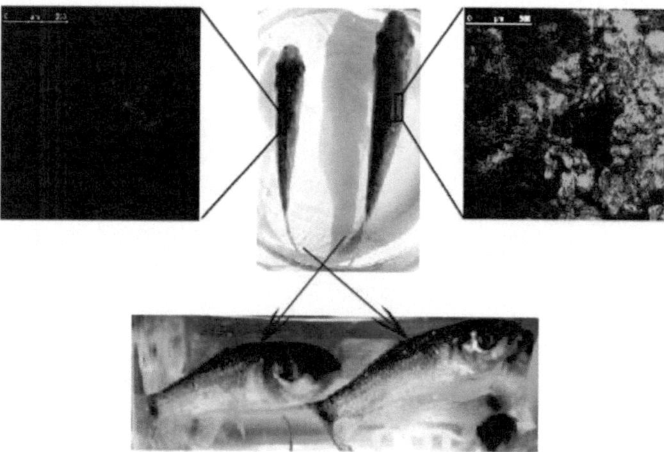

Fig. 4. Documented GFP expressions driven by the β-*actin* promoter in transgenic rohu (Reproduced from our publication, *Cellular & Molecular Biology Letters*, 20, DOI: 10.1515/cmble-2015-0010). *(See colour version on page 257)*

References

Barman H K, Das V, Mohanta R, Mohapatra C, Panda R P, Jayasankar P (2010) Expression analysis of β-actin promoter of rohu (*Labeo rohita*) by direct injection into muscle. Current Science 99: 1030-1032.

Barman HK, Mohanta R, Patra SK, Chakrapani V, Panda, RP, Nayak S, Jena S, Jayasankar P, Nandanpawar P (2015) The β-*actin* gene promoter of rohu carp (*Labeo rohita*) drove reporter gene expressions in transgenic rohu and various cell lines including spermatogonial stem cells. Cellular & Molecular Biology Letters 20, DOI: 10.1515/cmble-2015-0010.

Hamada K, Tamaki K, Sasado T, Watai Y, Kani S, Wakamatsu Y, Ozato K, Kinoshita M, Kohno R, Takagi S, Kimura M (1998) Usefulness of the medaka b-actin promoter investigated using a mutant GFP reporter gene in transgenic medaka (*Oryzias latipes*). Mol Mar Biol Biotech 7, 173-180.

Hwang GL, Rahman A, Razak SA, Shom F, Farahmand H, Smith A, Brooks C, Maclean N (2003) Isolation and characterisation of tilapia β-actin promoter and comparison of its activity with carp β-actin promoter. Biochim Biophys Acta 1625, 11–18.

Liu ZJ, Moav B, Faras AJ, Guise KS, Kapuscinski AR, Hackett PB (1990) Functional analysis of elements affecting expression of the beta-actin gene of carp. Mol Cell Biol 10, 3432–3440.

Mohanta R, Jayasankar P, Mahapatra KD, Saha JN, Barman H K (2014) Molecular cloning, characterization and functional assessment of the myosin light polypeptide chain 2 (*mylz2*) promoter of farmed carp, *Labeo rohita*. Transgenic Research 23(4): 601-607.

Nam YK, Noh JK, Cho YS, Cho HJ, Cho KN, Kim CG, Kim DS (2001) Dramatically accelerated growth and extraordinary gigantism of transgenic mud loach Misgurnus mizolepis. Transgenic Res 10, 353– 362.

Quitschke WW, Lin ZY, DePonti-Zilli L, Paterson BM (1989) The beta actin promoter. High levels of transcription depend upon a CCAAT binding factor. J Biol Chem 264, 9539–9546.

Takagi S, Sasado T, Tamiya G, Ozato K, Wakamatsu Y, Takeshita A, Kimura, M (1994) An efficient expression vector for transgenic medaka construction. Mol Mar Biol Biotechnol 3, 192–199.

Venugopal T, Anathy V, Kirankumar S, Pandian TJ (2004) Growth enhancement and food conversion efficiency of transgenic fish *Labeo rohita*. J Exp Zool A 301, 477–490.

13

Nutritional Management of Macro Minerals Disorders in Peri-parturient Dairy Animals

Vishal Mudgal

Senior Scientist, Mineral Nutrition Laboratory, Central Institute for Research on Bufaloes, Hisar-125 001, Haryana, India

R.K. Jain

Professor, Animal Nutrition, College of Veterinary Science and A.H., Mhow (MP)

Introduction

Mineral imbalance in the animal body produces several problems. Normal dairy animals experience constantly changing nutrient demands and environmental stress during pregnancy and lactation. In the first part of the cycle the negative balance must be held to minimum, later the reserves must be replenished through fine tuned nutritional support for optimum production of the dairy animals. Inadequate blood calcium (Ca), phosphorus (P), magnesium (Mg), or potassium (K) concentrations can cause a dairy animal to lose the ability to rise to her feet as these elements are necessary for nerve and muscle function and are therefore of particular concern in the newly calved dairy animal. Mechanisms for maintaining blood status of these elements concentrations perform efficiently most of the time but occasionally these homeostatic mechanisms fail and metabolic diseases such as milk fever occur. Understanding about cause and predisposing factors behind the same may be helpful to develop strategies to avoid these disorders.

Macro elements have a significant role in normal functioning of the body, including proper reproduction and production. Imbalance of these elements in the body of a peri parturient animal creates severe problems to the animal body and even the productivity of the animal gets seriously affected. Among the macro elements calcium, phosphorus and magnesium with cation-anion balancing elements (sodium, potassium and chlorine) play an important role in normal health of dairy animals during the parturition period.

Calcium

Blood Ca in the adult cow is maintained around 2.1–2.5 mmol/L. Bone/blood Ca is regulated by parathyroid hormone (PTH), which is produced by the signal of reduced blood Ca and maintains blood level of Ca through re-absorption from bone and even renal tubular re-absorption of Ca. However, a small amount of Ca can be recovered by reducing urinary Ca excretion. A second hormone, 1, 25-dihydroxy vitamin D_3, is required to stimulate the efficiency of dietary Ca absorption through the intestine. This hormone is synthesized in the kidney using Vitamin D_3in response to an increased blood PTH.

Milk fever is a common production disease usually occurring in high yielding dairy cows within 48 hrs of parturition especially in cows with third or later lactation (Horst *et al*., 1994). Usually the Ca requirement of an adult dairy cow is relativity low, resulting in lower absorption of Ca from the intestines (10-15%) as against 40-60%, when the animal is in milk and it remains the major predisposing cause for exposure of dairy animals for milk fever just after calving.

Factors impairing Ca homeostasis

Breed

Certain breeds of cattle *viz*. Swedish red and Jersey are more susceptible to milk fever than either breed. This may be due to the lesser receptors for 1, 25 dihydroxy vitamin D_3in the intestine of these breeds of cows. Lower receptors would result in a loss of target tissue sensitivity to 1, 25 $(OH)_2 D_3$.

Age

Cow rarely suffers from fever in the first lactation. However, by the third lactation this incidence increased very much and continued to increase in the subsequent lactation. The factors responsible for this age factor are increased milk production, decreased ability to mobilize calcium from bone, impaired production of 1, 25 $(OH)_2 D_3$ and decline in active transport of Ca in the intestine.

Diet

Manipulation of dietary Ca and P is known to have dramatic effects on the incidence of milk fever (Jorgensen, 1974). Feeding high Ca diet before parturition decreases active intestinal absorption and bone Ca resorption mechanism becomes quiescent and homeostatically depressed. Therefore, when increased Ca demand arises; these mechanisms take several days to be activated and severe hypocalcaemia results. The Ca:P ratio of the diet has been attributed to be responsible for milk fever, but Ca intake is a much more important factor than the Ca: P ratio.

Metabolic alkalosis

Recent studies have demonstrated that metabolic alkalosis is one of the underlying causes of milk fever. It has been seen that increased pH interferes with the response of cow's tissue to PTH, reducing the ability of the cow to draw bone Ca stores. Further production of 1, 25 $(OH)_2 D_3$that is needed for active Ca transport in the intestine is also impaired. Metabolic alkalosis is mainly due to the result of a diet that supplies more cations (K, sodium (Na), Ca, and Mg) than anions (chloride (Cl), sulphate (SO4), and phosphate (PO4)) to the blood.

Chronic Hypomagnesemia

Prolong feeding of Mg deficient diet is also considered to be a factor responsible to reduce Ca metabolism and predispose them to parturient paresis (Braak *et al*., 1987).

Hypomagnesemia affects Ca homeostasis in two ways: (1) by reducing PTH secretion in response to hypocalcemia and (2) by reducing tissue sensitivity to PTH. (Rude *et al.*, 1978; Littledike *et al.*, 1983). Field evidence suggests that blood Mg concentrations below 0.65 mmol/L in the periparturient cow will increase the susceptibility of cows to hypocalcemia and milk fever (van de Braak *et al.*, 1987).

Excessive blood phosphorus concentration

When blood P concentration is increased above the upper normal limit, around 2 mmol/L, the phosphate has a direct inhibitory effect on the renal enzyme converting 25-hydroxyvitamin D to 1,25-dihydroxyvitamin D. Therefore, even if PTH secretion occurs and the tissues recognize the PTH the cow will be unable to produce the hormone necessary for activation of intestinal Ca transport and the cow will suffer impaired Ca homeostasis (Barton, 1978; Kichura *et al.*, 1982).

Strategies to prevent hypocalcemia

However milk fever can be successfully treated by a slow intravenous injection of calcium borogluconate, which may have to be repeated if the symptoms reoccurs, a better choice is to prevent it by nutritional means. Prepartum feeding management with Ca-deficient diet, oral administration of soluble/gel calcium, feeding of chloride and sulphate salts of Ca, Mg and ammonium with decreased sodium and potassium without compromising ration palatability, administration of vitamin D, manipulation of dietary cation-anion balance (Goff *et al.*, 1995; Qetzel *et al.*, 1988; Tucker *et al.*, 1988; Hansen *et al.*, 2002 and Patel *et al.*, 2011) are the possible approach for reducing the incidence of milk fever in dairy cows.

Reducing diet cation–anion difference

Prevention of milk fever requires that the blood pH should be reduced to prevent metabolic alkalosis. Ender *et al.*, (1971) reported that the incidence of milk fever depended on the abundance of the cations, Na+ and K+ relative to the anions, Cl and SO^{-4}. Blood pH can be reduced by adding anions to the diets or by reducing the number of cations in the diet. Acid-base balance within the system depends on dietary absorption of anions and cations. If the quantity of absorbable ions (Cl and SO_4) increases in the diet, cows become acidotic resulting in lowered pH of blood and urine and reducing the incidence of milk fever. However, urine pH should be monitored and should not reduce to below 5.5; otherwise there is a risk of metabolic acidosis.

Proper care is required that a small amount of salt is added to the diet to prevent pica, but unlimited access to NaCl is to be avoided in late gestation because it will increase the risk of udder edema, not because it greatly affects acid–base status.

As per the level of different macro elements is concerned dietary Ca did not influence the degree of hypocalcemia experienced at calving or milk production in the subsequent lactation. It appears from various studies that close-up diet Ca concentration should be maintained between 8.5 and 10 g Ca/kg DM. Similarly, to ensure adequate concentrations of Mg in the blood of the periparturient cow so that PTH interacts effectively with its receptors on bone and kidney cells the dietary Mg concentration should be 3.5–4 g Mg/kg DM. This higher dietary Mg concentration allows the cow to take advantage of passive absorption of Mg across the rumen wall. Concentration of dietary P should be fed at a level to meet the NRC requirement for P in the late gestation cow (0.4 g P/kg DM). Level of dietary S must be kept above 2.2 g/kg DM for keeping adequate substrate for rumen microbial amino acid synthesis, while its should be kept below 4 g/kg DM to avoid possible neurological problems associated with S toxicity (Gould *et al.*, 1991). Calcium sulfate and Mg sulfate are good sources of sulfate anion that may also supply Mg and Ca if needed. For formulation purposes the concentration of Cl required in the diet to acidify the cow is approximately 5 g/kg DM, less than the concentration of K (about 10 g/kg DM).

Ca deficient diet to stimulate PTH secretion pre-calving

High dietary Ca before parturition predisposes to milk fever. Therefore, low dietary Ca, which keeps the mechanisms of active intestinal transport as well as bone calcium resorption (by stimulating PTH secretion), is the first preventive measure (Goings *et al.*, 1974; Green *et al.*, 1981). It is therefore recommended to restrict Ca supply (< 20g /day) at least two weeks before parturition. Studies have shown that feeding low Ca diets or adjusting the ratio of dietary Ca to P (1:3.3) lowered the incidence of milk fever (Boda and Cole, 1956).

Vitamin D supplementation

Vitamin D plays an important role in calcium absorption. Therefore, it is considered an important preventive measure of milk fever. A reasonable practice is to supplement the dry cow with 20–30,000 IU Vitamin D/day in the diet or parenteral administration of 10 million units of vitamin D_3, 2-8 days before to calving reduced the milk fever in cows with previous history (Julien *et al.*, 1977; Littledike and Horst, 1980). Use of Vitamin D_3 metabolites shows premising of being effective and practical, particularly in herds where excessive Ca is being fed during the dry period and Ca intake is difficult to reduce because of the feeding of legume forage.

Oral Ca treatments at calving

To prevent hypocalcaemia, efforts have been made to give soluble/gel forms of calcium before and just after parturition to maintain high levels of Ca in the extracellular fluid. Ca administered to the fresh cow may arguably be called a treatment rather than a preventative measure for hypocalcemia. Ca propionate has been recommended for this purpose with dual advantages that in addition to a source of Ca, it also acts as a glucogenic precursor at a time when the animal needs energy (Goff and Horst, 1993; Pehrson *et al.*, 1998). For best control of hypocalcemia a dose is given at calving and again 24 h later. The concept behind oral supplementation is that the cow's ability to utilize active transport of Ca across intestinal cells is inadequate to help her maintain normal blood Ca concentrations. Best results are obtained with doses of Ca between 50 and 125g Ca/dose. Ca chloride has been used but can be caustic. Large or repeated doses of calcium chloride can induce an uncompensated metabolic acidosis in the cow, especially if the cow is already being fed an acidogenic diet (Goff and Horst, 1993).

Magnesium

Mg is a major intracellular cation that is a necessary cofactor for enzymatic reactions vital to every major metabolic pathway. Extracellular Mg is vital to normal nerve conduction, muscle function, and bone mineral formation. Plasma Mg concentration in cow is normally between 1.8 and 2.4 mg/dl (0.75 and 1.0 mmol/L), while milk having approximately 5.2 mmol/L Mg and thus through milk high amount of Mg can rapidly withdraw resulting in hypo-magnesemia if not replaced. Bone did not work as a source of Mg that can be utilized in times of its deficiency, as bone resorption occurs in response to Ca homeostasis, not affected by Mg status. Maintenance of normal plasma Mg concentration is nearly dependent on a constant influx of Mg from the diet. Mg gets absorbed from the small intestine of young calves and lambs. As the rumen and reticulum develop these sites become the main, and perhaps the only, sites for net Mg absorption (Pfeffer *et al.*, 1970; Martens and Rayssiguier, 1980; Martens and Gabel, 1986). In adult ruminants the small intestine becomes a site of net secretion of Mg (Greene *et al.*, 1983). Mg absorption from rumen is dependent on its concentration in the rumen fluid and the integrity of the Mg transport mechanism, which is a Na-linked active transport process (Martens and Gabel, 1986). Solubility of Mg declines sharply when rumen pH rises above 6.5. Forages often contain 100– 200 mmol/kg of unsaturated palmitic, linoleic, and linolenic acids, which can form insoluble Mg salts in the rumen.

In low dietary Na addition of Na in the ration can improve Mg transport across the rumen when, though in high amounts it increases urinary excretion of Mg so that the benefit to the animal may be negated.

Grass tetany

It is not exactly synonyms of hypomagnesemic tetany, which occurs in both adult and young animals while the former usually occurs in older, lactating animals consuming lush, cool season grasses that have received some degree of intensive management *i.e.*, fertilization (Church, 2012). There are other synonyms like lactation tetany, grass staggers, wheat pasture poisoning *etc.* This disease is most common in Northern Europe and in the UK, Australia and New Zealand where the cows are not housed but have access to pasture overgrowth in the spring. It is a seasonal problem and occurs 5-10 days after cold and wet weather, when forages contain less than 2mg/kg DM and high concentration of N, K, organic acid, fatty acids, water and low concentration of total water soluble carbohydrates (Robinson *et al.*, 1989). Pregnant and adult lactating cows (first 2 months of lactation) and adult cattle of 4-7 years of age are most susceptible because of their increased Mg requirement. It is a complex metabolic disorder of ruminant animals that form a deficiency of available dietary Mg either due to decreased concentration in the diet or due to decreased alimentary absorption. These factors must be kept in mind to protect from grass tetany:

- High level of K in feed depresses blood Mg by depressing the Mg absorption High (Schonewille *et al.*, 1992).

- Early spring pasture (5-10 days after cold) is rich in protein, NPN substances (due to increased N-fertilization) elevates rumen NH_3levels which interfere with Mg absorption.
- Heavy top dressing of pasture with ammonium fertilizer decreases plant uptake of Mg and thus decreases availability at dietary level.
- Grasses with high ratio of K: Ca + Mg, low Mg pastures (wheat *etc.*) impaired Mg absorption from the rumen.
- High dietary aluminium and phytate effects Mg absorption from the rumen.
- Supplementation of higher fatty acids increases lipid content of young grass thus lowering Mg absorption.
- Low dietary soluble carbohydrate in lush green pasture contributes to an increased pH of rumen, which resulted in decreased Mg absorption.
- Calves fed on whole milk or milk replacer contain low levels of Mg and Ca.

Nutritional management

Hypomagnasemic tetany can be effectively managed nutritionally through provision of adequate delivery system (Mg mineral block salt lick, slow release Mg boluses, $MgCl_2$in drinking water (Martens *et al.*, 1991 and Dua and Care, 1995) dietary management to maintain optimum rumen acidity for better absorption (Robinson *et al.*, 1989), agronomic management practices (selection of soil forage species, liming and fertilization practices) (Robinson *et al.*, 1989, Majak *et al.*, 1995) use of ionophores (Dua and care, 1995) for better absorption *etc.*

- Mg supplements like MgO, Mg $(OH)_2$, $MgCO_3$, $MgCl_2$ and $MgSO_4$ *etc.* can be incorporated in the mineral mixture for the feeding of cows in suspected areas.
- Mg boluses (slow release of Mg in the rumen).
- Mg (1-2% $MgCl_2$) in drinking water is an efficient method of grass tetany prevention.
- Use of soluble carbohydrates like molasses, ground corn *etc.* to maintain optimum rumen acidity.
- Maintenance of serum Ca through Ca injection or supplements or supply of vitamin D_3may protect against grass tetany.
- Rumen microbial manipulation: *Selenomonas ruminantium* helps to prevent Mg deficiency by increasing rumen availability of Mg for absorption.
- Agronomic management practices aimed at selection of soil, selection of forage liming and fertilization practices *etc.*

Steps that can be taken to reduce the risk of grass tetany includes (Church, 2012):

- Delay grazing until grass is 4 to 6 inches tall.
- Plant grass/legume mixes in pastures.
- Feed legume hay during the winter feeding period prior to the grazing period.
- Feed a high magnesium mineral supplement.

- Avoid grazing cows that are nursing young calves, three months and under, on pastures where there is a risk of grass tetany.

Phosphorus

Plasma P concentration is normally 1.3–2.6 mmol/L. Maintaining the extracellular P pool involves replacing P removed for bone and muscle growth, endogenous fecal loss, urinary P loss, and milk production with P absorbed from the diet or reabsorbed from bone (Reinhardt *et al.*, 1988). During late gestation fetal skeletal development can withdraw up to 10 g P/day from the maternal P pools (House and Bell, 1993). About 0.3 g P is incorporated into each kg of body tissue (muscle) gained during growth of the animal (ARC, 1980; Bacon *et al.*, 1990). In the form of milk production, removes about 1 g P from the extracellular pool/kg of milk produced. Salivary glands remove between 30 and 90 g P from the extracellular P pool each day, which is a major buffer of rumen pH—most of this secreted P is reabsorbed in the small intestine to return to the extracellular pool.

Rumen microbes can digest phytic acid so that most of the phytate-bound P (35–70% of P in plants) is available for absorption in ruminants. P is primarily absorbed in the small intestine with active transport process and is responsive to 1,25-dihydroxyvitamin D. Intestinal P absorption efficiency can, in theory, be upregulated during periods of P deficiency as renal production of 1,25-dihydroxyvitamin D is directly stimulated by very low plasma P. However, the plasma P level must reach very low levels (0.3–0.6 mmol/L) to stimulate increased renal production of 1,25-dihydroxyvitamin D. Plasma P concentrations are generally well correlated with dietary P absorption. P absorbed in excess of needs is excreted in urine and saliva. PTH, secreted during periods of Ca stress, increases renal and salivary excretion of P (Wright *et al.*, 1984), which may be detrimental to maintenance of normal blood P concentrations. This is the likely reason that hypocalcemic animals tend to become hypophosphatemic. One might believe that prolonged PTH secretion would increase blood P concentration since it stimulates bone mineral resorption, but this effect is small when compared to the effect of PTH on P excretion. Since PTH stimulates the kidney to produce 1,25-dihydroxyvitamin D, it eventually can increase the efficiency of intestinal phosphate absorption, which should correct hypophosphatemia. However, it must be remembered that PTH is secreted in response to hypocalcemia, not hypophosphatemia.

Among the production disease, post parturient haemoglobinuria or red water disease causes a considerable loss, when diets are low in P or un-supplemented in dairy cattle. Sometimes feeding of cruciferous plants like beet pulp, turnips, rapeseed *etc.* has been associated with the disease (Mahmood *et al.*, 2012).

This disease usually occurs at 2-4 weeks after calving. High producing dairy cows and buffaloes especially in the age group of 3-6 lactation are mostly vulnerable to this disease. The disease is characterized by intravascular haemolysis, haemoglobinuria and anaemia. Phosphorus deficient soil, drought condition and prolonged hypophosphatemia are considered as predisposing causes. The same disease also occurs before parturition, various stages of lactation *etc.* it may be associated with grazing on pasture, which has grown on soil deficient in P, availability of P is also minimized by presence of excess Ca, Al and Fe. In India similar conditions accompanied with hypophosphatemia has been recorded in buffaloes in Hisar, sugar belt of Maharashtra, Malwa region of M.P. and certain hilly districts of Uttranchal.

Nutritional management

- Remove the animal from toxic feed, if any.
- Appropriate supply of P and Cu in feed.
- Usually P deficiency occurs in areas where P levels in soil, pasture and dietary intake are 0.002%, 0.2 and 20-25gm/day, respectively.
- Sodium acid phosphate @60-120g dissolved in 240ml of DW and mixed with 500 ml dextrose is given through injection. Most of the cows respond to treatment in 3-4 days. This is given in conjunction with blood transfusions.
- Cows and buffaloes are fed with leguminous straw (gram straw, masur straw *etc.*) during the advanced stage of pregnancy. It should be supplemented with wheat bran @ 2-3 kg /head/ day or with other suitable P supplemented *i.e.*, sodium acid phosphate @100-150 gm per head per day.
- Vitamin B_{12}, 5-10 ml with butaphosphan and supply of 120 g bone meal in the ration throughout the pregnancy period to prevent the condition.
- In bad cases whole blood transfusion @ 4-5 litre/450 kg body weight is recommended along with iron tonics containing ferrous gluconate 1-2 g, $CuSO_4$ 60 mg, and Cobalt sulphate 15mg, ascorbic acid 250 mg, molasses 30 ml to cattle.

Hypo-phosphatemia and downer cows

In late gestation, plasma P can decline precipitously as the growth of the fetus accelerates and removes substantial amounts of P from the maternal circulation. These animals often become recumbent and are unable to rise, though they appear fairly alert and will often eat feed placed in front of them. Cows carrying twins are most often affected. Hypophosphatemic downer cows are also often described as "alert" downers. The etiology of this disease is not clear. This occurs as a result of either the failure of cases of milk fever to respond or due to occurrence of relapse, which is expired within 48 hrs of first therapy. In most cases the animals are bright, alert with reduced appetite and remain in "forage leg attitude" and crawl on the ground popular name 'creeper cow'. They suffer from ischemic necrosis of thigh muscle due to heavy weight of animals and at the same time also suffer from damage of nerves of thigh region, due to tissue compression (Gunes, 2011).

Several factors have been identified as possible causes of downer cow syndrome including persistent hypocalcaemia, hypophosphatemia, hypomagnesaemia, muscular or nerve injury, myocardiosis (due to repeated Ca therapy), hepatosis or septic mastitis.

Nutritional Management

- Cow should not be over fatty through too much feeding during an advanced pregnancy.
- Cow should be made to stand within a short time following parturition.
- Periodical turning should be made in recumbent cows.
- Parental vitamin D_3 should be given in milk fever prone cows during pregnancy.
- Low Ca and high P diet should be given to stimulate parathyroid gland and thus to avoid hypocalcaemia.
- If possible, Ca metabolic profile test should be carried out in suspected cows of the dairy farm.
- There may be moderate ketonuria and proteinuria. The Ca, P, Mg and glucose levels of blood remain normal. Elevation of serum urea above 25 mmol/l and creatinine above 130 mmol/l has been described as a poor prognosis.
- Treatment of cows with phosphate containing solutions can affect recovery in some animals. Oral treatment restores normal blood P more slowly than intravenous treatment but the effect lasts much longer (Cheng *et al.*, 1998).

Potassium

Metabolism of K in cows is poorly researched since most diets provide more than ample supplies of K to the **cow**. However, severe hypokalemia occasionally develops which has been associated with muscle weakness and recumbency in cows. The majority of cases present with severe hypokalemia (plasma K below 2.5 mmol/L) and most cases occur secondary to prolonged inappetence, often secondary to other illnesses. Ketosis is commonly the factor precipitating the inappetence. Extracellular K concentration is normally 3.9–5.8 mmol/L and plays a vital role in osmotic equilibrium, and maintenance of acid–base balance. Intracellular K concentration is 150–160 mmol/L. Intracellular K is a co-factor of enzymes involved in protein synthesis and carbohydrate metabolism, and K plays a major role in intracellular osmotic and acid– base equilibrium. The ratio of intracellular: extracellular fluid K concentration is the main determinant of resting cell membrane potentials, which affects nerve and muscle cell excitability.

Effects of K on muscle function

K is the major determinant of nerve and muscle cell resting membrane potential since the majority of ion channels that are open in the resting cell membrane are K channels. Hypokalemia generally causes a loss of K conductance in cardiac muscle depolarization cardiac cell membranes (Schipperheyn, 1984).

Depletion of intracellular K reduces Ca release, which prevents effective interaction of actin and myosin molecules and reduced contractility of muscle (Meissner *et al.*, 1997).

Conclusion

It may be concluded that nutritional management of dairy animals is crucial during the peri-parturient period and proper attention and care may avoid various peri-parturient disorders which may ultimately prevent from huge economic losses to dairy farmers.

References

Agricultural Research Council (1980) The Nutrient Requirements of Ruminant Livestock. Commonwealth Agricultural Bureaux, Slough, England.

Bacon JA, Bell MC, Miller JK, Ramsey N, Mueller FJ (1990) Effect of magnesium administration route on plasma minerals in Holstein calves receiving either adequate or insufficient magnesium in their diets. J Dairy Sci 73, 470–473.

Barton BA (1978) Studies of Vitamin D, Calcium, and Phosphorus Metabolism of the Dairy Cow. Master's Thesis Dissertation. University of Wisconsin, Madison, WI. Boda J M, Cole HH (1956) Calcium metabolism with special reference to Parturient Paresis (Milk Fever) in dairy cattle: A Review. 39:1027-1054.

Braak VD, AE, Van KAT, Malestin A (1987) Influence of a deficient supply of magnesium during the dry period on the rate of calcium mobilization by dairy cows at parturition. Research in Veterinary Science 42, 101–108.

Cheng Y, Goff JP, Horst RL (1998) Restoring normal blood phosphorus concentrations in hypophosphatemic cattle with sodium phosphate. Vet Med 4, 383–386.

Church J (2012) Grass Tetany in Cattle. A beef cattle E–letter for area cattle producers. University of Idaho Extension p 1-3.

Dua K, Care A D (1995) Impaired absorption of magnesium in the aetiology of grass tetany. British Veterinary Journal 151: 4, 413-426.

Goff JP, Reinhardt TA, Horst RL (1995) Milk fever and dietary cation-anion balance effects on concentration of vitamin D receptor in tissue of periparturient dairy cows. Journal of Dairy Science 78: 2388–2394.

Goff JP, Horst RL (1993) Oral administration of calcium salts for treatment of hypocalcemia in cattle. J Dairy Sci 76, 101–108.

Goings RL, Jacobson NL, Beitz DC, Littledike ET, Wiggers KD (1974) Prevention of parturient paresis by a prepartum, calcium-deficient diet. J Dairy Sci 57, 1184–1188.

Gould DH, McAllister MM, Savage JC, Hamar DW (1991) High sulfide concentrations in rumen fluid associated with nutritionally induced polioencephalomalacia in calves. Am J Vet Res 52, 1164–1169.

Green HB, Horst RL, Beitz DC, Littledike ET (1981) Vitamin D metabolites in plasma of cows fed a prepartum low-calcium diet for prevention of parturient hypocalcemia. J Dairy Sci 64, 217–226.

Greene LW, Fontenot JP,Webb Jr, KE (1983) Site of magnesium and other macromineral absorption in steers fed high levels of potassium. J Anim Sci 57, 503–510.

Gunes V (2011) Downer Cow Syndrome: Review. Turkiye Klinikleri J Vet Sci 2(2):151-157.

Hansen T T, Jorgense RJ, Ostergaard S (2002) Milk Fever Control Principles: A Review Acta Vet Scand 43: 1-19.

Horst RL, Goff JP, Reinhardt TA (1994) Calcium and vitamin-D metabolism in the dairy cow. Journal of Dairy Science 77, 1936–1951.

House WA, Bell AW (1993) Mineral accretion in the fetus and adnexa during late gestation in Holstein cows. J Dairy Sci 76, 2999–3010.

Jorgensen NA (1974). Combating milk fever. J Dairy Sci 57:933-944.

Julien WE, Conrad HR, Hibbs JW, Crist WL (1977) Milk fever in dairy cows. VIII Effect of injected vitamin D3 and calcium and phosphorus intake on incidence. J Dairy Sci 60:431-436.

Kichura, T.S., Horst, R.L., Beitz, D.C., Littledike, E.T., 1982. Relationships between prepartal dietary calcium and phosphorus, Vitamin D metabolism, and parturient paresis in dairy cows. J. Nutr. 112, 480–487.

Littledike, E.T., Horst, R.L., 1980. Problems with Vitamin D injections for prevention of milk fever: toxicity of large doses and increased incidence of small doses. J. Dairy Sci. 63, 89. Littledike, E.T., Stuedemann, J.A., Wilkinson, S.R., Horst, R.L., 1983. Grass tetany syndrome. In: Role of Magnesium in Animal Nutrition. Virginia Polytechnic Institute and State University, Blacksburg, VA, p. 173.

Mahmood, A., Khan, M. A., Younus, M., Khan, M. A., Iqbal, H. J. and Ahad, A. (2012) Case Control Study of Parturient Hemoglobinuria in Buffaloes. Pak Vet J, 32(3): 375-377.

Majak, W., Hall, J. W. and McCaughey, W. P. (1995). Pasture management strategies for reducing the risk of legume bloat in cattle. J. Anim. Sci.73:1493-1498.

Martens, H., Lconard, S. and Gobel, G. (1991). In: Rumen microbial Metabolism and Ruminant Digestion, J. P. Jauony (Ed.). INRA Editions, Paris. pp 199-222.

Martens, H., Rayssiguier, Y., 1980. Magnesium metabolism and hypomagnesemia. In: Ruckebusch, Y., Thivend, P. (Eds.), Digestive Physiology and Metabolism in Ruminants. MTP Press, Lancaster, England.

Martens, H., Gabel, G., 1986. Pathogenesis and prevention of grass tetany from the physiologic viewpoint. DTW Dtsch. Tierarztl. Wochenschr. 93, 170.

Meissner, G., Rios, E., Tripathy, A., Pasek, D.A., 1997. Regulation of skeletal muscle Ca2+ release channel (ryanodine receptor) by Ca2+ and monovalent cations and anions. J. Biol. Chem. 272, 1628–1638.

Patel, V.R., Kansara, J.D., Patel, B.B., Patel, P.B., Patel, S.B. (2011). Prevention of Milk fever: Nutritional Approach. Vet World. 4(6): 278-280.

Pehrson, B., Svensson, C., Jonsson, M., 1998. A comparative study of the effectiveness of calcium propionate and calcium chloride for the prevention of parturient paresis in dairy cows. J. Dairy Sci. 81, 2011–2016.

Pfeffer, E., Thompson, A., Armstrong, D.G., 1970. Studies on intestinal digestion in the sheep 3. Net movement of certain inorganic elements in the digestive tract on rations containing different proportions of hay and rolled barley. Brit. J. Nutr. 24, 197–204.

Qetzel, G. R., Olson, J. D., Curtis, C. R. and Fettman, M. J. (1988). Ammonium chloride and ammonium sulphate for prevention of Parturient Paresis in dairy cows. J. Dairy Sci. 71:3302-3309.

Reinhardt, T.A., Horst, R.L., Goff, J.P., 1988. Calcium, phosphorus, and magnesium homeostasis in ruminants. Vet. Clin. North Am. Food Anim. Pract. 4, 331–350.

Robinson, D. L., Kappel, L. C. and Boling, J. A. (1989). Management practices to overcome the incidence of grass tetany. J. Anim. Sci. 67:3470-3484.

Rude, R.K., Oldham, S.B., Sharp Jr., C.F., Singer, F.R., 1978. Parathyroid hormone secretion in magnesium deficiency. J. Clin. Endocrinol. Metab. 47, 800–806.

Schipperheyn, J.J., 1984. The pathophysiology of potassium and magnesium disturbances. A cardiac perspective. Drugs 28 (Suppl. 1), 112–119.

Schonewille, J.T., van't Klooster, A.T., van Mosel, M., 1992. A comparative study of the *in vitro* solubility and availability of magnesium from various sources for cattle. Tijdschr. Diergeneeskd. 117, 105–108.

Tucker, W.B., Harrison, G.A., Hemken, R.W. (1988) *Influence of dietary cation-anion balance on milk, blood, urine, and rumen fluid in lactating dairy cattle. J. Dairy Sci.*71:346-354.

Van de Braak, A.E., van't Klooster, A.T., Malestein, A., 1987. Influence of a deficient supply of magnesium during the dry period on the rate of calcium mobilisation by dairy cows at parturition. Res. Vet. Sci. 42, 101–108.

Wright, R.D., Blair-West, J.R., Nelson, J.F., Tregear, G.W., Rosenblatt, M., 1984. Evaluation of the biological properties of parathyroid hormone and analogues in a vascularly isolated parotid gland-based assay. J. Endocrinol. 102, 375–379.

14

Hormonal Regulation of Partitioning of Nutrients in Bypass Fat Supplemented Animals

Mahendra Singh

Principal Scientist (Animal Physiology), National Dairy Research Institute Karnal-132001, Haryana

Introduction

During transition period and lactation, the high-producing dairy cows undergo a period of extensive tissue catabolism because of negative nutrient balance. Homeorrhetic mechanism at this stage ensures that nutrients are partitioned to favour the growth of fetus prepartum and meet the demand of nutrients in early lactation. Simultaneously the homeostasis secures survival of the animal body functions. However, a decline in feed intake in transition period leads to metabolic disturbances and low milk production in early lactation. The postpartum negative nutrient balance impairs immune and reproductive functions in dairy cows and buffaloes. The increased demand for nutrients and decreased dry matter intake results in low circulating glucose and insulin levels and elevated non-esterified fatty acids (NEFA) and ketone bodies postpartum. The energetic status of a cow or buffalo modulates the secretion of hormones that play key roles in growth of ovarian follicles, ovulation, corpus luteum (CL) formation, and oocyte competence. The NEBAL not only limits milk production potential but also has a detrimental effect on immune cells. Negative nutrient balance is associated with changes in the pattern of ovarian follicle growth and oocyte quality and alteration in endocrines. In addition, cows under negative nutrient balance have extended periods of anovulation. These changes could be minimized by supplementing energy rich supplements like prilled fat or any bypass fat preparations.

What is a Rumen Bypass Fat?

Rumen bypass or "protected" fats are essentially dry fats that naturally have high melting points, and are mostly insoluble at rumen body temperature. They have little impact on rumen fermentation. The most widely used and effective method for producing rumen bypass fat is to react vegetable fatty acids with calcium oxide to form insoluble calcium soaps. Within the feed industry, these calcium soaps, or salts, appear on feed labels as "calcium salts of long chain fatty acids." Fatty acids distilled from palm oil processing are most commonly used to make calcium salts, because these fatty acids are produced in the greatest quantity worldwide. By far, calcium salts

Palm fatty acids (PFA) are the highest quality and best understood bypass fat for dairy cattle. Although the primary reason for feeding fat is for its energy density, it is becoming increasingly evident that essential fatty acids supplied by fat may have an important role in the nutrition of the high-producing cow.

Few generalizations have been made regarding fat

- Vegetable fats have more value than animal fats.
- Animal fats have more saturated fatty acids, such as stearic acid, that are associated with reduced fat digestibility.
- Compared to animal fats, vegetable fats have very low levels of stearic acid and much higher levels of key essential fatty acids, linoleic and linolenic acid. Linoleic acid has favorable effects on reproductive performance.

Importance of bypass fat feeding

The modern dairy farming trend is leading to rearing of elite germplasm cattle and buffaloes which produce very high levels of milk production. Such animals need energy challenged rations. In early lactation, cows producing more than 20 kg of milk will actually lose a considerable amount of weight (10-15%), because energy intake is less than that needed to meet the nutrient demands of milk production in early lactation. As a result, cow mobilizes body nutrient reserves, particularly body fat, to meet energy demand. Considering its energy density, fat is a logical choice for boosting ration energy density. The additional advantage of feeding supplemental fat is that the detrimental effects (including acidosis and laminitis) of feeding high levels of grain can be avoided. Improving forage quality will always be the most economical and nutritionally safe way to balance high production rations. However, supplemental fat almost always has a place in the ration when high-quality forages are not readily available.

Thus productivity of lactating animals can be enhanced by strategic supplementation with energy, and energy density can be increased by incorporating fat into their diet. However, fats that are not protected causes physical and chemical changes in the microbial fermentation of feed that are generally negative. Feeding of free or unprotected fat above 1% level has a depressing effect on rumen cellulolytic microbial activity. Energy intake is directly related to production in milk-producing systems. Dairy cows in early lactation are usually in a negative energy balance. Supplementation of the diet with fat may be used to maintain a high dietary energy density while avoiding ruminal acidosis, which may result when excessive amounts of starch are provided.

Effect of bypass fat feeding on milk production

Feeding of prilled fat or bypass fat augments milk yield by 10-17% in lactating cows and buffaloes under field and farm conditions. The increase in milk yield was attributed to an increase in galactopoietic hormone levels such as GH, T3 and T3 in conjunction with higher dry matter intake in fat supplemented cows. The fat content of milk also increases in supplemented cows however milk protein, lactose and SNF content did not change.

The increase in milk yield is primarily due to the improved energy balance as such animals have more values of feed energy and milk energy. The BCS and body weight also gain while NEFA concentration declines which indicates restricted adipose tissue mobilization in prilled fat, a bypass fat, supplemented animals. However, the response of feeding on these parameters varies depending upon the milk yield and stage of lactation.

Effect of bypass fat on reproductive performance

The mechanism for resumption of ovulatory cycles seems to be associated with metabolic signals and regulatory hormones primarily insulin and insulin like growth factor (IGF-1), which link nutritional status with gonadotropin secretion, recoupling of the growth hormone-IGF system, and follicle maturation and ovulation. It is well accepted that supplemental fat benefits herd reproductive performance by minimizing body weight loss and accelerating body weight gain after calving. In addition, research strongly suggests that unsaturated vegetable fatty acids could have additive effects on reproductive parameters in the cows, including follicular size and hormone patterns. Linoleic acid has been identified as one of the essential fatty acids that may have direct effects on reproductive function. It has been found that calcium salts of palm fatty acids and feeding of prilled fat are very effective in improving reproductive performance of cows and buffaloes. The improved reproductive performance in terms of early onset of postpartum heat, less no. of AI/ conception and conception rate has been attributed to higher cholesterol levels which is a precursor of steroid hormone synthesis.

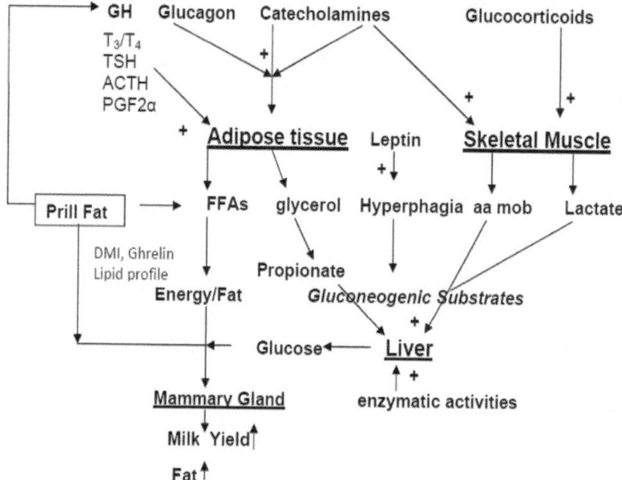

Fig. Role of hormones in partitioning of nutrients to augment lactation

Hormonal Regulation of Partitioning of Nutrients and Metabolic Modifications in Bypass Fed Animals

Metabolic modifications due to dietary fat intake have been reported to occur mainly at hepatic and adipose tissue levels. Alterations of blood concentrations of metabolic hormones have also been reported. Dietary fat supplementation did not affect plasma leptin and GH levels in the lactating cows. The levels of insulin-like growth factor- I and insulin was decreased with dietary fat supplementation in the lactating cows but remain unaffected in the growing steers, suggesting that responses to fat ingestion depend on the physiological state of the animal, including age and sex. Most studies have reported that dietary fat supplementation lowered or did not change the blood concentration of insulin-like growth factor I (IGF-I), however contradictory results has been obtained for serum growth hormone (GH) and insulin, their levels being reported as augmented, unchanged or, in the case of insulin, diminished. Leptin is an adipose-derived hormone that regulates a wide variety of physiological processes. As a signal from energy stores to the hypothalamus, it is involved in food-intake regulation and energy homeostasis. Reciprocally, there is long-term regulation of leptinemia by nutritional status and short-term regulation by food intake.

It has been shown that fat feeding increases plasma leptin concentration in rats, depending on total energy intake and type of fat. In ruminants, no effect of fat ingestion on leptin levels could be consistently demonstrated. The lowered leptin levels stimulate hyperphagia during early lactation to generate the gluconeogenic substance for glucose synthesis (Figure). Leptin is related to body fatness, food intake, and energy balance. Basal concentrations of the leptin hormone were higher in cows than in steers, despite the cows' lactational hyperleptinemia and the negative energy balance in early lactation, which likely contributed to the depression of leptin levels. Sexual differences in the circulating levels of leptin have previously been reported in rodents, primates (including humans), and ovines and have been attributed to the stimulating effect of estrogens and the inhibiting effect of androgens on leptin production, as well as to the differential distribution of subcutaneous and omental fat in males and females. Whereas fat mass is more important than age in determining blood leptin concentrations, differential effects of age and breed among the cows and steers. On the other hand, the higher basal levels of GH in the growing steers may have been involved in the lower leptin levels, as GH has been shown to inhibit leptin production in rodents. However, direct GH effects on leptinemia appear to be very low in cattle. The catabolic state during early lactation is governed by low insulin, IGF-I and higher GH levels which partition nutrients towards the mammary gland. At later stages of lactation catabolic state transforms to anabolic state and is indicated by higher IGF-I, insulin and lower GH levels. This an combination ensures better partitioning of energy during different stages of lactation.

The dietary addition of, or energy replacement by fat did not affect the circulating levels of leptin in the lactating cows. Similar results were observed in young heifers and lactating cows receiving a high-fat diet by means of sunflower seeds, calcium salts of palm oil or conjugated linoleic acids, corn oil or rumen-protected lin-oleic and linolenic acid, or linseed oil. When an aqueous emulsion of 18:2-rich oil was injected in the jugular vein of lactating cows, no effect was observed on leptin levels in early lactation, but an increase was reported in late lactation, suggesting different modulation of the hormone depending on the physiological status of the animal. Evidence indicates that bypass fat decreases plasma leptin concentration suggesting a strong inhibitory effect of fat intake on leptin production that overrides the likely increase in secretion of the hormone due to both the larger fat stores and the higher net energy intake.

Leptin is regulated by energy intake at 2 levels: a long-term effect that depends on adiposity and a short-term effect that is related to feeding level and diet composition. Therefore, plasma leptin concentrations are dependent on the amount of energy stored and strongly correlate with fat depots in humans, sheep, and cattle. A correlation between plasma leptin concentration and BCS was reported in dry late-pregnant cows than in early-lactation cows. Short-term fasting causes a rapid reduction in the plasma leptin concentration and that ref-feeding restores hormone levels in dairy cattle. Free fatty acids have been shown to down regulate leptin production in rat adipocytes in primary culture. The serum IGF-I level was also reported to be reduced in cows by the dietary administration of prilled saturated fatty acids or remain unchanged in lactating Jerseys given canola oil or oleamide supplements or Holsteins infused postruminally with canola oil suggesting that physiological state of the animal and the endocrine milieu determine the hormone response.

Dietary fats are partitioned in the liver between various possible metabolic pathways, depending on fatty acid composition and hormone regulation. When NEFA are mobilized from adipose tissue, they are partitioned to accumulate as triglycerides in the liver, which results in poor liver function in cows at calving and lower IGF-I secretion. However no increase in liver fat accumulation occurs during fat supplementation in early-lactating cows as dietary fatty acids are mainly absorbed in esterified form. The lower plasma insulin levels in early lactation are linked to lower energy balance and the lower plasma IGF-I levels in the fat-supplemented cows. Studies suggest that fat supplementation could have an inhibitory effect on circulating levels of insulin in early to peak lactation in cows. On the contrary, in nonlactating cows given supplementary saturated, polyunsaturated, or highly polyunsaturated fats, the serum insulin concentration markedly increased. The lowered insulin concentration is the result of decreased energy status as BW loss occurs during early lactation. High-fat diets sometimes decrease the molar proportion of ruminal propionate, which is a potent insulin secretagogue in ruminants. Plasma GH hormone which is important in partitioning of nutrients did not alter by dietary fat/ prilled fat supplementation. However few reports suggest an increase in GH concentration in lactating dairy cows. The different results are probably due to different fat sources, as well as differences in the animals used and in their physiological state. Thus dietary fat/ prilled fat has diverse effects on metabolic hormones, which depend on the sex, energy intake and balance, and physiological state of the animal.

References

Becú-Villalobos D, Tornadú IG, Shroeder G, Salado EE, Gagliostro G, Delavaud C, Chilliard Y, Lacau-Mengido IM (2007) Effect of fat supplementation on leptin, insulin-like growth factor I, growth hormone, and insulin in cattle. Canadian Journal of Veterinary Research 71(3): 218–225.

Bisinotto RS, LF Greco ES, Ribeiro N, Martinez FS, Lima CR, Staples WW, Thatcher JEP Santos (2002) Influences of nutrition and metabolism on fertility of dairy cows. Animal Reproduction 9 (3):260-272.

Bottger JD, Hess BW, Alexander BM, *et al.* (2002) Effects of supplementation with high linoleic or oleic cracked safflower seeds on postpartum reproduction and calf performance of primiparous beef heifers. Journal of Animal Sciences 80:2023–2030.

Cha MC, Jones PJ (1998) Dietary fat type and energy restriction interactively influence plasma leptin concentration in rats. Journal of Lipid Research 39:1655–1660.

Chilliard Y (1993) Dietary fat and adipose tissue metabolism in ruminants, pigs, and rodents: a review. Journal of Dairy Sciences 76:3897–3931.

Chilliard Y, Bonnet M, Delavaud C, *et al.* (2001) Leptin in ruminants. Gene expression in adipose tissue and mammary gland, and regulation of plasma concentration. Domest Animal Endocrinology 21:271–295.

Chelikani PK, Keisler DH, Kennelly, JJ (2003) Response of plasma leptin concentration to jugular infusion of glucose or lipid is dependent on the stage of lactation of Holstein cows. Journal of Nutrition 133:4163–4171.

Chelikani PK, Ambrose JD, Keisler DH, Kennelly JJ (2004) Effect of short-term fasting on plasma concentrations of leptin and other hormones and metabolites in dairy cattle. Domestic Animal Endocrinology 26:33–48.

Choi BR, Palmquist DL, Allen MS (2000) Cholecystokinin mediates depression of feed intake in dairy cattle fed high fat diets. Domest Animal Endocrinology19:159–175.

Delavaud C, Bocquier F, Chilliard Y, Keisler DH, Gertler A, Kann G (2000) Plasma leptin determination in ruminants: effect of nutritional status and body fatness on plasma leptin concentration assessed by a specific RIA in sheep. Journal of Endocrinology 165:519–526.

García MR, Amstalden M, Morrison CD, Keisler DH, Williams DH (2003) Age at puberty, total fat and conjugated linoleic acid content of carcass, and circulating metabolic hormones in beef heifers fed a diet high in linoleic acid beginning at four months of age. Journal of Animal Sciences 81:261–268.

Grum DE, Drackley JK, Hansen LR, Cremin JD Jr (1996) Production, digestion, and hepatic lipid metabolism of dairy cows fed increased energy from fat or concentrate. Journal of Dairy Science 79:1836–1849.

Grum DE, Drackley JK, Clark JH (2002) Fatty acid metabolism in liver of dairy cows fed supplemental fat and nicotinic acid during an entire lactation. Journal of Dairy Science 85:3026–3034.

Hocquette JF, Bauchart D (1999) Intestinal absorption, blood transport and hepatic and muscle metabolism of fatty acids in preruminant and ruminant animals. Reprod Nutr Dev 39:27–48.

Khorasani GR, De Boer G, Robinson PH, Kennelly JJ (1992) Effect of canola fat on ruminal and total tract digestion, plasma hormones, and metabolites in lactating dairy cows. Journal of Dairy Science 75:492–501.

Lammoglia MA, Bellows RA, Grings EE, *et al.* (2000) Effects of dietary fat and sire breed on puberty, weight, and reproductive traits of F_1 beef heifers. Journal of Animal Sciences 78:2244–2252.

Meikle A, Kulcsar M, Chilliard Y, *et al.* (2004) Effects of parity and body condition at parturition on endocrine and reproductive parameters of the cow. Reproduction 127:727–737.

Rajesh G, Singh M, Roy, AK, Singh S (2014) Effect of prilled fat supplementation on milk yield, composition and plasma hormones in early lactation crossbred cows J Bio Innov 3(4):216-224.

Robinson RS, Pushpakumara PGA, Cheng Z, Peters AR, Abayasekara DRE, Wathes DC (2012) Effects of dietary polyunsatu-rated fatty acids on ovarian and uterine function in lactating dairy cows. Reproduction 124:119–131.

Salado EE, Gagliostro G, Becú-Villalobos D, Lacau-Mengido IM (2004) Partial replacement of corn grain by hydrogenated oil in grazing dairy cows in early lactation. Journal of Dairy Science 87:1265–1278.

Shroeder GA, Gagliostro G, Becú-Villalobos D, Lacau-Mengido IM (2002) Supplementation with partially hydrogenated oil in grazing dairy cows in early lactation. Journal of Dairy Science 85:580–594.

Singh S (2015) Nutritional effects on metabolic profile and early lactation performance of Murrah buffaloes fed diets supplemented with prilled fat. Ph.D. Thesis submitted to National Dairy Research Institute (Deemed University), Karnal, Haryana, India

Singh M, Sehgal JP, Roy AK, Pandita S, Rajesh G (2014) Effect of prill fat supplementation on hormones, milk production and energy metabolites during mid lactation in crossbred cows. Veterinary World 2231-0916.

Sjogren K, Jansson JO, Isaksson OG, Ohlsson CA (2002) Model for tissue-specific inducible insulin-like growth factor-I (IGF-I) inactivation to determine the physiological role of liver-derived IGF-I. Endocrine 19:249–256.

Staples CR, Burke JM, Thatcher WW (1998) Influence of supplemental fats on reproductive tissues and performance of lactating cows. Journal of Dairy Science 81:856–871.

Thomas MG, Bao B, Williams GL (1997) Dietary fats varying in their fatty acid composition differentially influence follicular growth in cows fed isoenergetic diets. Journal of Animal Sciences 75:2512–2519.

Yadav GA, Roy K, Singh M (2015) Effect of prill fat supplementation on certain energy metabolites and milk production performance of crossbred cows. Indian Journal of Animal Nutrition (press).

Yildiz S, Blache D, Celebi F, *et al.* (2003) Effects of short-term high carbohydrate or fat intakes on leptin, growth hormone and luteinizing hormone secretions in prepubertal fat-tailed Tuj lambs. Reprod Domest Anim 38:182–186.

15

Nutrigenomics A New Concept in Animal Nutrition Tools and its Applications

Amrish Kumar Tyagi, Sachin Kumar and Ravindra Kumar Yogi

Dairy Cattle Nutrition Division, ICAR-National Dairy Research Institute Karnal-132001, Haryana

Introduction

"The new science of nutrigenomics teaches us what specific foods tell your genes. What you eat directly determines the genetic messages your body receives. These messages, in turn, control all the molecules that constitute your metabolism: the molecules that tell your body to burn calories or store them. If you can learn the language of your genes and control the messages and instructions they give your body and your metabolism, you can radically alter how food interacts with your body, lose weight, and optimize your health." (Mark Hyman 2006).

Nutrients have long been considered merely as fuel or cofactors however, it is accepted that diet and feeding strategies play an important role in determining the basic physiological processes that influence the health and wellbeing of animals and ultimately influence the efficiency of production. Traditional research related to animal nutrition mainly deals with either deficiency or excess of the particular nutrient which affects their health and productivity. Subsequently, it was appreciated that nutrients can themselves participate in the regulation of metabolic pathways, for instance through the allosteric regulation of specific enzymes, or by modulating hormone secretion. Shifting of balance between health and disease states involves the complex interplay of genes and the environment, which includes nutrients. The use of systems biology approach in nutrition has attracted both scientists and industrialists during recent decades and a link between diet and health is well established. However, it has often been difficult to easily evaluate the effects of specific nutrients, combinations of nutrients and nutrient interactions because of the lack of straightforward biological indicators that respond to even the simplest changes in nutrition or nutritional status. Renewed interest in which dietary components are biologically active and how they interact with genes to exert their effects is being propelled by the development of nutritional genomics. Nutrigenomics involves the characterization of gene products, their physiological function and their interactions. It focuses on the effect of nutrients on the genome, proteome, metabolome and explains the relationship between these specific nutrients and nutrient-regimes on health. New techniques like genomic, proteomic, metabolomic, and bioinformatics are now making their ways to solve the intervening puzzle between nutrients and genes.

Concept of Nutrigenomics

It is well-known fact that dietary deficiency, imbalance of nutrients and or excess of diet has a profound effect leads to ill health indicative that dietary compounds have direct effects on molecular processes which ultimately change the gene expression. Advancement in nutritional science discovered that nutrients or their metabolites can regulate the various bodily functions directly or indirectly by stimulating or inactivating specific regulators. Hence, to study the interaction between genomics and nutrition, nutrigenomics has been introduced in nutrition research (Mariman, 2006).

Nutrigenomics is the study of molecular relationships between nutritional stimuli and the response of the genes (Chavez *et al.*, 2003). Müller and Kersten (2003) defined nutrigenomics as 'the application of high-throughput genomic tools in nutrition research. Applied wisely, it will promote an increased understanding of how nutrition influences metabolic pathways and homeostatic control; how this regulation is disturbed in the early phase of diet-related disease, and to what extent individual sensitizing genotypes contribute to such disease. Many diseases and disorders are related to suboptimal nutrition in terms of essential nutrients, imbalance of macronutrients, or event toxic concentrations of certain food compounds. There are multietiological diseases that are due to the interaction of different nutrients along with several genes (Mariman, 2006). The functional integrity of genes mainly depends on metabolic signals that the nucleus receives from internal factors, e.g., hormones, and external factors, e.g. nutrients, which are among the most influential of environmental stimuli(Harland, 2005). Genomes evolve in response to many types of environmental stimuli, including nutrition. Therefore, the expression of genetic information can be highly regulated by nutrients, micronutrients, and phytochemicals found in food (Van Ommen, 2004).

Five tenets of Nutrigenomics

- Common dietary chemicals act on the human genome, either directly or indirectly, to alter gene expression or structure.
- Under certain circumstances and in some individuals, diet can be a serious risk factor for several diseases.
- Some diet-regulated genes are likely to play a role in the onset, incidence, progression, and/or severity of chronic diseases.
- The degree to which diet influences the balance between healthy and disease states may depend on an individual's genetic makeup.
- Dietary intervention based on knowledge of nutritional requirement, nutritional status, and genotype (*i.e.*, individualized nutrition) can be used to prevent, mitigate or cure chronic diseases.

Goals of Nutrigenomics

- The identification of transcription factors that function as nutrient sensors and the genes they target.

- The elucidation of the signaling pathways involved, and characterization of the main dietary signals.
- The measurement and validation of cell and organ specific gene expression signatures of the metabolic consequences of specific micronutrients and macronutrients.
- The elucidation of the interactions between nutrient-related regulatory pathways and pro-inflammatory stress pathways, to understand the process of metabolic dysregulation that leads to diet related diseases.
- The use of nutritional systems biology to develop biomarkers of early metabolic dysregulation and susceptibility (stress signatures) that are influenced by diet.

Nutrient - gene interaction

Metabolic signals that the nucleus receives from internal factors, e.g. hormones, and external factors, e.g. nutrients, which are among the most influential of environmental stimuli regulate the expression of genes (Harland, 2005). Early in evolutionary development, the nutrients that organisms ingested functioned as primitive signals that turned on and off pathways of synthesis or storage during periods of starvation or excess. Genomes evolve in response to many types of environmental stimuli, including nutrition. Therefore, the expression of genetic information can be highly dependent on and regulated by nutrients, micronutrients, and phytochemicals found in food (Kaput *et al.*, 2005). The shifting balance between health and disease states involves the complex interplay of genes and the environment, which includes diet.

In addition to the traditional essential nutrients, like carbohydrates, amino acids, fatty acids, calcium, zinc, selenium, folate, and vitamin A, C and E, there is a variety of nonessential bioactive components that seem to significantly influence health (Theulaz *et al.*, 2005 and Trujillo *et al.*, 2006). These bioactive food components are involved in modifying many metabolic processes associated with health and disease prevention, including carcinogen metabolism, hormonal balance, cell signaling, cell cycle control, apoptosis and angiogenesis. Nutrients can influence gene expression directly by acting as ligands for transcription factor receptors; or indirectly as metabolized products of various primary or secondary metabolic pathways (Kaput *et al.*, 2004; Kaput and Rodriguez 2004). That is why these dietary chemicals are considered to be signaling molecules that regulate numerous biochemical processes through appropriate cellular sensing mechanisms (Müller and Kersten 2003; Afman and Müller 2006).

Transcription factors are the main agents through which nutrients regulate gene expression (Müller and Kersten 2003, CorthésyTheulaz *et al.*, 2005, Afman and Müller 2006, Ordovas 2006). Numerous receptors in the nuclear receptor superfamily of transcription factors bind nutrients and their metabolites. For example, retinoic acid receptor (RAR) binds retinoic acid, vitamin D receptor (VDR) binds vitamin D, and peroxisome proliferator activated receptors (PPARs) bind fatty acids. By activating these receptors, nutrients can influence a wide array of specific genes and cellular functions. Nutrigenomics has been introduced for the research on the interaction of the genome with its nutritional environment.

Nutrigenomics and other 'omics technologies

Genomics

Genomics is the study of the genome; an approach of mapping, sequencing, and analysis of all genes present in the genome, focusing on resolving the variation in the genome between individuals. Genomics, genotyping, transcriptomics, proteomics and metabolomics, together with bioinformatics, constitute the discipline *functional genomics*, which is also referred to as *systems biology*. Functional genomics aims to uncover both the functional roles of different genes and how these genes interact with, and/or influence each other in the functional network underlying health and disease.

Nutrigenomics and nutrigenetics

Nutrigenomics aims to determine the influence of common dietary ingredients on the genome, and attempts to relate the resulting different phenotypes to differences in the cellular and/or genetic response of the biological system (Mutch *et al.*, 2005). More practically, nutrigenomics describes the use of functional genomic tools to probe a biological system following a nutritional stimulus that will permit an increased understanding of how nutritional molecules affect metabolic pathways and homeostatic control. *Nutrigenetics*, on the other hand, aims to understand how the genetic makeup of an individual coordinates their response to diet, and thus considers underlying genetic polymorphisms. It embodies the science of identifying and characterizing gene variants associated with differential responses to nutrients, and relating this variation to disease states.

Transcriptomics

The transcriptome is the complete set of RNA that can be produced from the genome. Transcriptomics is the study of the transcriptome, *i.e.*, gene expression at the level of the mRNA. Using either cDNA or oligonucleotide *microarray technology*, it describes the approach in which gene expression (mRNA) is analyzed in a biological sample at a given time under specific conditions. It is the most widely used of the 'omics technologies. Regulation of the rate of transcription of genes by food components represents an intriguing site for the regulation of an individual's phenotype (Trujillo *et al.*, 2006). Macronutrients, vitamins, minerals, and various phytochemicals can modify gene transcription and translation, which can alter biological responses such as metabolism, cell growth, and differentiation, all of which are important in health and disease development. This information should assist in the discovery of new biomarkers for disease diagnosis and prognosis prediction and of new therapeutic tools.

Microarrays have been described as "the hottest thing in biology and medicine since the advent of the polymerase chain reaction" (Page *et al.*, 2003). The best practices and standard operating procedures for microarray analyses in nutrigenomic studies have been defined by Garosi *et al* (2005). Microarrays represent a powerful tool for studies of diet-gene interactions.

Proteomics

Dietary components can also modify the translation of RNA to proteins and the posttranslational events, which can affect protein activity (Trujillo *et al.*, 2006). Just as the genome is the entire set of genes, the proteome is the set of proteins produced by a species. However, unlike the genome, the proteome is dynamic and varies according to the cell type and the functional state of the cell. Proteomics is the study of the proteome, and it addresses three categories of biological interest: protein expression, structure and function (Kussmann *et al*., 2006). It attempts to characterize all proteins in a biological sample, including their relative abundance, distribution, posttranslational modifications, functions, and interactions with other biological molecules. Proteomics is technically very challenging and the presence/absence of protein is not necessarily indicative of metabolic change. Currently, the most widely used technologies for proteomics are two dimensional (2D) gel electrophoresis to separate the proteins in a complex mixture isolated from cells or tissues, and specialized mass spectrometry techniques as protein identification tools (Fuchs *et al* 2005, Harland 2005, Kussmann *et al*., 2006, Mariman 2006, Wang *et al*., 2006).

Metabolomics

One of the newest "omics'' technologies in nutrition is metabolomics. It focuses on the analysis of metabolites, the metabolome. It tries to measure the level of all substances (other than DNA, RNA or protein) present in a sample; the metabolome comprises the complete set of metabolites synthesized by a biological system (Corthésy Theulaz *et al*., 2005, Gibney *et al*., 2005, Harland 2005). In common with transcriptomics and proteomics it involves the non-targeted determination of all metabolites present under specific environmental conditions. The analysis and interpretation of the data that is derived from the comparison of different cell conditions are achieved by the use of bioinformatics. Metabolomics is making great advances in this complex approach to nutrition research (German *et al*., 2004; Whitfield *et al*., 2004; Gibney *et al*., 2005 and Rochfort, 2005). This is partly because nuclear magnetic resonance (NMR) and mass spectroscopy (MS) are established techniques, but also because the application of pattern recognition statistics, such as principal component analysis, is conventional in this field.

Systems biology

The long-term aim of nutrigenomics is to understand how the whole body responds to real nutrients using an integrated approach termed 'systems biology'. Systems biology is an approach for studying biological systems that analyzes multiple macromolecular species (DNA polymorphisms, RNA, protein, metabolites, etc) in one experiment. In the relation between nutrition and health (unlike the relationship between nutrition and disease) it is necessary to develop a new concept for *biomarkers* (van Ommen & Stierum 2002). Single nutrients may have multiple known and unknown biochemical targets and physiological actions, which may not be easily addressed with classical biomarkers (*i.e.*, the single gene, protein or metabolite approach), usually under non-physiological conditions. In addition, the efficacy assessment of health effects of nutritional components is even further complicated by the fact that single dietary constituents are hardly consumed as separate entities, but are part of a dietary mixture. Thus, systems biology generates pathway information and provides the capacity to measure (small) perturbations of the pathway resulting from nutritional influences (van Ommen & Stierum 2002). Nutrition is chronic, constantly varying, and composed of a very large amount of known and unknown bioactive compounds. Thus, nutrition by its nature needs to be studied in an integrated way (Theulaz *et al.*, 2005).

Practical Applications

In ruminants

- There are several application of nutrigenomics in ruminants like,
- improves the ruminant health;
- improves production of milk protein and fats;
- improve fertility and reproductive performance.

When animals are fed with selenium deficiency feeds that cause alteration of protein synthesis at transcriptional level; selenium deficiency adverse effect is the enhancement of stress through up-regulation of specific gene expression and signaling pathways. Genes controlling the protection of oxidative damage, detoxification mechanism these consequences cause alteration of phenotype. The identification of the gene markers related to economically important traits like milk, meat, wool production *etc.* These traits can be improved by dietary regimens (Kore *et al.*, 2008).

The impact of diet supplementation with active yeast culture (Saccharomyces cerevisiae) on the expression of selected immune system genes in goat milk somatic cells (MSC) and on milk production traits like, BAC5, BAC7.5, HAMP, LF, Lyz, GBD1 and GBD2 genes expression levels were determined by qRT-PCR method (Bagnicka *et al.*, 2014). Genes encoding β2- defensin, bactenecin 7.5 and hepcidin were influenced by yeast diet supplementation resulting in their increased expression in MSC regardless of the amount of supplement (Bagnicka *et al.*, 2014). These findings support that β2-defensin, bactenecin 5, bactenecin 7.5 and hepcidin may play a role in maintaining the health of the goat mammary gland.

Nan *et al.*, (2014) studied the effects of lysine to methionine ratio on the expression of genes involved in milk protein transcription and translation and mammalian target of rapamycin (mTOR) -phosphorylation in bovine mammary cells. They found that peak concentration of casein at a supplemental 3:1 Lys: Met is driven in part via upregulation of the mRNA expression of components of the JAK-STAT and mTOR. Wang *et al.*, (2014) reported that arginine plays an important role in the transcriptional regulation of casein genes and mTOR-related genes in bovine mammary epithelial cells. They found that arginine increase the expression of gene involved in the synthesis of casein (CSN1S1, CSN1S2, CSN2, CSN3, JAK2, STAT5, mTOR and S6K gene was highest with arginine twice the control.

Mammary synthesis of milk fat continues. This can be regulated by bioactive fatty acids (FAs). The biodegradation theory established that diet induced milk fat depression (MFD) in the dairy cow is caused by an inhibition of mammary synthesis of milk fat by specific FAs produced during ruminal biodegradation. The first such shown to affect milk fat synthesis was trans-10, cis-12 conjugated linoleic acid and effect has been characterized by dose response relationship. During MFD lipogenic capacity and transcription of key mammary lipogenic genes are co-coordinately down regulated. Results provide strong evidence for sterol response element–binding protein-1(SREBP1) and Spot14 as biodegradation intermediate responsive lipogenic signaling pathway for ruminants and rodents. Rumen derived bioactive FAs regulate milk fat synthesis in ruminants (Bauman *et al.*, 2011). Mach *et al.*, (2011) reported that fat is the most variable component in the milk of dairy cows, with the amount and composition affected by genetic, physiological and environmental factors. It has been also shown that lipid metabolism in the mammary gland is highly controlled at the level of transcriptome. *Trans*-10*cis*-12 C18:2 FAs produced as intermediates in rumen biohydrogenation of unsaturated FA, reduce transcription of coordinated and concerted genes, including transcriptional regulators such as sterol response element-binding protein-1 (*SREPB1*), peroxisome proliferator-activated receptor gamma (*PPARG*) or Spot14. The effect of specific rumen-derived bioactive FAs on transcription, as well as post-transcriptional and translational modifications in major lipogenic gene networks in the bovine mammary gland, can provide insights for the development of methods to alter milk fat yield and improve its FA profile.

Reproduction performance in cattle and other species of livestock is based on dietary induced changes in specific genes function. It is possible to understand the relationship between nutrients and regulation of gene expression e.g. study of dietary selenium on gene expression in mice (Rao *et al.*,2001). Genes that were down-regulated are detoxification mechanisms, selenoprotein production, oxidative stress protection and lipid transport. These changes in gene expression can be used for outward phenotypic characteristics of selenium deficiencies (Rao *et al.*, 2001). This is revealed in genes influenced by selenium supplementation that 100 of these can be directly associated with reproductive function (Dawson *et al.*, 2006). Direct effect of dietary selenium on gene expression in key reproductive tissue yet to be examined however, these data can be used to identify candidate genes that are is regulated by various selenium supplementation.

Oxidative stress on the reproductive tissues leads to decreased reproductive efficiency and male infertility (Shalini and Bansal, 2005). Selenium yeast and sodium selenite added to diet has major impact on reproductive tissue, sperm quality and embryo development. This will provide a better understanding of dietary selenium on reproductive performance of animals (Dawson, 2006). Fertility in piglets is possible to regulate selenoprotein (anti-oxidant) by dietary chemicals to improve the fertility of livestock. Microarray analysis will undoubtedly revolutionize our basic understanding of cattle physiology and help new methods of managing animal nutrition and reproduction.

In poultry

Nutrigenomics can provide a systems biology approach to understanding how nutrients influence intestinal health through interaction with gut cells and the microbiota in the intestine (which in turn can change gut cell dynamics). The cellular mechanisms behind beneficial effects of probiotics and prebiotics on gut health and improved feed utilization efficiency has been elucidated utilizing nutrigenomics. For example, adding mannan oligosaccharides (MOS) to broiler diets not only increases the expression of mucin, an important component of the protective intestinal mucosal barrier, but also surprisingly down-regulates selected genes involved in cell turnover and proliferation, potentially conferring an energy-sparing effect (Brennan *et al.*, 2013b). The addition of MOS in broiler diet leads to differential expression of gene as compared to the control group (Xiao *et al.*, 2012). The pathway analysis indicated that 15 genes related to oxidativeü phosphorylation were upregulated in the jejunum and expression of genes important in cellular stress response, suchü as peroxiredoxin 1, superoxide dismutase 1 and thioredoxin, were also increased by MOS. Differential expression of genes associated with cellular immuneü processes, including lysozyme, lumican, β 2-microglobin, apolipoprotein A-1, and fibronectin 1, were also observed in MOS fed broilers (Xiao *et al.*, 2012) Similarly, probiotic bacteria introduced to poultry diets after bacterial challenge has been shown to down-regulate selected genes associated with intestinal- pathogens (Yang *et al.*, 2014).

An even newer area of research microbiomics uses molecular biology techniques, such as advanced DNA sequencing, to study the ecology of the GIT microbial communities (Yeoman *et al.*, 2012). Currently this field is in its infancy and research is limited to general characterization of the unique communities present in each segment of the intestine. Eventually molecular profiling should provide the data needed to equip us to optimize the microbiome through nutrition for improved bird health and production.

Nutrigenomics studies have shown that vitamin E acts as transcriptional regulator in lipid metabolism and oxidation, helping to further explain its beneficial effects to confer antioxidant benefits and to improve meat quality and shelf life in broiler (Li *et al.*, 2009). In other studies, nutrigenomics has been used to determine why different nutrients can sometimes have the same effects on physiological markers. For example, Xiao *et al.*, (2011) showed that a commercial algae-based antioxidant had effects similar to those of vitamin E on total antioxidant status of broilers and meat shelf life. Nutrigenomics data suggest that the antioxidant mimics vitamin E at a transcriptional level by inducing the expression of genes involved in lipid metabolism, cell morphology and cellular oxidation (Xiao *et al.*, 2011).

Nutrigenomics has also been used to determine the underlying reasons why we see a production response with one nutrient form but not with another (e.g., organic versus inorganic minerals). Hall *et al.*, (2012) found that different forms of zinc can differently regulate the expression of transport proteins in the intestine. For example, Brennan *et al.*, (2011 and 2012) showed that, in both male and female birds, different forms of selenium activate transcription of different functional groups of genes, explaining why organic selenium improves reproduction over inorganic selenium.

Over the past several years, researchers have begun to investigate how restricted, "programmed" nutrition during the neonatal and early-life periods can affect animals during adulthood. In chickens, for example, more than 24 h of fasting post-hatch has been shown to have unfavorable effects on weight gain, gut health and meat quality in adult broilers (Gonzales *et al.*, 2003, Halevy *et al.*, 2000). Conversely, feeding chicks post-hatch diets with reduced protein levels as been shown to benefit bird growth and development throughout adulthood, even after chicks are switched to a traditional diet (Everaert *et al.*, 2010). This is explained as delayed access to feed post-hatch has been shown to alter hepatic gene expression (Richards *et al.*, 2010).

Nutrigenomics can help us understand how nutritional programming works by revealing the gene expression patterns associated with early-life nutrition. For example, feeding 100% of the NRC recommendations (normal) for trace minerals for the first 96-h post-hatch can have positive effects on gene expression even after birds have switched to low (20% of the NRC recommendations) mineral diets (Brennan *et al.*, 2013a). In this study, higher levels of minerals fed during the post-hatch period were shown to increase the expression of genes such as Cyclin D1, which play a key role in cell cycle regulation, a biological function essential for gut mucosal growth and repair. The expression of solute carrier proteins, a family of transporters essential for the active and passive transport of nutrients in the small intestine, were up-regulated in adult birds that received the normal post-hatch diet, as was the expression of genes involved in the uptake of minerals and other nutrients

Conclusion

Nutrigenomics is a potential goldmine for the discovery of genes that are important as dietary targets. Nutrigenomics provides to understand the effects of nutrition on gene expression and the relationship between genes and nutrients. It should also have a pivotal role in elucidating nutrient signaling pathways that might contribute to certain diet-related diseases, such as cancer or metabolic syndrome. Various researches are carried out to determine the interaction between genes and feeds or nutrients affecting production and quality of meat, milk, semen, egg in livestock. The results obtained from research, opportunity has arisen to develop nutrition strategies using feed additives brought to the desired level of expression levels of a gene of interest on performance and quality of livestock product by changing nutrition. However, we should also be aware that merely accumulating microarray datasets alone cannot lead to important insights. These data must be gathered in conjunction with smart functional studies using the knowledge of nutrient signals and sensors, or systems-biology driven analysis of signatures, to define molecular biomarkers of dietary responses Although it seems that the contribution of nutrigenomics to animal production and health will be minor during the next few years, in the long-term, the field has the potential to make an important contribution. At some point, we will be able to solve the more sophisticated nutritional questions.

References

Afman L. and Müller M. (2006). Nutrigenomics: from molecular nutrition to prevention of disease. J Am Diet Assoc, 106: 569-576.

Bagnicka E., Jarczak J., Kościuczuk E., Kaba J., Jóźwik A., Czopowicz M., Strzałkowska N. and Krzyżewski J. (2014). Active Dry Yeast Culture Supplementation Effect on the Blood Biochemical Indicators of Dairy Goats. J Adv Dairy Res, 2014: 2:2.

Bauman, D. E., and Griinari, J. M. (2003). Nutritional regulation of milk fat synthesis. Ann Rev Nutr, 23(1): 203-227.

Brennan K. M., Crowdus C. A., Cantor A. H., Pescatore A. J., Barger J. L., Horgan K., Xiao R., Power R. F. and Dawson K. A. (2011). Anim Repro Sci, 125: 180-188. Brennan K. M., Graugnard D. E., Xiao R., Spry M. L., Pierce J. L., Lumpkins B. and Mathis G. F. (2013). Brit Poult Sci, 54: 238-246.

Brennan K. M., Pierce J. L., Cantor A. H., Pescatore A. J. and Power R. F. (2012). Biol Trace Elem Res, 145: 330-337.

Brennan K. M., Samuel R. S., Graugnard D. E., Ao T., Xiao R. and Pescatore A. J. (2013) Biol Trace Elem Res, 156: 166-174.

Chavez, A. and de Chávez, M. M. (2003). Nutrigenomics in public health nutrition: short-term perspectives. Eur J of Clin Nutr, 57: S97-S100.

CorthésyTheulaz I., den Dunnen J. T., Ferré P., Geurts J. M. W., Müller M., van Belzen N. and van Ommen B. (2005). Nutrigenomics: the impact of biomics technology on nutrition research. Ann Nutr Metab, 49: 355-265.

Dawson, K. A. (2006). Nutrigenomics: feeding the genes for improved fertility. Ani Repro Sci, 96(3): 312-322.

Everaert N., Swennen Q., Coustard S. M., Willemsen H., Careghi C., Buyse J., Bruggeman V., Decuypere E. and Tesseraud S. (2010). Br J of Nutr, 103: 206-211.

Fuchs D., Winkelmann I., Johnson I. T., Mariman E., Wenzel U. and Daniel H.(2005). Proteomics in nutrition research: principles, technologies and applications. Br J Nutr, 94: 302-314.

Garosi P., De Filippo C., van Erk M., Rocca Serra P., Sansone S. A. and Elliot R.(2005). Defining best practice for microarray analyses in nutrigenomics studies. Br J Nutr 93: 425-432.

Gibney M. J., Walsh M., Brennan L., Roche H. M., German B. and van Ommen B. (2005). Metabolomics in human nutrition: opportunities and challenges. Am J Clin Nutr, 82: 497-503.

Gonzales E., Kondo N., Saldanha E. S., Loddy M. M., Careghi C. and Decuypere E. (2003). Poult Sci, 82: 1250-1256.

Halevy O., Geyra A., Barak M., Uni Z. and Sklan D. (2000). J of Nutr, 130: 858-864.

Hall R. M., Brennan K. M., Spry M. L., Ford M. J. Ao T. and Pescatore AJ (2012). *World Poultry Congress* (poster).

Harland J. I. (2005). Nutrition and genetics. Mapping individual health. ILSI Europe Concise Monograph Series.

Hyman, Mark. "Clinical approaches to environmental inputs." *Textbook of functional medicine. Washington: Chapter Institute of Functional Medicine* (2006): 347-388.

Kaput J., Astley S., Renkema M., Ordovas J., van Ommen B. (2006). Harnessing nutrigenomics: development of web based communication, databases, resources, and tools. Genes and Nutr, 1: 512.

Kaput J., Ordovas J. M., Ferguson L. *et al*: 2005. The case for strategic international alliances to harness nutritional genomics for public and personal health. Br J Nutr, 94: 623-632. Kaput J., Rodriquez R. L. (2004). Nutritional genomics: the next frontier in the postgenomic era. Physiol Genomics, 16: 166-177.

Kore, K. B., Pathak, A. K., and Gadekar, Y. P. (2008). Nutrigenomics: Emerging face of molecular nutrition to improve animal health and production. Vet world, 1(9): 285-286.

Kussmann M., Raymond F. and Affolter M. (2006). OMICS driven biomarker discovery in nutrition and health. J Biotechnol 124: 758-787.

Kussmann M., Raymond F., Affolter M. (2006). OMICS driven biomarker discovery in nutrition and health. J Biotechnol 124: 758-787.

Li W.J., Zhao G.P., Chen J. L., Zheng M. Q. and Wen J. (2009). Brit Poult Sci 50: 188-198.

Mach, N., Jacobs, A. A. A., Kruijt, L., Van Baal, J. and Smits, M. A. (2011). Alteration of gene expression in mammary gland tissue of dairy cows in response to dietary unsaturated fatty acids. Animal, 5(08): 1217-1230.

Mariman E. C. M. (2006). Nutrigenomics and nutrigenetics: the 'omic' revolution in nutritional science. Biotechnol Appl Biochem, 44: 119-128.

Müller M. and Kersten S. (2003). Nutrigenomics: goals and strategies. Nat Rev Genet 4: 315-322.

Mutch D. M., Wahli W. and Williamson G. (2005). Nutrigenomics and nutrigenetics: the emerging faces of nutrition. FASEB J, 19: 1602-1616.

Nan X. M., Bu D. P., Li X. Y., Wang J. Q., Wei H. Y., Hu H., Zhou L. Y. and Loor J. J. (2014). Ratio of lysine to methionine alters expression of genes involved in milk protein transcription and translation and mTOR phosphorylation in bovine mammary cells. Physiol Genomics, 46: 268–275.

Ordovas J. M. (2006). Nutrigenetics, plasme lipids, and cardiovascular risk. J Am Diet Assoc 106: 1074-1081.

Page G. P., Edwards J. W., Barnes S., Weindruch R. and Allison D.B. (2003). A design and statistical perspective on microarray gene expression studies in nutrition: the need for playful creativity and scientific hardmindedness. Nutrition 19: 997-1000.

Rao, L., Puschner, B. and Prolla, T. A. (2001). Gene expression profiling of low selenium status in the mouse intestine: transcriptional activation of genes linked to DNA damage, cell cycle control and oxidative stress. The J of Nutr, 131(12), 3175-3181.

Richards M. P., Proszkowiec-Weglarz M., Rosebrough R. W., McMurtry J. P. and Angel R. R. (2010) Comp Bioch and Physiol, 157: 374-388.

Shalini, Sonia, and Bansal M. P. (2005). "Role of selenium in regulation of spermatogenesis: Involvement of activator protein 1." *Biofactors* 23.3: 151-162.

Trujillo E., Davis C., Milner J. (2006). Nutrigenomics, proteomics, metabolomics, and the practice of dietetics. J Am Diet Assoc, 106: 403-413.

van Ommen B. (2004). Nutrigenomics: exploiting systems biology in the nutrition and health arenas. Nutrition 20: 48.

van Ommen B. and Stierum R.(2002). Nutrigenomics: exploiting systems biology in the nutrition and health arena. Curr Opin Biotechnol, 13: 517-521.

Wang J., Li D., Dangott L. J. and Wu G. (2006). Proteomics and its role in nutrition research. J Nutr 136: 1759-1762.

Wang M., Xu B., Wang H., Bu D., Wang J. (2014). Effects of Arginine Concentration on the In Vitro Expression of Casein and mTOR Pathway Related Genes in Mammary Epithelial Cells from Dairy Cattle. PLoS ONE 9(5): e95985. doi:10.1371/journal.pone.0095985.

Whitfield P. D., German A. J., Nobel P. J. (2004). Metabolomics: an emerging postgenomic tool for nutrition. Br J Nutr 92: 549-555.

Xiao R., Power R. F., Mallonee D., Routt K., Spangler L., Pescatore A. J., Cantor A. H., AoT., Pierce J. L. and Dawson K. A. (2012). Effects of yeast cell wall-derived mannan oligosaccharides on jejunal gene expression in young broiler chickens. Poultry Science 91: 1660–1669.

Xiao, R., Power, R. F., Mallonee, D., Crowdus, C., Brennan, K. M., Ao, T. and Dawson, K. A. (2011). A comparative transcriptomic study of vitamin E and an algae-based antioxidant as antioxidative agents: Investigation of replacing vitamin E with the algae-based antioxidant in broiler diets. Poult Sci, 90(1): 136-146.

Yang, H. L., Xia, H. Q., Ye, Y. D., Zou, W. C., and Sun, Y. Z. (2014). Probiotic Bacillus pumilus SE5 shapes the intestinal microbiota and mucosal immunity in grouper Epinephelus coioides. Dis Aqua Org, 111(2): 119-127.

Yeoman, Ian. (2011). The changing behaviours of luxury consumption. J Rev and Pric Manag, 10.1: 47-50.

16

Effects of Plant Bioactives on Protein Metabolism and GI Parasite in Small Ruminants

Narayan Dutta
Centre of Advanced Faculty Training in Animal Nutrition, Indian Veterinary Research Institute, Izatnagar-243122, Uttar Pradesh

Avijit Dey
CIRB, Sirsa Road, Hisar-125001, Harayana

Introduction

Increasing public concern regarding the use of pharmaceuticals in livestock feeding due to the emergence of drug resistance has led to an enhanced interest to plant derived bioactive compounds as alternative means to improve livestock health and production. Plants bioactive compounds are the plant secondary metabolites having pharmacological or toxicological effects in animals. Secondary metabolites are formed within the plants as well the primary biosynthetic and metabolic routes for compounds associated with plant growth and development, and are considered as products of biochemical deviate in the plant cells and not required daily for the performance of the plant. Some of them are found to have various important functions such as protection, attraction or signaling in the plants. Most species of plants seem to be competent in synthesizing such compounds. Plants with potent bioactive compounds are often characterized as both poisonous and medicinal, and a beneficial or an adverse effect may depend on the quantity eaten by the animal. Some tropical tree leaves and typical food and feed plants with bioactive compounds with less prominent effects, their intakes are usually considered as advantageous.

Role of bioactive compounds in plants

Phyllogenetically, the secondary bioactive compounds in plants emerge to be accidentally synthesized but they are not worthless products. Some of them are found to have important functions in living plants. The flavonoids can protect against free radicals generated during photosynthesis. Terpenoids and phenyl propanoids may attract pollinators or seed dispersers, or inhibit competing plants. Alkaloids usually discourage herbivore animals or insect attacks (Phytoalexins). Other secondary metabolites function as cellular signalling molecules or have other functions in the plants. The plant bioactive compounds seem to be the rule rather than the exception.

Thus, most plants even common food and feed plants are capable of producing such compounds. However, the typical poisonous or medicinal plants contain higher concentrations of more effective bioactive compounds than common food and feed plants. The main bioactive compounds in plants like tannins and saponins with their toxicological and nutritional effects in animals will be discussed here under:

Tannins

Tannins are widely distributed in plant kingdom. The levels in plants vary greatly between species, within species, stage of development, from location and from year to year. They are found in the wood, bark, leaves and fruits of many species but are more abundant in some than others. It is found in higher concentration in tropical plants as light intensity and high temperature stress enhances synthesis. Tannins are generally divided in two groups: (1) the hydrolyzable tannins (HT) consist of a carbohydrate moiety, in which the hydroxyl groups are esterified with gallic acid or ellagic acid, and (2) condensed tannins (CT), also known as proanthocyanidins (PA), consist of oligomers of the flavan-3-ols and related flavanol residues linked by carbon-carbon bonds and produce anthocyanidins on acid degradation. The molecular weight of condensed tannins can range from 6000 to 12000 Dalton.

Saponins

The saponins are naturally occurring surface-active glycosides. They are mainly produced by plants, but also lower marine animals and some bacteria (Riguera, 1997; Yoshiki *et al.*, 1998). They derive their name from their ability to form stable, soap like foams in aqueous solutions. This easily observable character has attracted human interest from ancient times. Saponins consist of a sugar moiety usually containing glucose, galactose, glucuronic acid, xylose, rhamnose or methylpentose, glycosidically linked to a hydrophobic aglycone (sapogenin) which may be triterpenoid in nature. The aglycone may contain one or more unsaturated C–C bonds. The oligosaccharide chain is normally attached at the C3 position (monodesmosidic), but many saponins have an additional sugar moiety at the C26 or C28 position (bidesmosidic). The great complexity of saponin structure arises from the variability of the aglycone structure, the nature of the side chains and the position of attachment of these moieties on the aglycone. Experiments demonstrating the physiological, immunological and pharmacological properties of saponins have provoked considerable clinical interest in these substances.

CT and saponins may be used as plant bioactives/functional feed in the diet of ruminants but at certain levels begin to affect feed intake. This level varies considerably, depending on the chemical nature of plant secondary compounds and the animal species studied. The palatability of tropical tree leaves/ browse species was closely related to the concentration of tannins. There appears to be a threshold of tannin contents (about 5%) below which no adverse effect is observed (Waghorn *et al.*, 1994). CT protects the protein from microbial hydrolysis and deamination in the rumen and increases the proportion of dietary amino acids available for post-ruminal absorption. Over the last few years, the move towards organic farming systems has increased the stress for alternatives to chemoprophylaxis against GI parasitism.

The potential alternative methods include the use of tanniferous plants with anthelmintic properties in the diet of ruminants.

Condensed tannins as an organic protectant of proteins in the rumen

Protein in ruminants' diet is often poorly utilized because of extensive break-down in the rumen. CT can be used as an organic protectant of proteins, which facilitate the by-pass of protein that might otherwise be lost through microbial deamination in the rumen (Dey and Narayan Dutta, 2014). CT has the potential to modify rumen fermentation favourably, however, higher levels are reported to negatively affect rumen fermentation. An optimum concentration has been suggested to be 15 to 40 g/kg dry-matter (Dey *et al.*, 2008; Pathak *et al.*, 2013). When CT-containing herbage is masticated, CT-protein complexes are formed; these are stable over the pH range of 3.5-7.0 but dissociate in the abomasum and anterior duodenum. This protects the protein from microbial hydrolysis and deamination in the rumen and increases the proportion of dietary amino acids available for post-ruminal absorption, since the tannin-protein complex is assumed to dissociate at low pH of the abomasum. Supplementation of CT at graded levels (1–2%) from various tropical tree leaves in the substrate significantly reduced the *in vitro* nitrogen degradability (IVDN) of GNC. The leaves of *Ficus glomerata* and *Ficus infectoria* were found to be most effective and decreased 35-37% IVDN of GNC (92vs. 55%) (Dey *et al.*, 2006).

Table 1. Effect of graded levels of CT on IVDN of groundnut cake

Source of CT	IVDN at different CT levels (%)						SEM
	0	0.5	1.0	1.5	2.0	2.5	
Artocarpus heterophyllus	0.92^{d}	0.91^{d}	0.85^{cC}	0.75^{bC}	0.68^{aC}	0.66^{aC}	0.05
Ficus bengalensis	0.92^{d}	0.91^{d}	0.79^{cB}	0.68^{bB}	0.61^{aB}	0.58^{aB}	0.07
Ficus glomerata	0.92^{d}	0.91^{d}	0.71^{cA}	0.61^{bA}	0.57^{aA}	0.55^{aA}	0.08
Ficus infectoria	0.92^{d}	0.92^{d}	0.80^{cB}	0.67^{bB}	0.59^{aB}	0.57^{aAB}	0.07

$^{abcd/ABC}$ *means with different superscript within a row/ column differ significantly (P<0.01)*

Feeding of CT to lambs up to 2% of diet decreased the urinary N excretion (g/day) and significantly improved N-retention as compared to control (Table 2), which could have been due to better amino acid availability and apparent biological value of CT protected diets (Dey *et al.*, 2008). This protects the protein from microbial hydrolysis and deamination in the rumen and increases the proportion of dietary amino acids available for post-ruminal absorption. Studies indicated that the rumen protective effect of CT was much higher for essential amino acids than non-essential amino acids, which is likely to account for at least part of higher growth rates and N retention in sheep given diets containing condensed tannins (Dey *et al.*, 2008; Dubey *et al.*, 2013). The presence of CT has a potentially beneficial effect on protein nutrition to the host animal by altering partitioning of nutrients towards higher microbial yield rather than short chain fatty the acids (Pathak *et al.*, 2014b).

Table 2. Effect of CT supplementation on N balance by lambs

Attributes	Treatments*				SEM
	CT-0	CT-1.0	CT-1.5	CT-2.0	
Nitrogen balance (g per day)					
Intake	15.2[a]	15.9[ab]	17.0[b]	14.7[a]	0.37
Faecal loss	4.6[a]	6.0[ab]	6.6[b]	5.7[a]	0.15
Urinary loss	5.7[c]	5.0[bc]	4.7[b]	3.6[a]	0.21
Nitrogen excretion (% intake)					
Faecal	37.0	38.0	38.5	38.6	0.58
Urinary	37.4[c]	31.3[b]	27.5[ab]	25.5[a]	1.06
Retention (%)					
N intake	25.7[a]	30.7[b]	30.2[b]	37.0[c]	1.29
N absorbed	40.7[a]	49.3[b]	54.6[bc]	60.1[c]	1.75

* *CT-0: Control supplement, CT-1.0: 1% CT containing supplement, CT-1.5: 1.5% CT containing supplement, CT-2.0: 2% CT containing supplement.*

Improved protein utilization would always lead to an increase in host resilience, provided that the host continues to be offered access to a scarce food resource. The effect of improved protein utilization will be more dramatic in infections of young, naive hosts, which result in substantial patho-physiological changes and damage or loss of host tissue.

Condensed tannins as an anthelmintic agent

Anthelmintic properties of CT in ruminants are not only associated with improved nutrient supply to the lower GI tract, the positive effects of CT on GI nematodes also include lower faecal egg counts, decreased worm burdens, inhibition of egg hatch and larval development (Dutta *et al.*, 2012; Pathak, *et al.*, 2013). Butter *et al.*, (2001) suggested that dietary quebracho tannin might reduce nematode worm burdens through a toxic effect that requires direct contact between and tannins. This raises the possibility that feeding locally available plant material containing CT may be an alternative method for controlling parasite infections, especially in areas such as the tropics and subtropics. Similarly, Netpana *et al.*, (2001) showed that the faecal parasitic egg counts in cattle and buffaloes were significantly lower when fed with cassava hay that contained CT, and were similar to the group that had been drenched CT. The possible explanations are that the animals received supplemental proteins in protected form and /or that CT could have a direct toxic effect on the internal parasites. Possible mechanisms through which CT may reduce larval migration and development remain to be elucidated, but the effect may be mediated through ingestion of CT and interactions of CT with the external surface of the larvae. Pathak *et al.*, (2013) observed that aqueous defatted crude extracts of CT (freeze dried) from *Psidium guajava*, *Ficus glomerata*, *Eugenia jambolana*, *Artocarpus heterophyllus* and *Ficus infectoria* leaves possess the anthelmintic property and were found to be very effective (P<0.01) against *Haemonchus contortus*. They observed that after 2 hrs of incubation *H. contortus* became very sluggish in all the CT extracts except control, however, mortality of parasites was started after 4 hrs of incubation. The mortality of *H. contortus* after 12 hrs of incubation was significantly (P<0.01) higher in *Psidium guajava* (85%) followed by comparable values in *Ficus glomerata* (80%) and *Ficus infectoria* (80%), *Eugenia jambolana* (75%) and *Artocarpus heterophyllus* (60%), respectively. The adult *H. contortus* in control group were seen active throughout the incubation period (12 hrs). Max *et al.*, (2002) observed the effect of drenching quebracho extract (QT) (2.4g/kg L.W.) on worm burdens of parasitized sheep and observed two distinct egg profiles, while the faecal egg counts (FEC) of control group increased progressively throughout the 10-day monitoring period, the treated group started to decline two days after the first QT dose. Comparison of mean FEC on the day of slaughter (day 25 post infection) showed 91% reduction in faecal eggs. Madibela and Jansen (2003) observed that the incorporation of *V. verrucosum* in the diet of Tswana goats significantly decreased the faecal egg counts after four weeks of feeding while egg counts were increased in goats given *V. verrucosum* free diet. Dubey *et al.*, (2012) reported significantly lower faecal egg counts in kids fed diets containing CT at 1-2% of diet from a mixture of tropical tree leaves (Fig. 1). Supplementation of CT may enhance resistance against GI parasites through increases in tissue protein supply, which are prioritized for repair and immune response. The CT could form a complex with nutrients and inhibit nutrient availability for larval growth or decrease GI parasites metabolism directly through inhibition of oxidative phosphorylation (Scalbert, 1991), causing larval death. Inhibition of the electron transport system by CT was observed with *Photobacterium phosphoreum* (Scalbert, 1991). Molan *et al.*, (2002) have observed that CT extracts from several forages can disrupt the life cycle of nematodes by preventing their eggs from hatching and by preventing larval development to the infective stage. Since CT is not absorbed in the digestive tract, they become concentrated in the faeces and may be chemically active in the faeces. The CT may react directly with parasite larvae in the faecal pellet by binding to the cuticle of the larvae, which is high in glycoprotein, inhibiting larval development.

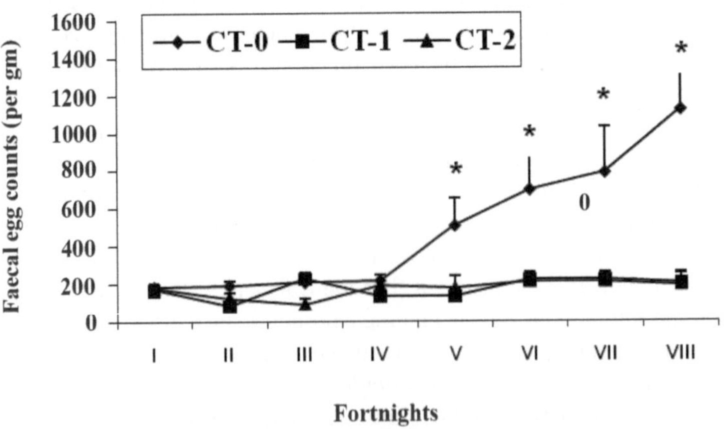

Fig. 14.1. Effect of CT supplementation on faecal egg counts by kids

Pathak *et al*., (2013) revealed the therapeutic role of CT against *H. contortus* infection in terms of reduced FECs, total worm counts and larval development in sheep. Moreover, CT supplementation in infected sheep had an inhibitory effect on intensity of *H. contortus* infection. Therefore, the tanniferous leaf meal mixture may be used as part of a sustainable strategy to control GI nematodes in sheep. Similarly, Kumar (2012) compared the effect of CT (1.5% of TMR) in GI infected lambs with dewormed lambs and found that CT from tanniferous tree leaves possess the anthelmintic and anticoccidial properties and decreased GI parasitic load in lambs. He further reported a perceptible positive impact on feed intake, growth rate, FCR, wool yield, metabolic profile and immune response.

Effect on immune response

Pathak *et al*., (2014a) reported that supplementation of CT from tropical tree leaves mixture at 1.5% of diet in *Haemonchus contortus* infected sheep improved humoral (Fig. 2) and cell mediated immune response and inhibited the different development stages of *H. contortus*. They further reported significantly lower adult worm count and no histopathological changes in CT fed animals as compared to control (Pathak *et al*., 2014c). Similarly, a noticeable impact on antioxidant status and humoral immune response was reported in kids and lambs given diet containing 1-2% CT from a leaf meal mixture (Dutta *et al*., 2012; Dey *et al*., 2015).

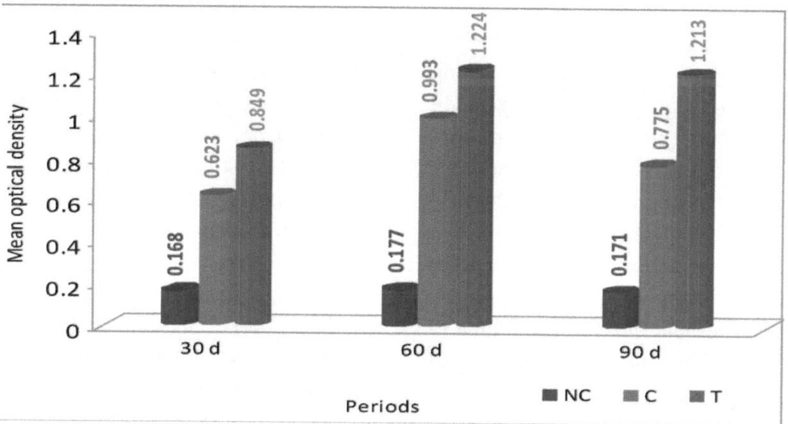

Fig.2. IgG response in *H. contortus* infected sheep fed CT supplemented diets

Effects of saponins on animal growth and feed intake

Animal nutritionists have generally considered saponins to be deleterious compounds. In ruminants and other domestic animals the dietary saponins have significant effects on all phases of metabolism, from the ingestion of feed to the excretion of wastes (Cheeke, 1996). Lucerne and soya beans are the main examples of saponin-rich plants that serve extensively in human, ruminant and poultry diets. *Y. schidigera* plant extract (the plant is common in south and central America where it is used as animal feed, like many other saponin-rich plants, as a herbal medicine has been found to improve growth, feed efficiency and health in ruminants (Mader and Brumm, 1987). Quillaja saponins increased the efficiency of *in vitro* rumen-microbial protein synthesis and decreased the degradability of feed protein (Makkar and Becker, 1996). Partially hydrolyzed lucerne saponins administered intra-ruminally resulted in a significant reduction in the total protozoa count in the rumen of sheep (Lu and Jorgensen, 1987), which may be the reason for the decrease in feed protein degradability. Saponins are considered to have detrimental effects on protozoa through their binding with sterols present on the protozoal surface. Sterols are absent on bacterial membranes. Yucca extract can also bind NH_4 when ruminal NH_4 concentrations are high, and release it again when ruminal NH_4 is low, providing a continuous and adequate supply of NH_4 for microbial protein synthesis (Hussain and Cheeke, 1995). A positive effect of Yucca saponins in ruminant nutrition was attributed to the enhancement of the entrapment of NH_4-N from urea-supplemented straw (Makkar *et al.*, 1999). This increases the availability of nutrients to rumen bacteria and reduces environmental damage by decreasing losses of NH_4 to the air. Supplementation of feed with leaves of *Sesbania sesban*, known for its high saponin content, has been found to have the potential to improve protein flow from the rumen by suppressing protozoal action there (Newbold *et al.*, 1997) but rumen bacteria were observed to be capable of metabolizing the antiprotozoal factor. Saponins may also be degraded by the saliva of sheep fed saponin-rich foods for a long time (Teferedegne, 2000). Ingested saponins were quickly hydrolyzed in the rumen to free sapogenins and, in part, epimerized at C3 into episapogenins. The absorption of free sapogenins appeared to occur in the jejunum. The concentration of sapogenins in faeces reached a plateau 108 h after dosing started. The positive effects of saponins were more pronounced when they were directly administered into the rumen rather than added to the feed (Odenyo *et al.*, 1997). Killeen *et al.*, (1998) proposed that a surfactant or flocculent action of saponins on the feed constituents that alters the rate of digestion would account for the substrate-dependent nature of the effect of *Y. schidigera* on rumen DM and N digestibility. This substrate-dependency might also be due to negative effects of saponins on specific bacterial populations (Hussain and Cheeke, 1995). Wang *et al.*, (2000a, b) observed that supplementation with Yucca extracts might be beneficial to ruminants fed a high-grain diet. Yucca saponins were found to have a direct negative effect on cellulolytic bacteria while being harmless to amylolytic bacteria, suggesting the possibility of using saponins for 'designing' the rumen population. The mechanism of action against bacteria remains unclear. Dietary saponins were often suspected of having a role in causing ruminant bloat (Cheeke, 1996; Sen *et al.*, 1998), but clear experimental proof for this is lacking in the literature. The absence of any positive effect in experiments where Yucca saponins were fed to ruminants (Wu *et al.*, 1994) might have been because animals with adapted rumen microbial populations were used.

Effects of saponins on the immune system

Saponin-based adjuvants have the unique ability to stimulate the cell-mediated immune system, as well as to enhance antibody production, and have the advantage that only a low dose is needed for adjuvant activity (Oda *et al.*, 2000). Quillaja and other saponins either as crude mixtures or as purified compounds have been reported to increase immune-cell proliferation *in vitro* (Plohmann *et al.*, 1997; Lacaille-Dubois *et al.*, 1999). Purified Quillaja saponins boosted antibody production without producing any reaginic antibodies (So *et al.*, 1997). The mechanisms of immune-stimulating action of saponins have not been clearly understood, but many explanations have been put forward. Saponins reportedly induced production of cytokines such as interleukins and interferons that might mediate their immunostimulant effects (Jie *et al.*, 1984; Kensil, 1996). It is likely that they interact with antigen-presenting cells to induce many of these responses (Barr *et al.*, 1998). The incorporation of the saponins into cell or endosomal membranes might expose the incorporated antigen to cytosolic proteases.

Conclusions

It may be concluded that condensed tannins and saponins may be used as functional feed and desirable concentration of condensed tannins and saponins in ruminants' diet represents a balance between the positive and negative effects of these compounds. Condensed tannins can also improve animal health by improving bioavailability of protein in the rumen and overcoming effects of GI nematodes. Supplementation of condensed tannins from tanniferous tree leaves at 1-2% of diet may be beneficial for ruminants and can be integrated in small-holder farming systems.

References

Barr IG, Sjolander A, Cox JC (1998) Advanced Drug Delivery Reviews, 32: 247–271.

Butter NL, Dawson J M, Wakelin D, Buttery PJ (2001) The Journal Agricultural Science, 137(4): 461-469.

Cheeke PR (1996) In: Saponins used in Food and Agriculture, pp. 377–386 [GR Waller and Y Yamasaki, editors]. New York: *Plenum Press.*

Dey A, Narayan Dutta (2014) Universal Journal of Pharmacy, 3 (2): 20-25.

Dey A, Dutta N, Sharma, K, Pattanaik AK (2006) Animal Nutrition. Feed Technology, 6 (2):215-222.

Dey A, Dutta N, Sharma K, Pattanaik AK (2008) Small Ruminant Research, 75: 105- 114.

Dey A, Narayan Dutta, Pattanaik AK and Sharma K. 2015. Japanese Journal of Veterinary Research, 63 (1): 15-24.

Dubey M (2007) Strategic use of tanniferous tree leaves on nutrient utilization growth and GI parasites in goats. M.V. Sc. Thesis submitted to Deemed University IVRI, Izatnagar. UP, India

Dubey M, Narayan Dutta, Banerjee PS, Pattanaik AK, Sharma K, Singh M (2012) Animal Nutrition and Feed Technology, 12: 91-102

Dutta, N., Dubey, M., Banerjee, P. S., Pattanaik, A. K., Sharma, K., Kumar, P. and Narang, A.2012. *Livestock Research for Rural Development*, Volume 24 (2), http://www.lrrd. org/lrrd24/2/dutt24035.htm.

Hussain I, Cheeke PR (1995) Animal Feed Science and Technology, 51: 231–242.

Jie YH, Cammisuli S, Baggiolini M (1984) Agents and Actions, 15: 386–391.

Kensil CR (1996) Critical Reviews in Therapeutic Drug Carrier Systems, 13: 1–55.

Killeen GF, Madigan CA, Connolly CR, Walsh GA, Clark C, Hynes MJ, Timmins BF, James P Headon DR, Power RF (1998). Journal of Agricultural and Food Chemistry, 46: 3178–3186.

Kumar S (2012) Anthelmintic effect of tanniferous tree leaves in lambs. Thesis submitted to Deemed University IVRI, Izatnagar. UP, India.

Lacaille-Dubois MA, Hanquet B, Cui ZH, Lou ZC, Wagner H (1999) Journal of Natural Products, 62: 133–136.

Lu CD, Jorgensen NA (1987) Journal of Nutrition, 117: 919–927.

Mader TL, Brumm MC (1987) Journal of Animal Science. 65: 9–15.

Madibela OR, Jansen K (2003). Livestock Research and Rural Development, 15(9) Retrieved, from http:// www.cipav.org.co/lrrd/lrrd 15/9/lin 2.htm

Makkar HPS, Becker K (1996) Effect of Quillaja saponins on invitro rumen fermentation. In Saponins used in Food and Agriculture, pp. 377–386 [GR Waller and Y Yamasaki, editors]. *New York,: Plenum Press.*

Makkar HPS, Aregheore EM, Becker K (1999) Journal of Agricultural Science, 132: 313–321.

Max RA, Wakelin D, Buttery PJ, Kimambo, AE, Kassuku AA, Mtenga LA (2002) Proceedings: of an Int. Conf. on Responding to the Increasing Global Demand for Animal Products, 12-15 November 2002. Merida, Mexico. pp 89.

Molan AL, Waghorn GC, McNabb WC (2002) *Veterinary Recordord*, 150: 65-69.

Netpana N, Wanapat M, Toburan W (2001) Proceedings of International Workshop on Tannins in Livestock and Human Nutrition (Ed J D Brooker), ACIAR Proceedings No.92: 171pp.

Newbold CJ, El Hassan SM, Wang J, Ortega ME, Wallace RJ (1997) British Journal of Nutrition, 78: 237–249.

Oda K, Matsuda H, Murakami T, Katayama S, Ohgitani T, Yoshikawa M (2000) Biological Chemistry, 381: 67–74.

Odenyo AA, Osuji PO, Karanfil O (1997) Animal Feed Science and Technology, 67: 169–180.

Pathak AK (2010) Influence of tanniferous tree leaves on gastrointestinal parasites, methane emission and performance of lambs. Ph.D. Thesis submitted to Deemed University IVRI, Izatnagar. UP, India.

Pathak AK, Narayan Dutta, Sharma, K (2014b) International Journal of Biology and Biological Sciences, 2 (3): 209-224.

Pathak AK, Narayan Dutta, Banerjee PS, Goswami TK, Sharma K (2014a) Journal of Parasitic Diseases, DOI 10.1007/s12639-014-0455-1.

Pathak AK, Narayan Dutta, Banerjee PS, Pattanaik AK, Sharma K (2013) Asian Australasian Journal of Animal Sciences, 26 (10): 1446-58.

Pathak AK, Narayan Dutta, Banerjee PS, Sharma K, Pattanaik AK (2013) Veterinary Practitioner, 14 (1): 127-29.

Pathak AK, Narayan Dutta, Pawaiya RVS, Sharma K (2014c) Indian Journal of Veterinary Pathology, 38(4): 231-234.

Plohmann B, Bader G, Hiller K, Franz G (1997) Pharmazie, 52: 953–957.

Riguera R (1997) Journal of Marine Biotechnology, 5: 187–193

Scabert A (1991) Phytochemistry, 30: 3875-3883.

Sen S, Makkar HPS, Becker K (1998) Journal of Agricultural and Food Chemistry, 46: 131–140.

So HS, Yoon HS, Kwoon YS, Sung JH, Lee TG, Park EN, Cho HS, Lee BM, Cho JM, Ryu WS (1997) Molecular Biology of Cells, 7: 176–186.

Teferedegne B (2000) Proceedings of the Nutrition Society, 59: 209–214.

Waghorn GC, Shelton ID, McNabb WC (1994) The Journal of Agricultural Science–(Cambridge), 123: 99–107.

Wang Y, McAllister TA, Yanke LJ, Cheeke PR (2000a) Journal of Applied Microbiology, 88: 887–896.

Wang YX, McAllister TA, Yanke LJ, Xu ZJ, Cheeke PR, Cheng KJ (2000b) Journal of the Science of Food and Agriculture, 80: 2114–2122.

Wu, Z., Sadik, M. and Sleiman, F.T. 1994. *Journal of Animal Science*, 72: 1038–1042.

Yoshiki Y, Kudou S, Okubo K (1998) Bioscience Biotechnology and Biochemistry, 62: 2291–2299.

17

Molecular Breeding to Enhance Production in Livestock

G.K. Gaur, Triveni Dutt, P.K. Bharti, BHM Patel and Mukesh Singh
Livestock Production and Management Section, Indian Veterinary Research Institute, Izatnagar-243122, Uttar Pradesh

Introduction

Genetic programs in livestock have been extensively used to improve their productivity over the last 50 years. The traditional approach of breeding, based on quantitative genetics principle, has been very successful (Schaeffer, 2006), without knowledge of genes increasing or decreasing in herds. Effective progeny testing program and use of genetically proven bulls have made drastic genetic improvement in livestock populations. Further advances in computation for genetic merit have further added to improvement process. Livestock producers presently are focusing on overall development of livestock with improved health, production, reproduction and longevity and therefore, the traits are becoming the part of selection program (Decker *et al*., 2009). Advancement in molecular biology along with high-throughput genotyping has led to discovery of a number of single nucleotide polymorphisms (SNPs) in livestock (Van Tassell *et al*., 2008). SNP arrays covering the entire genome may explain most of the genetic variation in important traits of livestock (Meuwissen *et al*., 2001). These SNPs may act as molecular markers and be used as a substitute for phenotypic selection. This process, in a broad sense is known as molecular or marker-assisted breeding and describes selection strategies including marker-assisted selection (MAS) and genome wide selection (GWS) or genomic selection (GS). GS refers to selection criteria based on genomic estimated breeding values (GEBV), which are computed using SNP/ genotypic data and phenotypic data with the objective to increase the accuracy of prediction of breeding and genotypic values.

Knowledge of markers without phenotypic information has changed standard practices of genetic improvement of quantitative traits in livestock. Cost of marker technology is now continuously reducing with an increase in the number of markers. GS increases genetic gain per unit of time (Meuwissen *et al*., 2001; Boichard *et al*., 2006) and allows identification of genetically superior animals at the earliest age. Animals with DNA test information receive accurate GEBV before sexual maturity. Hence, it is believed that GS will replace traditional breeding systems in near future.

Single nucleotide polymorphic (SNP) markers

SNP markers consist of one genetic letter with two different forms in entire population. Millions of SNP markers have been investigated in different livestock covering entire genome. All markers may be studied simultaneously in one step process, known as typing or high-density and high-throughput genotyping. The process is done in laboratory through a chip carrying various markers. A small amount of DNA is used for typing. Out of many markers over the entire genome, at least one marker is expected to be close to every gene, influencing the trait.

The first high-density and high-throughput genotyping assay was 10K single nucleotide polymorphism (SNP) chip commercialized by Affymetrix (The Bovine HapMap Consortium, 2009). This density of SNPs was however insufficient for many genomic studies including whole genomic selection and genome-wide association analyses. Accordingly, Illumina BovineSNP50 chip was developed by a consortium of animal scientists using SNP discovery populations in Holstein, Angus and mixed breeds of beef cattle (Van Tassell *et al.*, 2008), which provided higher density (~50,000 SNPs per animal). This assay became the international standard for genomic selection and genome-wide association studies in livestock (Decker *et al.*, 2009; MacEachern *et al.*, 2009). Though, Illumina BovineSNP50 was useful for many genomic studies, however, higher density assays were realized to build models for genomic selection across the breeds. A new high-density SNP genotyping chip was introduced in 2010 by Illumina utilizing bead technology and single base extension chemistry similar to Bovine SNP50K chip. This chip is capable to genotype approximately 700K SNPs simultaneously.

Illumina BovineSNP50 was performed using DNA samples of Angus, Holsteins and other important US beef breeds. Accordingly, this assay may perform slightly better in these breeds. SNP discovery of Illumina 700K panel was however performed by sequencing a large number of animals from other breeds including *Bos taurus* and *Bos indicus* to minimize the bias in SNP information across the breeds.

How to execute whole genome selection

Different genes and their effects on performance traits are not known. The SNP samples need to be correlated with known production traits to find out the SNPs effects, *i.e.*, the association between markers and trait. Animals with known genetic production may be daughters of proven bulls. The population used for this analysis is called training sample. The training sample/set is therefore, a reference population in which the marker effects are estimated. It contains phenotypic information of breeding germplasm and molecular marker score. Marker effects are estimated based on advanced statistical methods. It is to be ensured that the reference population is updated over the generations; otherwise predictive ability will decrease over time (Meuwisen *et al.*, 2001). The number of animals to be genotyped depends on heritability of the trait and rate of genetic gain. Best and worst, both animals need to be genotyped for a given trait.

Marker effects obtained from training sample are thereafter used for calculation of genomic breeding values of other animals, which do not have reliable breeding value information. These animals refer to target/validation sample/set and contain the candidates for selection. Animals from the target sample have their genotypic information but no phenotypic information and as a result selection is practiced based on marker effects estimated in the training set.

Statistical analysis of genomic selection (Meuwissen *et al.*, 2001) is carried out to know the effect of all alleles/markers on performance traits (breeding goal traits). There are many ways to analyze genomic selection data *i.e.*, Least Squares Method, Best Linear Unbiased Prediction (BLUP) and Bayesian Estimation Method. In least squares method, all the markers are tested one by one for their statistical significance and the effect of non-significant markers is set to zero. Subsequently, significant markers are taken in the model simultaneously for analysis. Best linear unbiased prediction method fits the allelic effects as random instead of fixed. The fitting of random effect does not require degree of freedom and thus all allelic effects are estimated simultaneously. The random effect however requires an estimate of the variance of the allelic effect. The method assumes similar variance for all the markers. The bayesian estimation method is similar to BLUP except that the variance of allelic effects is assumed different for every marker and is estimated using a prior distribution for the variance.

Marker estimated breeding value (MEBV) or genomic estimated breeding value (GEBV) is predicted by $MEBV_i/GEBV_i = \sum M_{ij}$, where M_{ij} is the estimate of the effect of the jth allele/haplotype of animal i. The development of statistical models dealing with GS to get accurate estimates, however needs to be considered. The GenSel Program (Fernando and Garrick, 2009), which is based on Bayesian approach is being extensively used for estimation of GEBVs of animals under selection, incorporating SNP data of large number of markers and the phenotype of interest.

Whole genome selection in livestock

Genomic selection has modified the concept of traditional livestock breeding. Though, concept of molecular markers to improve genetic gain is not very new (Smith, 1967; Soller and Beckman, 1983) but its application has certain limitations. Large numbers of loci affect the quantitative traits and each locus captures a limited proportion of total genetic variance (Hayes and Goddard, 2001; VanRaden *et al.*, 2009). Furthermore, small gains may only be expected with few markers having high genotyping costs. Computation advancement with respect to genetic worth using marker information also restricted marker-assisted selection in livestock. Sequencing of bovine genome, discovery SNPs and reduction in cost of genotyping however brought revolution in genomic selection scheme. Therefore, accurate selection decisions based on dense marker data became possible (Meuwissen *et al.*, 2001).

Schaeffer (2006) suggested that GS should be used for the selection of young bulls and progeny tests should be given less priority. Additionally, nucleus breeding herd especially cows need to be selected by GS. Lillehammer *et al.*, (2011) performed computer simulation of GS cattle breeding schemes and found an increase in genetic improvement by 13%. Pryce *et al.*, (2010) observed that genetic gain through GS may increase between 60 and 120%, depending on the age of breeding males and females.

The accuracy of GEBV has been worked out for dairy cattle, beef cattle, sheep, and pigs. Meuwissen *et al.*, (2001) demonstrated that accuracies of predicted breeding values from markers alone may be achieved to the level of 0.85. Similarly, Kolbehdari *et al.*, (2006) obtained a high correlation between GEBV and true breeding values (0.80) in a simulation study using different heritabilities and evenly or randomly spaced QTLs. The simulation results suggest that the accuracy of the GEBV for a bull calf at birth may be as high as the accuracy of an EBV of progeny test. Consequently, genomic selection may lead to double rate of genetic gain (Schaeffer, 2006) as compared to 5-19% improvement in genetic response through marker assisted selection (Boichard *et al.*, 2006). Furthermore, avoiding progeny testing, bull breeding programs may save up to 92% of their costs (Schaeffer, 2006), however, some of these savings may be offset by investment on genotyping. Spelman *et al.*, (2006) reported accuracy of DNA based BVs varying from 0.45 to 0.60 for the production traits in validated population of Holstein-Friesian breed. They further predicted that selection based on genomic information will increase the rate of genetic gain in New Zealand by 50-70%. Berry (2007) in Irish Holstein–Friesian dairy cows expected genetic gain through genomic selection @ 0.539 genetic standard deviations per year with accuracy of selection of 0.75 against 0.199 genetic standard deviations per year under the current scheme of progeny testing.

Harris *et al.*, (2008) reported reliabilities of GEBV in New Zealand dairy cattle. Reliabilities of GEBV for young bulls with no daughter information ranged from 50 to 67% for milk production traits, live body weight, fertility, somatic cell count and longevity; compared with an average 34% for parental average breeding values. Furthermore, Bayesian methods gave slightly greater (2 to 3%) reliabilities than the BLUP approach, whereas the regression methods performed poorly. Hayes *et al* (2009) reviewed results of genomic selection in Australia. Reliability of genomic breeding values at the time of birth ranged from 0.18 (fertility) to 0.53 (Australian Profit Ranking) in BLUP method and from 0.14 (fertility) to 0.55 (Australian Profit Ranking) in Bayesian method. The reliability of the fertility GEBV was substantially lower than the reliability of other traits. The Bayesian method gave small increases in reliability for all traits except fertility (2 to 7%). VanRaden *et al.*, (2009) reported reliabilities of GEBV for US and Canadian young bulls. Across the traits, the GEBV had reliability of 50%, compared with 27% from the parent average alone. Using BLUP in place of Bayesian approach gave slightly (1%) reduced reliability. Fernanda *et al.*, (2011) observed that accuracy of GEBV increased significantly with the increase in number of bulls in the training set (480, 960 or 1920), trait h^2(0.10, 0.25 or 0.40) and marker densities (40 k or 800 k).

Hayes *et al.*, (2009) reviewed results of genomic selection in the Netherlands. The increase in reliability of GEBV over parent average EBV at the time of birth was 33% (fat percentage), 19% (kilograms of protein), 15% (feet and legs), 13% (udder depth, SCS), and 9% (fertility). They concluded that having a larger number of bulls in their reference population would increase the reliability of GEBV in their selection candidates substantially. The effect of different breeding structures was investigated by Duthie *et al.*, (2010). It was realized that including genomic information increases the economic response to selection in both breeding structures.

Berry and Crowley (2013) reviewed that feed efficiency may also be estimated as residual feed intake (RFI), which is the difference between actual and predicted feed (or energy) intake. RFI was measured in 2000 growing Holstein heifers and genotyping was done with 625 000 SNPs (Pryce *et al.*, 2012) to examine the feasibility of genomic selection. Prediction equation for RFI was developed in training data set. Accuracy of genomic selection was estimated as the correlation between genomic breeding value and phenotypic value of RFI. Accuracy averaged 0.37 and 0.31 in the validation data set of Australia and New Zealand (Pryce *et al.*, 2012). Furthermore, the Bayesian method (0.42) had the highest accuracy of prediction among all the methods. Lower accuracy for RFI as compared to production traits may be due to lower heritability of the trait and lesser availability of phenotypic and genotypic data. Both factors may be the main limitations for achieving high accuracy for RFI using genomic selection (Daetwyler *et al.*, 2008). Hence, data of different research groups on RFI, across the laboratories/states/countries need to be shared to improve the accuracy of genomic prediction.

Genomic selection is an attractive strategy for dairy sheep, because rams can be selected for milk production and other traits' GEBV, which are not expressed earlier in life. Duchemin *et al.*, (2012) in French Lacaune dairy sheep noticed that for young rams with no progeny test records, accuracies of EBV for milk yield, fat content, and somatic cell scores may be improved by 18–25% by including DNA marker information. The advantages of genomic selection are relatively less for meat and wool sheep. However, additional genetic gain @ 20–30% may be obtained through the application of GS (Banks and Van Der Werf, 2009). Accuracies of genomic breeding values were high (>0.6) for wool traits such as fleece weight and fiber diameter (Daetwyler *et al.*, 2012) but lower for traits like lean-meat yield. These lower accuracies were however still higher than those estimated based on pedigree alone (Daetwyler *et al.*, 2012). Accuracies of genomic selection in beef cattle, evaluated using cross-validation technique for growth and carcass traits were reported up to 0.42 and 0.65 (Weber *et al.*, 2012).

GS offered great opportunities for selection in pigs. Target trait for the genomic selection in pigs is feed conversion ratio (FCR) because this trait is expensive to measure. Christensen *et al.*, (2012) estimated accuracy of GEBV for FCR using 60,000 SNPs in Danish Duroc pigs and concluded that GEBVs were significantly accurate than pedigree EBV. Forni *et al.*, (2010) in litter size of pigs noticed 68% increase in accuracy of the breeding values of the training population through GS over traditional selection (BLUP). Simianer (2009) showed the potential of GS for litter size in two breed scheme and reported that the genetic progress per year could be increased by 37% compared to the conventional scenario.

Conclusion

Molecular breeding in general describes breeding of livestock based on molecular markers and covers selection strategies, especially genome-wide selection or genomic selection. Whole genome selection has a major impact on livestock breeding goals, especially for the traits that are complicated to select. It provides accurate estimates of breeding value earlier in life with optimum selection accuracy and lower generation interval. The rate of genetic improvement may increase from 20 to 100% in different herds of livestock using genomic selection. Major breakthrough in molecular biology including discovery of DNA-markers, sequencing and genome mapping of farm animal species has created new avenues to apply genomic selection in livestock. Conventional livestock breeding systems are therefore being reshaped due to the availability of powerful tools in molecular biology. Genomic selection has become the an important method in many countries for selecting genetically meritorious cows and bulls for production, reproduction and feed efficiency parameters. It is believed that it will soon completely replace all the traditional genetic evaluation systems of livestock not only in developed countries but also in developing countries.

References

Banks RG, Van Der Werf JHJ (2009) Economic evaluation of whole genome selection using meat sheep as a case study. Proc. Assoc. Adv. Anim. Breed. Genet. 18:430–33.

Berry D (2007) Report on the potential of genomic selection in Irish dairy cattle. Draft Paper I (available on internet).

Berry DP and Crowley JJ (2013) Genetics of feed efficiency in dairy and beef cattle. Journal of Animal Science 91, 1594–1613.

Boichard D, Fritz S, Rossignol MN, Guillume F, Colleu JJ, Druet T (2006) Proceedings of the 8thWorld Congress on Genetics Applied to Livestock Production (available on internet).

Christensen OF, Madsen P, Nielsen B, Ostersen T, Su G (2012) Single-step methods for genomic evaluation in pigs. Animal 5:1–7

Daetwyler HD, Kemper KE, van der Werf JH, Hayes BJ (2012) Components of the accuracy of genomic prediction in a multi-breed sheep population. J. Anim. Sci. 90(10): 3375–84.

Daetwyler HD, Villanueva B, Woolliams JA 2008. Accuracy of predicting genetic risk of disease using a genome-wide approach. doi:10.1371/journal.pone.0003395.

Decker JE, Pires JC, Conant GC, McKay SD, Heaton MP, Chen K, Cooper A, Taylor JJF (2009) Resolving the evolution of extant and extinct ruminants with high throughput phylogenomics. Proc. Natl. Acad. Sci. 106(44):18644-9.

Duchemin SI, Colombani C, Legarra A, Baloche G, Larroque H (2012) Genomic selection in the French Lacaune dairy sheep breed. J. Dairy Sci. 95(5):2723–33

Duthie C, Sawalha R, Navajas E, Roehe R, Roughsedge T (2010) Economic response that can be achieved from including genomic information to the terminal sire index of beef cattle. Presented to the British Society of Animal Science Annual Conference, April 12 to 14, 2010, Queen's University, Belfast.

Fernanda V Brito, José Braccini Neto, Mehdi Sargolzaei, Jaime A Cobuci and Flavio S Schenkel (2011) Accuracy of genomic selection in simulated populations mimicking the extent of linkage disequilibrium in beef cattle. BMC Genetics, 12:80

Fernando R, Garrick D (2009) GenSel- User Manual for a portfolio of Genomic Selection related Analyses. (http://taurus. ansci. iastate. Edu /Site /Welcome_files /GenSel%20 Manual% 20v2. pdf)

Fornis S, Aguilar I, Misztal I, Deeb N (2010) Genomic relationships and biases in the evaluation of sow litter size. Proc 9th World Congress on Genetics Applied to Livestock Production, Liepzig, Germany. Aug 2-6, p. 266.

Georges M, Massey JM (1991) Velogenetics, or the synergistic use of marker assisted selection and germ-line manipulation. Theriogenology 35: 151–59

Harris BL, Johnson DL, Spelman RJ (2008) Genomic selection in New Zealand and the implications for national genetic evaluation. Proc. Interbull Meeting, Niagara Falls, Canada (available on internet).

Hayes BJ, Goddard, ME (2001) The distribution of the effects of genes affecting quantitative traits in livestock. Genet. Sel. Evol. 33: 209–229.

Hayes BJ, Bowman PJ, Chamberlain, AJ, Goddard, ME (2009) Invited review: Genomic selection in dairy cattle: Progress and challenges. J. Dairy Sci. 2009. 92: 433-443.

Kolbehdari D, Wang Z, Grant JR, Murdoch B, Prasad A, Xiu Z, Marques E, Stothard P, Moore SS (2009) A whole genome scan approach to map QTL for milk production traits and somatic cell score in Canadian Holstein bulls. J. Anim. Breed. Genet. 126(3): 216-72.

Lillehammer M, Meuwissen TH, Sonesson AK (2011) A comparison of dairy cattle breeding designs that use genomic selection. J. Dairy Sci. 94: 493–500.

MacEachern S, McEwan J, McCulloch A, Mather A, Savin K, Goddard, M (2009) Molecular evolution of the Bovini tribe (Bovidae, Bovinae): is there evidence of rapid evolution or reduced selective constraint in Domestic cattle? BMC Genom. 10: 179.

Matukumalli LK, Lawley CT, Schnabel, RD, Taylor JF, Allan MF, Heaton MP, O'Connell J, Moore SS, Smith TPL, Sonstegard, TS, Van Tassell, CP (2009) Development and characterization of a high density SNP genotyping assay for cattle. PLoS One 4:e5350.

Meuwissen THE, Hayes BJ, Goddard, ME (2001) Prediction of total genetic value using genome-wide dense marker maps. Genetics 157: 1819–1829.

Meuwissen TH, Goddard ME (2004) Mapping multiple QTL using linkage disequilibrium and linkage analysis information and multitrait data. Genet. Sel. Evol. 36: 261–279. Peippo J, Viitala S, Virta J, Räty M, Tammiranta N, *et al.* (2007) Birth of correctly genotyped calves after multiplex marker detection from bovine embryo microblade biopsies. Mol. Reprod. Dev. 74(11):1373–78.

Pryce JE, Arias J, Bowman PJ, Davis SR, Macdonald KA, Waghorn GC, Wales WJ, Williams YJ, Spelman RJ, Hayes BJ (2012) Accuracy of genomic predictions of residual feed intake and 250 day bodyweight in growing heifers using 625,000 SNP markers. Journal of Dairy Science 95, 2108–2119.

Pryce JE, Goddard ME, Raadsma HW, Hayes BJ (2010) Deterministic models of breeding scheme designs that incorporate genomic selection. J. Dairy Sci. 93(11):5455–66.

Schaeffer LR (2006) Strategy for applying genome-wide selection in dairy cattle. J. Anim. Breed. Genet. 123: 218–223.

Simianer H (2009) The potential of genomic selection to improve litter size in pig breeding programs. Proc 60th Annual meeting of the European Association of Animal Production, Barcelona, Spain. Pp. 210

Smith C (1967) Improvement of metric traits through specific genetic loci. Anim. Prod. 9: 349–358.

Soller M, Beckmann, JS (1983) Genetic polymorphism in variety identification and genetic improvement. Theor. Appl. Genet. 67: 25–33.

Spelman RJ, Arias J, Keehan M, Obolonkin V (2006) Application of genomic information in dairy cattle. Draft Paper (available on net).

VanRaden PM, Van Tassell CP, Wiggans GR, Sonstegard TS, Schnabel RD, Taylor JF, Schenkel F (2009) Invited review: Reliability of genomic predictions for North American Holstein bulls. J. Dairy Sci. 92: 16–24.

Van Tassell CP, SmithTPL, Matukumalli LK, Taylor JF, Schnabel RD, Lawley CT, Haudenschild CD, Moore SS, Warren WC, Sonstegard, TS (2008) Simultaneous SNP discovery and allele frequency estimation by high throughput sequencing of reduced representation genomic libraries. Nat. Meth. 5: 247-52.

Weber KL, Thallman RM, Keele JW, Snelling WM, Bennett GL *et al.* (2012) Accuracy of genomic breeding values in multibreed beef cattle populations derived from deregressed breeding values and phenotypes. J. Anim. Sci. 90: 4177–90.

18

Water Footprints of Dairy Cattle Husbandry

R.K. Sharma, Nazam Khan, Ankur Rastogiand Zulfqarul Haq
Faculty of Veterinary Sciences & Animal Husbandry, SKUAST-J, R. S. Pura Jammu-181102, Jammu and Kashmir

Introduction

Water resource is imperative for the survival of all life-forms on planet earth and defines the limits of sustainable development, without any substitute. Only 2.5% of all water on the earth is freshwater, and of that, around 0.5% is accessible through ground or surface water supplies. The increasing world population, industrialization and climate change is putting additional pressure on water resources. This is also true for livestock sector. As per prediction equations, the requirement of water for livestock will rise from 2.3 billion m^3 in 2000 to 2.8 billion m^3in 2025 and 3.2 billion m^3 in 2050 (Hedge, 2012).

The balance between humanity's demands and the quantity available is already precarious (Karin *et al.*, 2002). Additionally, climate change poses a serious threat to water resources as the climate system and the hydrological cycles are intimately linked, and any variability in climate affects the hydrological cycle. The World Bank report on the water and climate change inter-linkages also reiterated that climate change could profoundly alter future patterns of both water availability and use, thereby increasing levels of water stress and insecurity, both at the global scale and in sectors that depend on water (Alavian *et al.*, 2009). India is also bound to face severe scarcity of water in the near future, because the potential for increasing the volume of utilization of water is hardly 5-10% (GOI, 2009).

Concept of water footprint

The concept of water footprint has been developed to have an indicator of water use in relation to consumption. The water footprint of an individual, business or nation is defined as "the total volume of freshwater used to produce the goods and services consumed by the individual, business or nation" (Chapagain and Hoekstra, 2004). This concept is closely linked to the virtual water concept which is defined as the"volume of water used to produce a commodity, measured at the place where the commodity is produced" (Allan, 1994). The inverse of the virtual water content is known as the water productivity of the commodity. In line with the concept of virtual water, the concept of the water footprint has been introduced to create a consumption based indicator of water use (Hoekstra and Chapagain, 2007). From the perspective of a nation, the water footprint is defined as the volume of water needed for the production of the goods and services consumed by the inhabitants of a country. It can be assessed by taking the use of domestic water resources, subtracting the virtual water flow that leaves the country and adding the virtual water flow that enters the country. From the commodity perspective, its water footprint is the Consumptive Water Use (CWU) in the process of production of a commodity (Hoekstra, 2003).

Water footprint in Dairy sector

The water footprint or CWU in the production process of primary commodities has three components namely, blue water footprint (includes irrigation, both groundwater and surface water), green water footprint (includes rainwater), greywater footprint (deteriorated water due to contamination by animal wastes, chemical fertilizers, *etc.*). In milk production, the CWU is both, direct (drinking, bathing and servicing) and indirect (through feed and fodder intake). In the case of stall-fed animals, the direct water requirement is entirely met from groundwater and /or surface water sources; hence it comes under blue component of water footprint (Sejian *et al.*, 2013). For animals partly or fully under grazing system, rainwater may also partly account for water use by animals for drinking and bathing. But in the absence of data on the proportion of rain: groundwater use, the entire volume of water is considered under the blue component.

In feed and fodder production, there is CWU from irrigation and effective rainfall. Also virtual water content of livestock products is higher than that of crop products. This is because a live animal consumes a lot of feed crops, drinking water and service water in its lifetime before it produces some output. Let us consider an example of beef produced in an industrial farming system. An animal takes on an average 3 years before it is slaughtered to produce about 200 kg of boneless beef. It consumes nearly 1300 kg of grains (wheat, oats, barley, corn, dry peas, soybean meal and other small grains), 7200 kg of roughages (pasture, dry hay, silage and other roughages), 24 cubic meters of water for drinking and 7 cubic meters of water for servicing. This means that to produce one kilogram of boneless beef, we use about 6.5 kg of grain, 36 kg of roughages, and 155 litres of water (only for drinking and servicing). On producing the above said amount of feed, on average 15,340 litres of water is required. With every step of food processing we lose part of the material as a result of selection and inefficiencies. The higher we go up in the product chain, the higher will be the virtual water content of the product.

To sensitize about the issue of water use efficiency in livestock sector, the estimation methodology of dairy water footprint is presented underneath:

Estimation of direct water use

The reported estimates of direct water use by dairy cattle vary widely from 64 litres/day (Chapagainand Hoekstra, 2003) to 100 litres/day (Singh *et al.*, 2004). The estimation of this component at the research stations/organized farms is easy, but it is tedious at farmer's field. The information on water use for drinking, servicing and bathing can be collected partly from observation and partly through farmer's interviews or can be proxied from related information like, the diameter of water pipe used for serving and bathing, time period of water flow and number of animals in the enclosure at farm household. Similarly, data about drinking water can be approximated from the information on the volume of bucket/water trough used and number of times in a day the same was filled by the farmer.

DW = DW (in litres) + Bathing and Servicing (in litres)

Where DWU is direct water use, DW is drinking water

CWU m3/ton = DMU/Av. milk yield (litres/day)

Where CWU is consumptive water use

Estimation of Indirect water use

The calculation of indirect water footprint consists of calculation of water use of feed and fodder crops and calculation of CWU of animals through feed and fodder. The starting point in this methodology is the calculation of consumptive water use of a crop which is estimated as follows:

Calculation of crop water requirement

There are four periods in the crop growth *i.e.*, initial, development, mid- and late stage, so the crop water requirement is the actual evapo-transpiration (ETp) of these four growth periods (Allen *et al.*, 1998) and is calculated by the equation present underneath

$$ETp = \sum_{i=1}^{4} ki \times \sum_{\text{month j in } i^{th} \text{ growth period}} d_{ij} ET_0^{ij}$$

Where,

ki = crop coefficient of ith growth period

dij = Number of days of the jth month in the ith crop growth period

ET_0^{ij} = Reference evapo-tranpiration of the jth month in the ith crop growth period

The above equation is used if rainfall meets the full crop water requirement;in this case, CWU from effective rainfall is equal to actual evapo-transpiration. But if rainfall is insufficient to meet full crop water requirement, then it is equal to the effective part of rainfall at the root zone (P_{eff}), where,

$$P_{eff} = \sum_{i=1}^{4} \sum_{\text{month } j \text{ in } i^{th} \text{ growth period}} \frac{d_{ij}}{n_{ij}} P_{eff}^{ij}$$

Whereas

$$P_{eff}^{ij} = \left\{ P75^{ij} \times \frac{(125 - 0.2 \times P75^{ij})}{125} \right\} \text{ if } P75^{ij} \leq 250 \text{ mm}$$

But if, $P75^{ij} > 250$ mm, then

$$P_{\text{eff}}^{ij} = \left\{ P75^{ij} \times \frac{(125 + 0.1 \times P75^{ij})}{125} \right\}$$

Where, $P75^{ij}$ = daily 75% exceedance probability of rainfall
n = total number of days in the jth month of the ith crop growth period
$CWU^{\text{effective rainfall}}$ = Min (ETp, P_{eff}), green water footprint

When irrigation meets part of the deficit crop water requirement, the irrigation CWU is the net evapotranspiration, that is the difference between the actual evapotranspiration (ETp) and P_{eff} $CWU^{\text{irrigation}} = ETp - P_{ef}$, blue water footprint

In India, as the livestock are fed on crop-residues (eg. wheat straw, rice straw, *etc.*) and by-products of crop (*e.g.*, oilseed cakes), the CWU in crops is apportioned on main and by-product. The data requirement for the same is(i) conversion ratios of main: by-product (ii) prices of main: by product.

The conversion ratios can be region and crop-variety specific. There is a lot of difference in the prices of the main and by-products; hence the prevailing market price should be taken into consideration. The CWU(m³/ha) of by-product is

$$CWU^{\text{by product}} = a^{i} CWU^{\text{crop}}$$

Where $\alpha_i = q_i p_i / \Sigma q_j p_j$ and q_i, p_i are conversion ratios and prices of the main product or by-products(conversion ratio of the main product is 1). By using the conversion ratios, the yield of main and by-product can be worked out and dividing the $CWU^{\text{by product}}$ by its respective yield gives the water use on per tonne basis.

Calculation of CWU of animals through feed and fodder

After estimating the blue and green CWU in prevalent feed and fodder crops, the next step is to collect data on their intake by the dairy animals. There are vast seasonal varieties in the feed and fodder, and therefore, to capture the same, the data should be collected on seasonal basis, preferable for three seasons *i.e.*, hot-humid/rainy, winter and summer. Intake of each type of feed and fodder is then multiplied by the CWU (inm³/kg) of respective crop to get the indirect water use by animals. Thus,

$$\text{Indirect Water Use} = \sum_i x_i CWU_i$$

Where, x_i is the intake of '*i*' feed/fodder by the animal and CWU_i is the consumptive water use of '*i*' feed/fodder resource. By adding up the direct and indirect water use, the total water footprint can be ruled out.

Virtual water exports from livestock products

Another related concept is the virtual water use as a commodity. India has been reported to be among the top-ten net exporter of virtual in the world (Hoekstra and Hung, 2002; Chapagain and Hoekstra, 2003, 2004). During 1997-2001, the average gross exports of virtual water from the country were estimated to be 42.6 Gm³/year, of which about 8% (3.4 Gm³/year) was attributable to livestock and livestock exports (Chapagain and Hoekstra, 2004). However recent reports suggested that India's gross export of virtual water from livestock and livestock products has shown more than three fold increase over the last decade.

Among livestock products, meat and its preparations have the predominant share in the Indian export basket and hence, in terms of virtual water exports also, their share is the largest followed by dairy exports. The gross virtual water outflow is high not only because of the volume of exports, but because Indian export basket contains the products that have high virtual water content per unit of the product. The comparison of virtual water content in Indian livestock products and global averages show an astonishing situation. The virtual water content of Indian products is very high as compared to the global averages, - difference being strikingly sharp in eggs where the difference in the average percent of virtual water content was more than 450% and milk powder whose virtual water content was around 141% higher than that of the global average. Even for the bovine meat products, the water content is 35 to 55%higher in comparison to world average.

The virtual water content of each livestock product is assessed by analysis of the direct and indirect water consumption of different kinds of animals in its life cycle and then various livestock products that originate from a particular animal type are delineated, to apportion the total water use among the livestock products. The distribution of the virtual water content of a live animal is done in such a way among the animal products that neither double counting nor un-accounting occurs. In processed products, the water used in processing is also taken into account.

Calculation of the virtual water content of live animals

The virtual water content of an animal at the end of its life span is defined as the total volume of water that was used to grow and process its feed, to provide its drinking water, and to clean its housing and the like (Chapagain and Hoekstra, 2003) and is calculated by the equation

$$VWC \propto [e, a] = VWC_{feed}[e, a] + VWC_{drink}[e, a] + VWC_{serv}[e, a]$$

Where, $VWC\alpha\,[e,a]$ represents the virtual water content of animal a in exporting country and e is expressed in cubicmetres of water per ton of live animal. VWC_{feed}, VWC_{drink} and VWC_{serv} are the virtual water contents from feeding, drinking and servicing respectively in terms of cubic metres of water per tonne of live animals.

Components of virtual water content of live animal

There are three components of virtual water content of live animals:

- Virtual water content from feed consumed
- Virtual water content from drinking water:
- Virtual water content from service water

Virtual water content from feed consumed

The virtual water content of an animal from the feed consumed has two parts. The first is the actual water that is required to prepare the feed mix and the second is the virtual water incorporated in the various feed ingredients (Chapagain and Hoekstra., 2003).

The virtual water content from feeding an animal at the end of its life span is calculated as follows:

$$VWC_{feed[e,a]} = \frac{\int_{\text{birth}}^{\text{slaughter}} \left\{ q_{\text{mixing}} e_a + \sum_{c=1}^{n_c} SWD[e,c] \times C[e,a,c] \right\} [dt]}{W_a[e,a]}$$

Where $VWC_{feed}[e, a]$ is expressed in cubic metres of water per ton of live animal. The variable q_{mixing} $[e, a]$represents the volume of water required for mixing the feed of animal$a$ in exporting country e (m^3/day).

$C[e,a,c]$ is the quantity of feed crop c consumed by animal a in exporting country e, expressed in tons per day.

$W_a[e,a]$is the average live weight of animal a in exporting country e at the end of its life span, expressed in tons.

$SWD[e,c]$ is the specific water demand of crop c in exporting country e, expressed in m^3 per ton of crop.

$$\text{SWD}[e,c] = \frac{\text{CWR}[e,c]}{\text{CY}[e,c]}$$

Here $CWR[e,c]$ represents the crop water requirement of crop c in country e (m^3/ha) and $CY[e,c]$ is the crop yield(ton/ha).

In calculating the crop water requirements the CROPWAT model developed by the FAO can be used. The climate data needed for the crop water requirement calculations need to be recorded whereas; other crop parameters are taken as in-built in the CROPWAT model.

Virtual water content from drinking water

The virtual water content of an animal originating from drinking is equal to the total volume of water used as drinking water supply, calculated over the entire life span of the animal. We express the virtual water content here in terms of volume of water per ton of live animal, and thus calculate the virtual water content from drinking (Chapagain and Hoekstra., 2003) as

$$VWC_{drink}[e,a] = \frac{\int_{\text{birth}}^{\text{slaughter}} q_d[e,a]dt}{W_a[e,a]}$$

Here $q_d[e,a]$ is the daily drinking water requirement of animal a in exporting country e (m^3/day). $Wa[e,a]$ is the live weight of the animal at the end of its lifetime.

Virtual water content from service water

The virtual water content of an animal from the service water used is equal to the total volume of water used to clean the farmyard, wash the animal and other services necessary to maintain the environment during the entire life span of the animal. The virtual water content from service water is calculated as:

$$VWC_{\text{serv}}[e,a] = \frac{\int_{\text{birth}}^{\text{slaughter}} q_{\text{serv}}[e,a]dt}{W_a[e,a]}$$

Where, *VWCserv*[*e*,*a*] represents the virtual water content of animal *a* in exporting country *e* and is expressed in cubic metres of water per ton of live animal,$q_{serv}[e,a]$ is the daily service water requirement (m^3/day) of animal *a* in exporting country *e*.

Conclusion

Water is the most vital nutrient required by animals, and has utmost importance while establishing a dairy venture. Its deficiency affects productivity and health of animals both directly and through indirect means. For achieving sustainable livestock development, an innovative and practical solution is required to manage accessible water for livestock. Most adapted species of livestock, feeding strategies (xerophytes and succulent feed resources) and water resource management could be considered in water scarcity zones. Also external water footprint can be increased by judiciously importing products rich in virtual water. An intensive research is required in the area of water management and its impact on availability of water for livestock and its efficient use for sustainable production.

References

Alavian V, Qaddumi HM, Dickson E, Diez SM, Danilenko AV, Hirji RF, Puz G, Pizarro C, Jacobsen M, Blankespoor B (2009) 'Water and Climate Change: Understanding the Risks and Making Climate-Smart Investment Decisions', the World Bank Report.

Allan JA (1994) 'Overall perspectives on countries and regions' In: Rogers P, Lydon P *Water in the Arab World: perspectives and prognoses*, Harvard University Press, Cambridge, Massachusetts, pp. 65-100.

Allen RG, Pereira LS, Raes D, Smith M (1998) '*Crop evapotranspiration - Guidelines for computing crop water requirements - FAO Irrigation and drainage paper 56'*. Food and Agriculture Organization of the United Nations, Rome, Italy. *http://www.fao.org/ docrep/ X0490E/x0490e00.htm* 1 April 2004.

Govt. of India (2009) Background note for consultation meeting with Policy makers on review of National Water Policy. Ministry of Water Resources. Pp. 50.

Hegde NG, Sharad Krishi. 2012. Water Scarcity and Security in India.Centre for International Trade in Agriculture & Agro-based Industries, Pune, Pp. 18-20.

Hoekstra AY, Chapagain AK (2007) 'Water footprints of nations: water use by people as a function of their consumption pattern', Water Resources Management, 21(1), pp. 35–48.

Hoekstra AY (2003) (ed) '*Virtual water trade: Proceedings of the International Expert Meeting on Virtual Water Trade*', Value of Water Research Report Series No. 12, UNESCO-IHE Institute for Water Education, Delft, Netherlands.

Hoekstra AY, Hung PQ (2002) '*A quantification of virtual water flows between nations in relation to international crop trade*', Value of Water Research Report Series No. 11, UNESCO-IHE Institute for Water Education, Delft, Netherlands.

Sejian V, Mech A, Roy KS, Kolte AP, Prasad CS (2013) Climate change and Abiotic stress management in livestock: Basic concepts and amelioration measures. National Institute of Animal Nutrition and Physiology, Bangalore, Pp. 255-260.

Singh OP, Sharma A, Singh R, Shah T (2004) Virtual water trade in dairy economy: Irrigation water productivity in Gujarat. Economic and Political Weekly, 39(31): 3492-3497.

19

Formulation and Supplementation of Urea Molasses Mineral Blocks for Improving Animal Production

Putan Singh
CAFT in Animal Nutrition, ICAR-IVRI, Izatnagar-243 122, Uttar Pradesh

Introduction

In developing countries, ruminants thrive mainly on poor quality feeds and pastures, whose nutritive value is poor. They are having a low content of nitrogen, energy, minerals and vitamins and high content of lignin and silica, which limit their efficient utilization by ruminants. Therefore, these poor quality feeds and fodder needs to be upgraded in terms of their nutritive value using various treatments like physical, chemical, physico chemical and biological methods to improve intake and utilization of nutrients from poor quality roughages. However, supplementation of critical nutrients like energy, protein, minerals, vitamins also improved the productivity and health of the ruminants (Dass *et al.*, 2011). Availability of oil cakes as protein supplement in developing countries is very poor and at a very high price, This has led to use of non-protein nitrogen source as urea, to compensate for the nitrogen deficiency of fibrous feeds (Dutta *et al.*, 2009). Thus, enhancing intake, digestibility and availability of nutrients from poor quality roughages are only possible through optimization of rumen fermentation. The use of solid multi-nutrient block supplementation /urea-molasses blocks/ multi nutrients blocks/ *pashu chocolates* to provide optimum levels of various nutrients primarily for better growth of rumen micro organisms. They need rich sources of fermentable nitrogen, minerals and vitamins, which are lacking in the fibrous feeds like cereal straws (Sahoo *et al*, 2009). This offer several advantages such as easy transport, storage and handling, and reduced risks of poisoning as compared with other approaches, such as giving a small amount of urea in drinking water, sprinkling of urea solution on fibrous feeds before feeding, or urea-ammonization of crop residues (Dutta *et al* ., 2009). If the block is too soft, it will be licked out rapidly and if it is too hard it may not be consumed at all. A binder is necessary to solidify the blocks, in that bentonite has many advantages over other binders. Bentonite is one of the common natural clays used in animal diets to improve digestibility of nutrients and daily gain and feed intake. Bentonite can absorb toxic products of digestion and decreases the accumulation of toxic substances in tissues, thus decreasing the incidence of internal disorders. The addition of bentonite to the diet can also partly equalize the supply of nitrogen to the rumen microorganisms. Urea and molasses are well known constituents for improving the utilization of straw based diets (Sihag *et al.*, 2008). However, this is not adopted as a common practice by farmers because of constraints associated with their use. Urea toxicity due to improper mixing (Mehra *et al.*, 1987) and limited availability of molasses are the major constraints. To overcome these constraints, UMMB is formed by mixing urea, molasses, binders and minerals. These blocks are being used, to replace the concentrate mixture at maintenance level and UMMB can safely be stored for a year at all temperatures (15-45°C) with relative humidity (RH) up to 65% without any visible fungal or mould growth (Sihag *et al.*, 2007).

Formulation of urea molasses multi-nutrients blocks/ solid multi-nutrients blocks

Keeping this fact in mind, urea containing blocks known as urea molasses mineral block (UMMB) are developed to supplement the diet of ruminants fed on poor quality roughages (Hosamani *et al.*, 2003). The main problem with the supplementation of block lick is great diurnal variation in its lick by animals. The variation may be due to the composition and degree of hardness of the block (Leng, 1984; Hande, 1989). It is not only the texture of the block but also the energy and protein content of the basal diet which may also influence the daily block intake (Ali and Mirja, 1986). Investigations have led to the formulation of UMMB using locally available ingredients namely sugarcane molasses, urea, common salt and wheat bran (Misra *et al.*, 2007). Other ingredients such as minerals, vitamins and a source of good quality protein like cottonseed cake or soya bean meal are readily available in the local market (Malek *et al.*, 2008). The system for preparing an ideal block should not involve complicated processing. It should be easy to handle and to be managed with an exceptionally high keeping quality. The proportion of ingredients used in the manufacture of three sets of UMMB, A, B and C, using different amounts of molasses, wheat bran, urea and cement is shown Table 1. The level of cement as a binding agent is adjusted to obtain blocks of good texture and hardness that regulate intake by the animals. To obtain a good setting, cement needs a minimal quantity of water, just enough to make a paste for proper mixing.

Table 1. Proportion of ingredients used in the manufacture of UMMB

Ingredients	% by weight (fresh basis)		
	Block A (IAEA)	Block B (IAEA)	Block C (IVRI)*
Molasses (>80°Brix)	40	45	40
Wheat Bran	20	24	38
Cement	17	12	10
Urea	10	8	10
Cottonseed Cake	5	6	--
Mineral Mixture	5	3	1
Common Salt	3	2	1

Ratio of water: cement is 2:5; *10g vitablend/Quintal

All ingredients should be weighed accurately before mixing. Mixing can be done either manually for small quantities, or mechanically using a concrete mixer, or a horizontal paddle mixer for large quantities. The sequence in which the ingredients are mixed is very important. Urea is first added to the molasses and thoroughly mixed. All lumps should be broken down to ensure proper mixing and to avoid toxicity problems when fed to animals. Mineral mixture, cottonseed cake and half of the amount of salt are then added, while mixing continuously. The remaining half of the salt is mixed with cement and water to make a paste, which is then added to the molasses mixture and thoroughly stirred to obtain a consistent paste. Wheat bran is added last, a little at a time and thoroughly mixed until the product is homogeneous. This product is then ready to be placed in moulds.

Moulding and Drying: Moulds can be made of wood, plastic, iron or carton boxes, which may be of any shape and size. A plastic sheet placed in the mould or an oil film prevents the block from sticking to the wall and allows easy removal from the mould. Once the mixture is placed in the mould, it should be left in a well ventilated room to set. The mixture takes about 48 hours to set, after which the blocks are ready to be utilized. For cattle, 10-kg blocks seem to be convenient. Blocks wrapped in a plastic sheet or left in carton boxes can be stored in a dry place for several months. Table 2 indicates the chemical composition of the three sets of UMMB, A, B and C.

Table 2. Chemical composition of UMMB (% fresh matter basis)

Attributes	A	B	C*
Crude protein	27.5	30.5	32.0
Carbohydrates, sugars, *etc.*	22.1	26.7	46.29
Crude fibre	2.2	2.1	3.66
Fats	1.4	0.3	0.94
Calcium (as Ca)	5.5	4.8	5.50
Phosphorus (as P2O5)	1.4	2.1	1.91
Ash	17.6	16.9	13.36

*UMMB prepared at IVRI

The dry matter (DM) content of blocks A, B and C is 77.7, 83.2 and 79.23%, respectively. The mean calculated metabolizable energy (ME) of the supplements A, B and C are 10.9, 11.0 and 10.6 MJ/kgDM, respectively. Urea molasses multi-nutrient blocks (UMMB) as a feed supplement for ruminants is very much useful to provide deficit nutrients of crop residues to optimize rumen fermentation.

Different processes as namely hot and cold processes have been tried to prepare the solidified urea molasses mineral blocks using various ingredients in numerous permutations and combinations. In case of hot process which was first developed in Australia, molasses and urea were heated with binding agents at a temperature of 100-120°C for about 10 minutes, cooled to 70°C and afterwards other ingredients were added by stirring and left to cool further. It settled after some hours. The cold process is a simple gelling process and all the ingredients are mixed at ambient temperature.

In this process usually calcium oxide and mono-sodium phosphate are used as binding agents. A lick prepared by cold process appeared to be the best from cost and quality point of view (Brar and Nanda, 2003). At first urea molasses, mineral mixture and vitamins are mixed properly and then other ingredients are added along with binding agents. The mixed material is transferred to mold for solidification which takes place within 12-15 hours depending on composition of the block. It is time consuming process and the end product is hygroscopic. The advantages in cold process are of saving energy which is important aspect for most developing countries, simplicity of manufacturing and also avoiding loss of nutrients due to maillard reaction.

The various binding agents to solidify the urea molasses mineral block are bentonite, calcium oxide, magnesium oxide, calcium carbonate, cement, calcium hydroxide *etc.* (Raman *et al* ., 2010). A successful block preparation needs selection of the most suitable binding agents and also the methods of its use so that the properties of these agents may be optimally utilized without any harmful effect. Cement is used as a binding agent. Studies conducted in Canada and USA on the utilization of cement and its by-products as minerals for animals did not reveal any negative effect when fed up to a maximum of 3% of the total daily dry matter intake (Aarts *et al*., 1990). Molasses is a readily available energy source and urea, a readily available nitrogen source in livestock feeding (Preston and Leng, 1990). When made in the form of multi-nutrient feed blocks with cement as a binder, it ensures slow release of the molasses and urea when fed in their readily available state. Recently, Sankar (2013) used the binding materials for the solidification of blocks are mainly cement (10%) alone and cement with bentonite in combination (5% each). SMB prepared using 10% cement or 5% cement and 5% bentonite as the binder showed similar compressive strength (kg/cm2). All blocks found negative for aflatoxin B1 content at 3, 6 and 9 months interval of storage.

Performance of animals

Various reports indicate that there was improvement in growth and production of animals due to urea molasses feeding. A significant increase was observed in the growth of buffalo calves fed urea molasses liquid diet (Sahoo *et al*.,1991) and with blocks (Elangovan *et al.,1991*). Sarkar (1991) found significant increase in growth and improvement in milk production in cows with ammoniated rice straw along with blocks. Saddul and Bodoo (2001) reported better response in terms of daily live weight gain in weaned kids fed on UMMB. Vatta *et al*., (2007) and Ali (1992) observed an increased body weight by urea feeding in goats. The use of supplementary UMMB increased the milk yield of dairy cows by 6.7% and the daily gains of heifers by 15.5% (Chen *et al*.,1993). Supplementation of UMMB increased DM intake, nutrient digestibility and nitrogen balances in crossbred cows fed wheat straw (Srinivas *et al*., 1997). Alam *et al*., (2006) observed that UMMB supplementation has a positive effect on milk yield and reproductive performance of cows maintained on straw based diets due to supply of nitrogen resulting in more intake and utilization of straw. Kang *et al*., (2005) also recorded higher conception rate in buffaloes supplemented with UMMB than un supplemented group. The UMMB Supplementation to wheat straw based diets could supply nutrients (over and above) to adequately meet the maintenance requirement of buffaloes (Sihag *et al.*, 2007). Brar and Nanda (2008) also reported average increase of 25% in fodder intake, 8% in milk yield and 7% in milk fat, following UMMB supplementation for 4 weeks to anoestrus buffalo in Punjab state. UMMB supplementation helped in inducing estrus in 83.33% buffaloes and 66.66% cows compared to the control groups with zero percent of estrus induction. Yadav *et al.*, (2011) reported that the supplementation of UMMB along with a balanced concentrate mixture was beneficial for lactating buffaloes. The milk components like fat and SNF content of the animals fed with UMMB were improved significantly ($p<0.01$) over control groups (Ramesh *et al.*, 2009). In contrast, Zile *et al.*, (2005) concluded that there was no improvement in any of the milk components in UMMB fed groups in buffaloes.

Intake and digestibility of nutrients

The aim of urea molasses mineral block supplementation is to increase the roughage intake as well as its utilization. There was a significant increase in DM intake due to block feeding on straw based ration in buffaloes (Tiwari *et al.*,1990) and in crossbred calves. Singh *et al.*, (1991) observed 24% increase in DM intake due to block feeding on wheat straw based diet in crossbred cattle. Meenakshi *et al.*, (1988) reported that supplementation with urea molasses mineral block (UMMB) significantly ($p>0.01$) increased daily dry matter intake in buffalo calves. Sudhakar *et al.*, (2002) observed significant difference ($p>0.01$) in average daily dry matter intake in buffaloes fed UMMB supplemented ration. Chauhan *et al.* (1997) reported that the intake of straw based ration was more pronounced in UMMB supplied groups. The total DMI was statistically different in UMMB fed groups, whereas Zile *et al.*(2007) reported no change in the total DMI in UMMB fed groups maintained on wheat straw and sorghum fodder. The daily dry matter intake was significantly ($p<0.05$) higher in UMMB fed groups maintained on wheat straw in buffaloes (Sihag *et al.*, 2008). Mohini (1991) reported that dry matter intake was not significant in buffaloes fed on UMMB and indicated that supplementation of UMMB in the ration over and above the normal requirements did not affect the voluntary intake.

Digestibility of crude protein, crude fiber, ether extract, organic matter and total carbohydrates increased significantly ($p<0.01$) in buffaloes due to block feeding on wheat straw diet. Mohini (1991) observed even significant enhancement in the digestibility of nitrogen-free extract (NFE) with UMMB supplemented to buffaloe calves in paddy-straw-based diets. NDF and ADF digestibility were significantly higher in buffaloes due to block feeding on wheat straw based diet (Hosamani, 1992). Dry matter (DM) digestibility increased significantly ($p< 0.01$) in UMMB-fed groups with or without concentrate supplementation in crossbred cattle. Digestibility of DM, CP and CF were higher in buffaloes fed UMMB supplemented rations in comparison to control rations (Sudhakar *et al.*, 2002). Toppo *et al.*, (1997) revealed that 15 g urea supplementation is sufficient to maintain the optimum intake of UMMB with higher CP digestibility and higher positive N balance as compared to control in adult crossbred cattle. Sihag *et al.*, (2007) also reported that DM and CF digestibility were significantly higher in UMMB fed group than control groups of lactating buffaloes. The digestibility of CP, CF, EE and NFE was found to be higher in cold process compared to hot process in calves (Sharma *et al.*, 2008). DM, OM, CP, CF, NFE digestibility was increased significantly ($p < 0.01$) in buffaloes and non significant in cows fed on UMMB supplementation (Ramesh *et al.*, 2009). Hosamani *et al.*, (1998) found that supplementation of more than 80 percent energy had no extra benefit on lick intake and nutrient utilization in buffaloes. Feeding of UMMB established a conducive environment in rumen of buffaloes with optimum production of volatile fatty acids, which was essential for better nutrient utilization. Recently, Sankar (2013) conducted experiments on 24 crossbred male calves of about 9-12 months of age; divided into 4 groups of six animals in each group. All animals were fed wheat straw *ad libitum* and 70% CP requirement through concentrate mixture (ICAR, 1998). Animals of groups I, II, III and IV were offered *ad libitum* UMMB, SMB-A,SMB-B, and SMB-C. The feeding trial was continued for 120 days. There was no significant difference in ADG, FCR and digestibility of nutrients among the 4 groups. The block intake was significantly ($P<0.01$) lower in group IV as compared to the other groups. The excretion of calcium through faeces and calcium balance was non-significant among the groups. The feeding cost per kg body weight gain (₹) was higher in group I followed by III, II and IV, respectively. In phase III, SMB was selected from phase II, based on animal performance and SMB vary in the mineral mixture levels. In phase-III, 24 crossbred male calves of about 14-17 months of age were divided in to four groups of six animals in each. In group I animals were fed 100% CP requirement through concentrate mixture and wheat straw *ad libitum* whereas, in group II, III and IV animals were fed *ad libitum* wheat straw,(SMB-I, II, III) and 70% CP requirement through concentrate mixture (ICAR,1998). The feeding trial was continued for 150 days. There was no significant difference in intake and digestibility of DM, OM, EE, NDF, and ADF among the 4 groups. The CP intake was significantly higher in group II, III and IV than that of group I. There was no significant difference in intake of DCP and TDN; ADG, FCR and blood biochemical parameters among the 4 groups. Serum calcium and iron level was significantly ($P < 0.01$) higher level in the groups receiving SMB than group I. All the animals in four groups were on positive nitrogen, calcium and phosphorus balance. The net cost benefit was ₹12.2, 9.3 and 16.2, respectively higher than that of group I in groups II, III and IV.

Conclusion

From the literature, it may be deduced that supplementation of SMB/UMMB in the roughage based diet of ruminants can improve productivity (growth and milk) and reproductive performance *vis-à-vis* can also replace 25–30% crude protein of concentrate mixture without affecting the performance.

References

Aarts G, Sansoucy R, Levieux GP (1990) Guidelines for the manufacture and utilization of molasses-urea blocks. Anim. Production and Health Div. FAO, Rome.

Brar PS, Nanda AS (2008) Indian J. Anim. Sci. 78: 606-608.

Chen YZ, Wen H, Ma X, Li Y, Gao Z, Peterson MA (1993) Livestock Res. Rural Dev, 53: 60-63.

Dass RS, Mendiratta SK, Bhadane KP, Mudgal V, Lakshmanan V (2011) Anim. Nutr. Feed Tech. 11: 221-231.

Dutta N, Sharma K, Pattanaik AK, Singh M (2009) Anim. Nutr. Feed Tech. 9: 185-193.

Elangovan AV, Mehra UR, Singh UB, Sahoo A (1991) Indian J. Dairy Sci., 44: 543-546.

Hande SP (1989) M.V.Sc. Thesis, IVRI, Izatnagar, U.P., India.

Hosamani SV, Mehra UR, Dass RS (2003) Asian Aust. J. Anim. Sci. 16: 818-822.

Kang RS, Nanda AS, Brar PS (2005) Indian J. Anim. Sci. 75: 1261-65.

Leng RA (1984) The potential of solidified molasses based blocks for the correction of multi nutritional deficiencies in buffaloes and other ruminants fed low quality agro-industrial byproducts. The Use of Nuclear Techniques to improve domestic buffalo production in Asia IAEA, Vienna, pp. 135-150.

Malek MA, Khan MJ, Islam KM (2008) Indian J. Anim. Sci. 78 (12): 1404-1407.

Meenakshi G, Kapoor PD, Nangia OP (1988) Ind. Vet. J. 65 (4): 320-324.

Mehra UR, Singh UB, Pathak NN, Singh RP (1987) J. Vety. Physiol. & Allied Sci. 6: 19-24.

Misra AK, Subrahmanyam KV, Ramakrishna YS (2007) Indian J. Anim. Nutr. 77 (5): 405-410.

Mohini M (1991) Ph.D. Thesis, NDRI, Karnal, India.

Mondal S, Samanta CC, Bairagi B, Biswas P (2009) Anim. Nutr. Feed Tech. 9: 45-50.

Preston, T. R. and Leng. R. A. 1990. Matching ruminant production systems with available resources in the Tropics and Sub-tropics. CTA, Netherlands.

Raman RS, Chahal SM, Sihag ZS (2010) Indian J. Anim. Nutr. 27 (2): 159-163.

Ramesh BK, Thirumalesh T, Suresh BN (2009) Indian J. Anim. Nutr. 26 (4): 322-326.

Robinson PH, Swanepoel N, Evans E (2010) Anim. Feed Sci. Tech. 161: 75-84.

Saddul S, Bodoo AA (2001) Food and Agri. Res. Council, Reduit, Mauritus, pp. 245.

Sahoo B, Vishwanath C, Bhushan J, Kwatra, Agarwal A (2009). Anim. Nutr. Feed Tech. 9: 171-178.

Sankar V (2013) Ph.D. Thesis, Deemed University IVRI, Izatnagar.

Sharma V K, Rajvinder S, Chauhan JS (2008) Indian J. Anim. Sci. 78 (1): 80-84.

Sihag ZS, Berwal RS, Sihag S, Nand Kishore (2008) Indian J. Anim. Nutr. 25 (1): 43-46.

Sihag ZS, Punia BS, Nand Kishore (2007) Indian J. Anim. Nutr. 24 (1): 24-26.

Singh GP, Gupta BN, Kunju PJG (1991) Proceedings of 1st International Animal Nutrition Research Workers' Conference for Asia and Pacific, Sept. 23-28, Bangalore, India, Compendium II. Abst. No. 13.

Srinivas B, Gupta BN (1997) Austr. J. of Anim. Sci. 10: 47-53.

Sudhakar K, Reddy GVK, Krishna N (2002) Indian J. Anim.Nutr. 19 (4): 301-305.

Tiwari SP, Singh UB, Mehra UR (1990) Anim. Feed Sci. Tech. 29 (3): 333-341.

Toppo S, Verma AK, Dass RS, Mehra UR (1997) Anim. Feed Sci. Tech. 64: 101- 112.

Vatta AF, de Villiers JF, Gumede SA, Smith MF, Stenson MO, Harrison LJ (2007) Kwazulu-Natal Province, South Africa, 78 (2): 81-89.

Yadav CM, Khan PM, Naagar KC, Meena RH, Meena RR (2011) Indian J. Anim. Nutr. 28 (1): 47-50.

Zile S, Sihag S, Punia BS, Nand Kishore (2005) Indian Buffalo J. 3: 39-42.

20

An Overview of Impact of Climate Change on Vector-Borne Zoonotic Diseases

Sandip Khurana

ICAR-National Research Centre on Equines, Hisar-125001, Haryana

Introduction

Global warming is chiefly due to combustion of fossil fuels for multifarious energy needs, causing emission of greenhouse gases which trap energy from the sun leading to warming. These climate changes bring in variation in patterns and emergence of new zoonotic diseases to newer areas. These changes sometimes create conducive conditions for the propagation of insect vectors. History shows that most of the diseases have a direct correlation with climatic changes. The survival and propagation of pathogens are directly related to temperature and humidity *etc*. Extreme shifts in weather patterns resulting from global warming and climate changes adversely affect the ecosystem resulting in new diseases, re-emergence of earlier diseases including emergence of zoonotic diseases. The emergence of the new cholera strain O: 139 and outbreaks of Dengue, West Nile virus and Rift Valley fever in newer and non-endemic areas have been linked with the El Nino effect. The spread of disease agents may be facilitated by factors including environmental conditions, the presence and availability of suitable hosts, the arthropod's feeding behavior and host preferences.

Vector-borne zoonotic diseases are becoming major problems worldwide in recent times. Several vector-borne pathogens have appeared in new and non-endemic areas recently. Several endemic diseases have recorded a spurt in incidence. There has been re-emergence of some vector borne zoonoses also after a gap of many years in many regions. These have possibly resulted from changes in climate creating favourable conditions for the survival and propagation of vectors, alterations in transmission pattern, cycles and periods, intrusion of vectors and reservoirs in newer areas. Extreme alterations in weather patterns resulting from global warming in turn alter the ecosystem and biodiversity leading to emergence of new diseases, re-emergence of some diseases and expansion of geographical areas of existing diseases, majority of such diseases may be zoonotic and vector-borne. Vector-borne zoonoses probably would be a major public health threat worldwide in future. A comprehensive effort is essential to create multidisciplinary and interdisciplinary relations to study the vector-borne zoonoses for devising appropriate strategies for prevention, control and eradication of these diseases.

Kilpatrick *et al.* (2012) have described some non-traditional approaches for prevention, control and eradication of such diseases.

Vector–borne zoonoses in relation to climate change

Vector-borne diseases are spread by the bite of infected arthropod vectors that carry disease agents. The insects/vectors act as an essential stage in the transmission of the infectious agent from person to person or from animals to human beings. Vector-borne zoonotic diseases assume greater importance in the subtropical and tropical regions of the world (McMichael, 2015). Several varied etiologies *viz.* viral, rickettsial, bacterial and parasitic diseases can be transmitted by vectors. Global warming directly affects the transmission of the disease by shifting the geographic range and increasing reproductive and biting rates of vectors leading to the shortening of incubation period. Several vectors especially mosquito species namely *Aedes*, *Anopheles* and *Culex* are sensitive to fluctuations in the atmospheric temperature (Githeko *et al.*, 2000). Larvae of these mosquitoes in water take less time at higher temperatures to develop into adults, thus shortening their life cycle, thereby increasing the probability of disease occurrence (Watts *et al.*, 1987).

During warmer periods there is an increase in digestion of blood in female mosquitoes, increasing the egg laying capacity (Rueda *et al.*, 1990). Evolution occurs in almost all species of life. For example, *Aedes aegypti aegypti* has acclimatized to the waters preserved by humans in the household, leading to spread of diseases from wild animals to humans (Tabachnick, 2010). Human and animal susceptibility to infection might be further compounded by malnutrition due to crop and pasture failure caused by climate stress. Impact of climate change on some of the important vector-borne zoonotic diseases is explained here.

Eastern Equine Encephalitis Virus (EEEV) infection

EEEV isolation was first reported from horses in 1933. The virus propagates in nature between birds and mosquitos. The virus causes encephalitis with a case-fatality rate of up to 70% in human beings. The incubation period is 4-10 days, fever, headache, vomiting, respiratory distress, seizures and coma may occur in human encephalitis cases. A trend towards milder winters and hotter summers along with extremes in both precipitation and drought in the northeastern United States, rainfall and accumulated groundwater increase the population of mosquitoes by creating suitable conditions for larval development. These environmental changes have the potential to alter disease risk by increasing the abundance and distribution of the vector, lengthening the virus transmission season and increasing the intensity.

Western Equine Encephalitis Virus (WEEV) infection

WEEV was first isolated from the brain of a horse (Meyer *et al.*, 1931). The first human WEEV was confirmed in 1938. WEEV is maintained in nature between passerine birds and mosquito vectors in endemic areas. Climate change plays a crucial role in the transmission of WEEV among animals and humans. At temperatures above usual, there is a decline in the survival of larvae and adult mosquitoes hence the virus adapts itself to complete its cycle in the adult before it dies. Mosquitoes will restrict the development of WEEV when the environmental temperature goes past 32°C (Sutherst, 2004). Reisen *et al.*, (2010) have studied the effect of climate change on extension of mosquito season which is related to vector-borne zoonoses including WEEV infection.

Venezuelan Equine Encephalitis Virus (VEEV) infection

VEEV is propagated naturally between rodents and mosquito vectors in enzootic cycles. Epidemics result when mosquitoes transmit the virus to human beings and equids. Horses, donkeys and mules can transmit the infection through mosquitoes. Humans may also transmit the infection especially in urban settings as suggested in some reports (Watts *et al.*, 1997, 1998; Morrison *et al.*, 2008).

Japanese encephalitis (JE)

Japanese encephalitis is a very important mosquito-borne Flavivirus causing encephalitis and is a major public health problem in Asian countries. JEV is transmitted by *Culex tritaeniorhynchus*, *C annulus*, *C annulirostris* and *Aedis* mosquitoes (Rosen, 1986). Pigs and aquatic birds are amplifying hosts and act as a source of infection for mosquitoes (Rosen, 1986). The disease affects primarily human beings, pigs and horses. Abortions and stillbirths are common manifestations in pigs, whereas, it is usually subclinical with fever, depression, tremors and ataxia in horses (Khurana *et al.*, 2015). The incidence is related to hot and humid climate. Heavy rainfalls increase the incidence of disease.

West Nile Fever

West Nile fever is caused by the West Nile Virus, a member of the family *Flaviviridae*. The virus mainly infects birds and infrequently humans through the bite of an infected *Culex* mosquito. The virus has been isolated from mosquitoes, wild rodents, migrating birds, hard ticks, horses and humans. Data from the West Nile fever outbreak in 2000, suggested a significant linkage between the aggressiveness of the vector (*Culex modestus*) and temperature, humidity, rainfall and sunshine related to the epidemic period (Ludwig *et al.*, 2005). The outbreaks in 1996-97 in southeastern Romania and in Israel in 2000 were both associated with a heat wave (Paz, 2000). A warming trend exists in the Mediterranean basin with changes in rainfall patterns and it is expected that vector-borne diseases will be influenced by climate change since weather conditions influence their emergence which has been proved in the case of West Nile virus (Negev *et al.*, 2015)

Rift Valley Fever

Rift valley fever is an acute febrile zoonotic disease caused by Rift valley virus belonging to genus Phlebovirus of *Bunyaviridae* family. It is primarily a zoonotic infection but humans are infected either through exposure to the blood, body fluids or tissues of animals that have been bitten by infected mosquitoes or directly from bites from infected mosquitoes. Climate change has resulted in several outbreaks of this disease in East Africa in the last ten years including the outbreaks in 1997-98 and the recent epidemic which affected Kenya, Somalia, Tanzania and Sudan in 2006-2007. Outbreaks of the disease are usually associated with heavy rainfall and warm temperatures (Steven, 2009).

Dengue fever

Dengue is a mosquito-borne disease caused by the Dengue virus belonging to the Genus Flavivirus and transmitted by *Aedes aegypti*. During the last 15 years, another vector *Aedes albopictus* has spread this disease to many countries of Europe due to global warming (Paz, 2000). The expansion of dengue related to both precipitation and temperature. Egg laying rate of *Aedes* mosquitoes declined when monthly mean temperature reduced to 16.5°C and no eggs were found below 14.8°C. Approximately, one-third of the world population lives in the hot and humid tropical and subtropical regions of the world where climate is ideal for propagation of mosquitoes. Since 1980, dengue has increased dramatically in tropical regions especially countries in the Caribbean, Central and South America, Pacific Islands, Asia and Africa. Current *Aedes albopictus* distributions were predicted by simple climatic indicators and northward range expansion was predicted for the future with climate change in North America (Ogden *et al*., 2014).

Chikungunya fever

Chikungunya fever is caused by a virus belonging to the genus Alphavirus in the family *Togaviridae*. It is transmitted to human beings by mosquitoes mainly *Aedes aegypti* and *Aedes albopictus*. Several epidemics of Chikungunya fever in recent times are the result of climate change. Dry and warm climate commonly precedes an outbreak. After several years of continuous drought conditions, Chikungunya affected 500,000 people in East Africa in 2004 (Steven 2009). The first Chikungunya outbreak in Europe had occurred in north-eastern Italy (Rezza *et al*., 2007).

Yellow Fever

Yellow fever is caused by an RNA virus belonging to the genus Flavivirus and depends on mosquitoes for transmission. As mosquitoes shift due to changes in water availability, yellow fever will appear in new areas. The disease affects primates as well as humans. Yusa *et al*., (2015) have done a very exhaustive study on public health impacts of droughts due to climate change and have found a spurt in vector-borne zoonoses including yellow fever due to unusually hot climates.

Tick-borne encephalitis (TBE)

Tick-borne encephalitis is caused by an Arbovirus of the family *Flaviviridae* and is transmitted by ticks predominantly *Ixodes ricinus*. An increase in temperature accelerates the developmental cycle, egg production, population density and distribution of ticks. *Ixodes ricinus* has expanded into higher altitudes in the Czech Republic over the last two decades due to an increase in average temperatures.

Crimean-Congo hemorrhagic fever

Crimean-Congo hemorrhagic fever (CCHF) is caused by an RNA virus of the Bunyaviridae family and is transmitted by Hyalomma spp ticks. The virus is the most widespread tick-borne arbovirus and is found in the Eastern Mediterranean where there have been a series of outbreaks in Bulgaria in 2002 and 2003, in Albania and in Kosovo in 2001. Milder weather conditions, favouring tick reproduction may influence CCHF distribution. For example, an outbreak in Turkey was linked to a milder spring season in the year before the outbreak. However, other factors such as land use and demographic changes have also been implicated (Ergonul, 2006). The emergence of CCHF in Iran probably due to environmental factors (Keshtkar-Jahromi *et al.*, 2013).

Kyasanur Forest disease

Kyasanur forest disease (KFD), a viral disease caused by the Flavivirus of *Flaviviridae* family. Natural hosts include black-faced langur (*Presbytis entellus*), red-faced bonnet monkey (*Macaca radiata*), striped forest squirrel (*Funambulus tristriatus tristriatus*), Blandford rat (*Rattus blanfordi*) and house shrew (*Suncus murinus*), transmitted by the tick vector, *Haemaphysalis spinigera* (Dobler, 2010). Due to deforestation and the movement of humans into areas of wild has led to the species jumping of this deadly virus. This viral disease has been currently reported more from southern parts of India mainly from Karnataka.

Plague

The plague is caused by *Yersinia pestis*. The World has suffered from three pandemics of plague and it still occurs in patches in parts of the world (Xu *et al.*, 2014). Rodents act as the reservoir of the bacterium and aids in the spread of the organism. Wild animals have also played their part in the spread of plague to humans during outbreaks in parts of central Asia. Vector namely *Xenopsylla cheopis*, oriental rat flea is involved in transmission of this bacilli to humans from the rodents. Several workers have earlier reported that temperature and humidity play a crucial role in the transmission of plague during outbreaks in India (Rogers, 1928). Later several workers showed different findings like plague outbreak was lesser in Africa when the temperature was above 27°C and below 15°C (Davis, 1953). Similarly in Vietnam plague outbreak increased after the heavy rainfall season in the dry climatic situation (Cavanaugh and Marshall, 1972). These findings are related to the life cycle of fleas that are involved in transmission of the bacteria (Krasnov *et al.*, 2001).

Lyme disease

Lyme disease is caused by a spirochete *Borrelia burgdorferi* which is transmitted to humans by blood-sucking hard ticks of the genus *Ixodes*. Berglund *et al.*, (1996) expressed the possibility of expansion of Lyme disease in higher regions of Sweden due to milder winter temperatures caused by climate change. Climate warming may have resulted in the emergence of Lyme disease in northeastern North America, and in the future may expand to new regions and increase tick-borne disease risk (Ogden *et al.*, 2014).

Tularemia

Tularemia is caused by *Francisella tularensis*, occurring mostly in the Northern parts of the world. Vectors involved in the transmission of this bacterium from its natural hosts, rabbits and hares are *Dermacentor andersoni*, *Amblyomma americanum*, *D variabilis*, and *Chrysops discalis*. Though tularemia is an example of direct zoonosis, the role played by vector transmission cannot be underestimated (Ellis *et al*., 2002). Research suggests that summer conditions when temperature is warmer favours tularemia outbreak while winter months shows lesser incidences.

Rocky Mountain spotted fever

Rocky Mountain spotted fever is caused by *Rickettsia rickettsii*, affecting the dogs mainly (Alvarez *et al*., 2014). Transmission of this pathogen to naïve dogs and also to humans from affected dogs is usually through the vectors namely, *Dermacentor variabilis*, *Dermacentor andersoni*, *Amblyomma cajennense* and *Rhipicephalus sanguineus* (Drexler *et al*., 2014). Though the dog ticks play a major role in transmission of the agent, these ticks are found mostly on the soil, between the cracks and crevices of walls rather than on the pet's body. Climate changes have led to changes in the habitat of ticks, risking human lives by causing severe infection.

Anaplasmosis

Human Anaplasmosis is caused by *Anaplasma phagocytohilum*, transmitted to human beings by *Ixodes ricinus* tick. In Europe, this disease was known to cause fever in goats, sheep and cattle till it emerged as a disease of human beings in 1996. It has now shifted to new geographical areas throughout Europe, and migrating birds have been implicated in its expansion.

Simian Malaria

Malaria is a deadly disease caused by protozoa of the genus Plasmodium, which are transmitted by anopheline mosquitoes. It is estimated that 30-500 million people are infected with Plasmodium spp. Worldwide, and that 1.5-2.7 million people a year die from the infection (Garcia, 2010). Traditionally, human malaria has been attributed to four Plasmodium species, *i.e*., *Plasmodium vivax*, *Plasmodium malariae* and *Plasmodium ovale*. Since 2004, a simian malaria parasite, *Plasmodium knowlesi*, has been implicated in human disease. Specifically, *P. knowlesi* has been confirmed in several human cases of malaria diagnosed from Malaysian Borneo, Thailand, Myanmar and the Philippines. Certainly, simian malaria is an emerging problem in Southeast Asia and in this new scenario the identification of malaria parasites to the species level becomes critical (Garcia, 2010). The zoonotic potential of *P. knowlesi* is emphasized because of its transmission by the forest-dwelling *Anopheles lateens*, a mosquito species that feeds on both the monkey natural host as well as on humans. Deforestation may raise the temperature by 3-4°C thereby increasing the breeding, development of mosquito vectors and increasing the incidence of this disease.

Leishmaniasis

Leishmaniasis is a protozoan parasitic infection caused by *Leishmania infantum* which is transmitted to human beings through the bite of an infected female phlebotomine sandfly that have previously fed on an infected host, usually a wild animal. Temperature influences the biting activity rates of the vector, diapause and maturation of the protozoan parasite in the vector. The biting activity of sandflies is seasonal, and it is prominent in summers (Rioux and Lanotte, 1990), earlier cutaneous leishmaniasis was thought to be an endemic disease confined to the north-western region of India (NICD, 2006). However, since 2003 from new foci infections have been reported from various parts of southern India. The ecology of phlebotomine sand flies is directly influenced by climate and other environmental variables. Recent studies have highlighted the spreading of the leishmaniases to northern Italy and from northern to southern Brazil (Tomaz-Soccol *et al*., 2009). Indeed, canine leishmaniasis is now well established in South America as far south as northern Argentina (Salomon *et al*., 2008; Dantas Torres, 2009). Global warming could lead to establishment of canine leishmaniasis in areas such as the United Kingdom, where the vectors are currently absent, but where *Leishmania infantum*-infected dogs that had traveled to endemic areas are present. Interestingly, cases of cutaneous leishmaniasis by an undescribed species of Leishmania were diagnosed in Northern Australian macropods and day feeding midges have been incriminated as potential vectors (Dougall *et al*., 2011).

***Thelazia callipaeda* infestation**

Over the last decade, an apparent invasion by a vector-borne nematode infestation has taken place in the western European countries, known as *T. callipaeda* infesting the eyes of humans (Otranto and Dutto, 2008) as well as domestic (dogs and cats) and wild carnivores, including foxes, wolves, beech martens and wild cats. Because of its earlier known distribution in the former Soviet Republics and many far eastern countries including India, Thailand, China and Japan, this nematode has long been known as the "oriental eye worm". In the last decade, *T. callipaeda* has proved to be widespread among dogs and cats in Italy. Following these first reports in Italy, new cases of the thelaziosis have also been recorded in France and Germany in dogs that had spent some time mostly during summer, in northern Italy.

Way Forward and Future Outlook

Global warming is mainly the result of increasing combustion of organic fuel and changes in land use which are anthropogenic factors. These climate changes have resulted in the emergence of new zoonotic diseases in newer and non-endemic areas. The changes in climate have created apt conditions for the propagation of vectors, alterations in transmission period, introduction of vectors and vertebrate reservoirs in non-endemic areas. IPCC, several governmental and non-governmental agencies, environmentalists, scientists and common people are contributing in their efforts to control the changes in climate. Sincere and dedicated efforts are needed to study and analyze the complex interaction of host vectors, reservoirs, disease agents and environmental factors with an aim of prevention, control and eradication of vector borne zoonoses.

Infectious diseases will indeed continue to emerge, re-emerge and spread due to human-induced environmental changes. Therefore, to avoid such harmful effects of global warming, changes in lifestyle are essentially required. The present scenario is indicating that within the next few decades environmental conditions may become more conductive for the entry of unwanted harmful agents in the biosphere; hence there is an urgent need to envisage a full-proof strategy to mitigate changes due to fluctuating climatic conditions.

References

Alvarez G, Rosales C and Sepulveda R (2014) Rocky Mountain Spotted Fever, a Reemerging Disease in Arizona and Sonora - Case Study. J Case Rep Stud 2(3): 301.

Berglund J, Eitrem R, Norrby SR (1996) Long-term study of Lyme borreliosis in an endemc area in Sweden. Scandinavian Journal of Infectious Diseases 28: 473.

Cavanaugh DC and Marshall JD. 1972. The influence of climate on the seasonal prevalence of plague in the Republic of Vietnam. J Wildl Dis 8: 85–94.

Dantas-Torres F (2009) Canine leishmaniosis in South America. Parasites Vectors 2 (Suppl. 1), S1.

Davis DH (1953) Plague in Africa from 1935 to 1949; a survey of wild rodents in African territories. Bull World Health Organ 5: 665–700.

Dobler G (2010) Zoonotic tick-borne flaviviruses. Veterinary Microbiology 140: 221–228.

Dougall AM, Alexander B, Holt DC, Harris T, Sultan AH, Bates PA, Rose K, Walton SF, (2011) Evidence incriminating midges (Diptera: Ceratopogonidae) as potential vectors of Leishmania in Australia. International Journal of Parasitology 41: 571–579.

Drexler N, Miller M, Gerding J, Todd S, Adams L, Dahlgren FS, Bryant N, Weis E, Herrick K, Francies J, Komatsu K, Piontkowski S, Velascosoltero J, Shelhamer T, Hamilton B, Eribes C, Brock A, Sneezy P, Goseyun C, Bendle H, Hovet R, Williams V, Massung R, McQuiston JH (2014) Community-Based Control of the Brown Dog Tick in a Region with High Rates of Rocky Mountain Spotted Fever, 2012–2013. PLoS ONE 9(12): e112368.

Ellis J, Oyston PC, Green M, Titball RW (2002) Tularemia. Clin Microbiol Rev 15 (4): 631–646.

Ergonul O (2006) Crimean-Congo hemorrhagic fever. Lancet Infectious Diseases, 6:203 Garcia, L.S., 2010. Malaria. Clin. Lab. Med. 30, 93–129.

Gascon J, Bern C, Pinazo MJ (2010) Chagas disease in Spain, the United States and other non-endemic countries. Acta Tropica 115: 22–27.

Githeko AK, Lindsay SW, Confalonieri UE, Patz JA (2000) Climate change and vector borne diseases: a regional analysis. Bulletin of the World Health Organization. 78 (9): 1136-1147.

Keshtkar-Jahromi M, Sajadi MM, Ansari H, Mardani M, Naieni KH (2013) Crimean-Congo hemorrhagic fever in Iran. Antiviral Research 100(1): 20–28. http://doi.org/10.1016/j.antiviral.2013.07.007

Khurana SK, Dhama K, Prasad M, Karthik K, Tiwari R (2015). Zoonotic pathogens transmitted from equines: diagnosis and control. Adv Anim Vet Sci 3(2s): 32-53.

Kilpatrick AM, Randolph SE (2012) Drivers, dynamics, and control of emerging vector-borne zoonotic diseases. Lancet. 380(9857): 1946-1955. Doi10.1016/S0140-6736(12)611151-9.

Krasnov BR, Khokhlova IS, Fielden LJ, Burdelova NV (2001) Development rates of two Xenopsylla flea species in relation to air temperature and humidity. Med Vet Entomol 15: 249–258.

Ludwig A, Biocout D, Chalvet-Monfray K, Sabatier P (2005). Modeling the of the Culex modestus, possible vector of West Nile fever in Camargue, as a function of meteorological data. Environ. Risque Santie. 4:109.

McMichael AJ (2015) Extreme weather events and infectious disease outbreaks, Virulence 6(6): 1-5.

Meyer KF, Haring CM, Howitt B (1931). The etiology of epizootic encephalomyelitis in horses in San Joachin Valley, 1930. Science. 74(1913): 227-228.

Morrison AC, Forshey BM, Notyce D, Astete H, Lopez V, Rocha C, Carrion R, Carey C, Eza D, Mongomery JM, Kochel TJ (2008). Venezuelan equine encephalitis virus in Iquitos, Peru: urban transmission of sylvatic strain. PLoS. Negl. Trop. Dis. 2: e349.

Negev M, Paz S, Clermont A, Pri-Or NG, Shalom U, Yeger T, Green MS (2015) Impacts of Climate Change on Vector Borne Diseases in the Mediterranean Basin - Implications for Preparedness and Adaptation Policy. International Journal of Environmental Research and Public Health, 12(6): 6745–6770. http://doi.org/10.3390/ijerph120606745

NICD (2006). Leishmaniasis and its control. NICD Monthly Newsletter, National Institute of Cummunicable Diseases. India. 10:1.

Ogden NH, Milka R, Caminade C, Gachon P (2014) Recent and projected future climatic suitability of North America for the Asian tiger mosquito Aedes albopictus. Parasites and Vectors 7:532. doi: 10.1186/s13071-014-0532-4.

Otranto D, Dutto M (2008) Human thelaziasis, Europe. Emerg. Infect. Dis. 4, 647–649.

Paz S (2000) The West Nile Virus outbreak in Israel from a new perspective: the regional impact of climate change. Int. J. Environ. Health Res., 16:1

Reisen WK, Thiemann T, Barker CM, Lu H, Carroll B, Fang Y, Lothrop HD (2010). Effects of warm winter temperature on the abundance and gonotrophic activity of Culex (Diptera: Culicidae) in California. J Med Entomol. 47(2):230-7.

Rezza G, Nicoletti L, Angelini R, Romi R, Finarelli AC, Panning M, Cordioli P, Fortuna C, Boros S, Magurano F, Silvi G, Angelini P, Ciufolini MG, Majori GC, Cassone A (2007) Infection with Chikungunya virus in Italy: an outbreak in a temperate region. Lancet. 370: 1840.

Rioux JA, Lanotte G (1990) Leishmania infantum as a cause of cutaneous leishmaniasis. Trans. R. Soc.Trop. Med. Hyg. 84:898.

Rogers L (1928) The yearly variations in plague in India in relation to climate: forecasting epidemics. Proc Roy Soc Ser B 103: 42–72.

Rosen L (1986) The natural history of japanese encephalitis virus. Annu. Rev. Microbiol. 40:395-414.

Rueda LM, Patel KJ, Axtell RC, Stinner RE (1990) Temperature-dependent development and survival rates of *Culex quinquefasciatus* and *Aedes aegypti* (Diptera: Culicidae). Journal of Medical Entomology 27: 892–898.

Salomon O, Sinagra A, Nevot M, Barberian G, Paulin P, Estevez J, Riarte A, Estevez J (2008) First visceral leishmaniasis focus in Argentina. Mem. Inst. Oswaldo Cruz 103, 109–111.

Steven VS (2009) The impact of climate change on health in the East, Central and Southern Africa (ECSA) region. Regional case study. Commonwealth Minister ECSA Health Community, Arusha, Tanzania, 40.

Sutherst RW (2004) Global change and human vulnerability to vectorborne diseases. Clin Microbiol Rev 17: 136–173.

Tabachnick WJ (2010) Challenges in predicting climate and environmental effects on vector borne disease episystems in a changing world. Journal of Experimental Biology 213: 946–954.

Tomaz-Soccol V, Castro EA, Navarro IT, de Farias MR, de Souza LM, Carvalho Y, Bispo S, Membrive NA, Minozzo JC, Truppel J, Bueno W, Luz E (2009) Allochthonous cases of canine visceral leishmaniasis in Paraná, Brazil: epidemiological implications. Rev Bras Parasitol Vet 18: 46–51.

Watts DM, Burke DS, Harrison BA, Whitmire RE, Nisalak A (1987) Effect of temperature on the vector efficiency of *Aedes aegypti* for dengue 2 virus. American Journal of Tropical Medicine and Hygiene 36: 143–152.

Watts DM, Callahan J, Rossi C, Oberste MS, Roehrig JT, Wooster MT, Smith JF, Cropp CB, Gentrau EM, Karabatsos N, Gubler DJ, Hayes CG (1998) Venezuelan equine encephalitis febrile cases among humans in the Peruvian Amazon river region. Am J Trop Med Hyg 58(1): 35-40.

Xu L, Stige LC, Kausrud KL, Ari TB, Wang S, Fang X, Schmid BV, Liu Q, Stenseth NC, Zhang Z (2014) Wet climate and transportation routes accelerate spread of human plague. Proc. R. Soc. B 281: 20133159.

Yusa A, Berry P, Cheng JJ, Ogden N, Bonsal B, Stewart R, Waldick R (2015). Climate Change, Drought and Human Health in Canada. International Journal of Environmental Research and Public Health 12(7): 8359–8412. http://doi.org/10.3390/ijerph120708359

21

Toxicopathology of Important Plants of North-Western Himalayan Region of India

Rinku Sharma, Devi Gopinath, Gauri Jairath, Ajayta Rialch
Uma Shankar Pati, Birbal Singh, Gorakh Mal and Sudesh Radotra
ICAR-Indian Veterinary Research Institute, Regional Station, Palampur-176061
Himachal Pradesh

Livestock poisoning by plants is often a result of management errors, range conditions, or the type of animal, rather than just the presence of poisonous plants. Forage availability can be influenced by drought, overgrazing and snow storms, or altered grazing patterns. Animals can become overly hungry during transportation or other management activities that deprive them of food and water for extended periods of time, thus making them more likely to graze toxic plants. Grazing during the wrong season may compromise an animal's ability to select adequate and non-toxic forages (James, 1994).

The toxicity of plants varies with environmental factors such as site, temperature, precipitation, and light, time of day and stage of growth. For example, mature oak leaves are less toxic than young leaves. Cyanogenic plants such as arrow grass are more toxic following a frost or drought condition. Nitrates can be higher in plants following heavy nitrogen fertilisation or during a drought. Certain animal factors must also be considered in livestock poisoning by plants. For example, goats are considered to be comparatively resistant to lantana poisoning than cattle. A hungry animal is more susceptible to poisoning than a full one. A full rumen slows consumption and also dilutes the toxin. Though the animals are exposed to a large number of toxic plants when they are left for grazing, five will be discussed in detail in this chapter. These include lantana, ageratum, eupatorium, oak and ferns (James, 1994).

Lantana

Lantana camara Linn. (common name *lantana*, wild sage; locally known as *bara phulnoo* in Himachal Pradesh), an ornamental shrub, belongs to the family Verbenaceae (Fig.1A). The most prevalent and most noxious variety of *L. camara* is red flower variety (*L. camara* var. *aculeata*), which causes severe toxicity in grazing animals (Sharma *et al.*, 2007). Lantana readily invades disturbed or neglected areas and where native woodlands have been thinned or cleared for grazing. The genus *Lantana* consists of many species that are native to the Americas and Africa, and has become naturalized as a noxious weed in tropical, subtropical, and warm temperate countries (Day *et al*., 2003). It is considered that Mexico and Central America is the generic epicenter of *L.camara* (Spies, 1984) from where it was introduced to the rest of the world via Europe (Stirton, 1977).

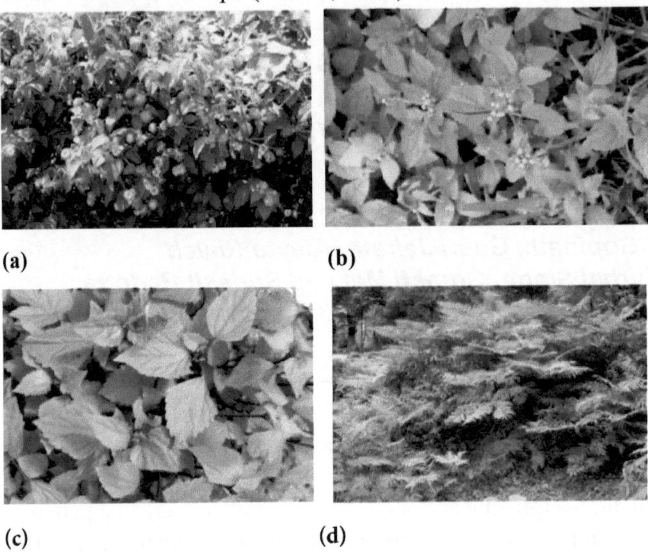

Fig. 1. (a) Lantana camara **(b)** Ageratum conyzoides **(c)** Eupatorium **(d)** Fern
(See colour version on page 258)

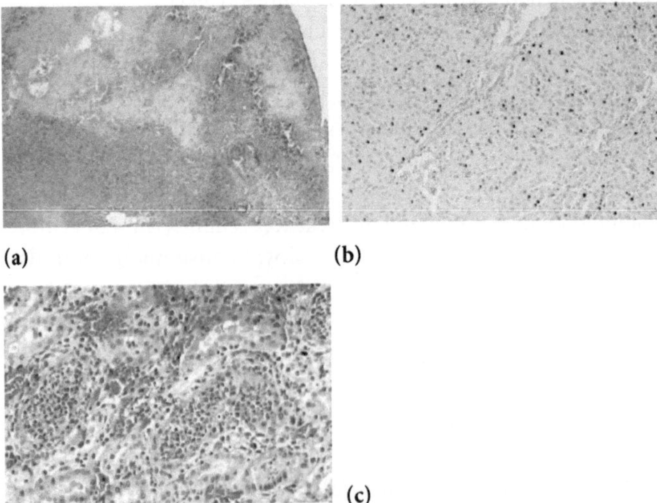

Fig. 2. Lantana intoxicated guinea pig: **(A)** Liver showing large area of coagulative necrosis, haemorrhages, infiltration of heterophils and proliferation of bile ducts. HE ×40. **(B)** Liver showing TUNEL positive apoptotic hepatocytes. Substrate, DAB; Counter stain, Mayer's Haematoxylin; TUNEL assay ×10. **(C)** Kidneys showing necrosis of the lining tubular epithelium and occlusion of the tubular lumen with inflammatory cells mainly heterophils. Degenerative changes in kidney tubules leading to formation casts in the lumen are also visible. HE x20
(See colour version on page 258)

Lantana is a principal weed in 12 countries and has been found in nearly 50 countries (Ghisalberti, 2000). It has been listed as one of the nine declared noxious weeds of the north coast of Australia (Dayson, 1989). *Lantana camara* toxicity caused by lantadenes is characterized by intrahepatic cholestasis, associated liver damage and photosensitization. Both ruminants including cattle, sheep, buffaloes, goats, and non ruminants like horses, guinea pigs, rabbits, female rats are susceptible to lantana toxicity. Goats were reported to be less vulnerable than other animals (Lal and Kalra, 1960). Guinea pigs, from a non-ruminant group, exhibited the most typical symptoms comparable to experimental or field cases of lantana toxicosis in ruminants (Sharma *et al.*, 1992).

L. camara causes substantial losses to farmers in India and Australia, where livestock contributes significantly to the economy (Sharma *et al.*, 2007). On consuming this plant, grazing animals suffer from hepatotoxicity and this is an important cause of livestock morbidity and mortality in lantana-infested regions (Sharma and Makkar, 1981). *L. camara* is spread widely over Kangra valley in Himachal Pradesh (Sharma and Makkar, 1981) and many other parts of the country. In a survey of the Kangra valley of Himachal Pradesh in India, Sharma and Makkar (1981) observed lantana poisoning as the main cause for loss of livestock. The incidence was maximum during summer months, April to June, before the onset of the rainy season, when there is a scarcity of green forage (Sharma and Makkar, 1981; Sharma, 1994).

The toxic compounds of *L. camara* are lantadenes which are pentacyclic triterpenoids in nature. The major constituents of the leaves of the red flower variety are lantadene A (LA), lantadene B (LB), lantadene C (LC) and lantadene D (LD). Reduced lantadene A (RLA) and reduced lantadene B (RLB) are the minor constituents (Sharma *et al.*, 2007).

The triterpenoids can be absorbed from all the regions of the digestive tract but most rapidly from the small intestine. It is reported that bile is not important for the absorption of lantana toxin (Pass *et al.*, 1981). Features of the mechanism of lantana toxicity which are important in determining the onset and the progression of disease in ruminants have been identified. These include: 1) Only a small proportion of triterpenoids are absorbed from the digestive tract. 2) Continuous absorption of toxins is necessary for the disease to develop and to be maintained (Pass, 1991). 3) Ruminal stasis occurs and results in retention of toxins in the rumen for a long period. The stasis of rumen in lantana intoxicated animals is initially due to inhibitory neural impulses arising from damaged liver and to the effect of anorexia (McSweeney and Pass, 1983). 4) Absorption of toxins from the rumen maintains the liver injury. 5) Injury to the bile canalicular membrane is a prominent finding in affected liver damage.

In ruminants, *L. camara* toxicity primarily attacks liver and kidney and also causes photosensitization. Inappetence and constipation within 24 h of dosing followed by ictericity and photosensitization are typical signs of lantana toxicity (Sharma *et al.*, 1992). The dose determines the severity of ictericity (Gopinath and Ford, 1969).

Rumination is suspended or ceases completely. Other signs may include sluggishness, weakness and transient, sometimes bloody diarrhea. In acute cases, death occurs in 2 to 4 days. Signs of photosensitization are observed in animals which continue to take green fodders. These are in the form of swollen and oedematous ears and eyelids with cracks and fissures on muzzle and other non-hairy parts, reddening and discharge from the eyes (conjunctivitis), ulceration of the tip and under surface of the tongue (if unpigmented), *etc.* Signs of jaundice include pale conjunctival, vulvar, or vaginal mucous membranes and sclera of eye. At necropsy, the subcutaneous tissue and fat show yellow discoloration. The liver exhibits swelling and rounding of edges. Liver is pale yellow and fragile. Gall bladder is 3–4 times distended. Kidneys are pale and swollen (Seawright and Allen, 1972). Normally, phylloerythrin is excreted via bile, but because of intrahepatic cholestasis by lantadenes, there is retention of phylloerythrin (a degradation product of chlorophyll), which results in photosensitization.

In guinea pigs, lantadene at the dose of 500 mg/kg BW (equivalent to approximately 1 kg green leaves) resulted in acute toxicity characterized by inactivity, dullness and depression within 24 h. The animals showed a reduction in body weight, anorexia, severe icteric index, and constipation, and all became moribund within 24–36 h of lantadene administration. At necropsy, severe yellow discoloration of subcutaneous tissue, severe congestion, hemorrhages, and pinpoint necrotic foci in the liver and inspissated, greenish-black tarry gall bladder contents were observed. Kidneys appeared swollen and markedly pale (Parimoo *et al.*, 2015). Lantadenes when administered at the dose of 100 mg/kg BW, also resulted in acute toxicity within 48-72 hrs with a significantly reduced total erythrocyte count, heterophilia and the resultant lymphocytopenia (Parimoo and Sharma, 2014). Studies have shown that administration of lantadenes at higher doses, *i.e.*, 100 and 50 mg/kg bw (equivalent to approximately 200 and 100 g green leaves, respectively), lead to development of signs, characteristic of acute lantana poisoning. At 100 mg/kg BW animals became moribund within 48–72 h of dosing while at 50 mg/kg BW they became moribund within the second week of initial administration. The animals showed a significant elevation in total serum bilirubin levels which corroborated with the gross pathomorphological changes, including severe yellowish discolorations of the subcutaneous tissue and renal medulla.

Sub-acute poisoning is more common in field conditions and may result in death after 1 to 3 weeks of illness and weight loss (http://www.library.illinois.edu/vex/toxic/lantana/lantana.htm). In a study, the dose of 25 mg/kg BW of lantadenes (equivalent to approximately 50 g green leaves) did not result in mortality, produced typical gross and histopathological changes in liver and kidneys, and resulted in the highest levels of serum liver marker enzymes *i.e.*, alanine aminotransferase, aspartate aminotransferase and alkaline phosphatase. These findings were characteristic of sub acute toxicity of lantadenes in guinea pigs. Elevated lipid peroxidation levels and decreased levels of superoxide dismutase and catalase indicated free-radical-induced damage by lantadenes. Grossly, the liver surface showed presence of large, whitish yellow, necrotic mass embedded deep into parenchyma, and multiple, pinpoint to linear necrotic areas, and generalized hemorrhages. The kidneys showed slight pale discoloration. Histopathological alterations revealed marked multifocal coagulative necrosis with fibrotic capsule, bile duct proliferation, and severe leukocyte infiltration in parenchyma and around necrotic foci. The kidneys revealed mild cortical congestion, degenerative changes, leukocyte infiltration, increased cytoplasmic eosinophilia, and nuclear pyknosis in the lining tubular epithelial cells (Parimoo *et al.*, 2015). Quantitative reverse-transcriptase polymerase chain reaction (qRT-PCR) analysis of the liver of animals during subacute exposure to lantadenes at the dose of 25 mg/kg bw revealed elevated expression of pro-inflammatory cytokines *viz.*, TNFα, TGFβ, IL-1, IL-6 and COX-2 (Kharwal, 2017).

The above sub-acute toxicity studies in guinea pigs suggested that lantadenes have two pronged effects on the liver; one at the level of bile canaliculi membrane and other at the level of hepatocytes. Interaction of lantadenes with the bile canalicular membrane resulted in intrahepatic cholestasis which in turn led to ictericity and severe pathological changes in gallbladder and finally led to death of guinea pigs. Lantadenes also targeted the hepatocytes, thereby leading to cellular degenerative changes and hepatic necrosis. The results indicated that the animals which were administered a lower dose of lantadenes developed some compensatory mechanism at the level of bile canalicular membrane level for the excretion of bilirubin, thereby escaping the primary effect of lantadenes, *i.e.*, ictericia and pathological changes of gallbladder. But, the sub-acute toxic dose of lantadenes continued to produce their secondary effect, *i.e.*, cellular degenerative changes in hepatocytes and hepatic necrosis. Because of this secondary effect, a severe degree of hepatic necrosis was produced in animals which were administered lower doses of lantadenes (Parimoo *et al.*, 2015). In another study, the toxicopathological effects of subchronic (90 days) administration of lantadenes in guinea pig models were investigated. The results of gross pathology, histopathology, serum marker enzyme values, oxidation stress levels, confirmation of fibrous tissue by Masson's Trichrome stain and ultrasonography revealed that the various doses of lantadenes showed a dose-dependent toxicity in decreasing order with the highest dose (24 mg/kg BW) producing maximum lesions and the lowest-dose (6 mg/kg BW) producing minimum alterations. Lantadenes produced maximum damage in kidneys followed by liver and stomach during subchronic exposure (Kumar, 2015).

Ageratum

Ageratum spp. is a tropical plant that is very common in West Africa, Australia, parts of Asia and South America (Fig. 1B). The plant grows commonly in waste and on ruined sites. It has a peculiar odour like that of a male goat, hence its name 'goat weed' or 'billy goat weed'. It is one of the most noxious weeds in many crops in the lower hills of Himachal Pradesh and adjoining areas (Negi, 1988). The species which are most prevalent in Kangra valley are *A. conyzoides* and *A. houstonianum* (Sharma, 1994). *A. conyzoides* contains flavonoids, alkaloids, coumarins, tannins and essential oils. Fifty one terpenoid compounds including precocene I and precocene II have been identified. The plant has also been found to be poisonous to rabbits due to the presence of HCN and coumarin (Ekundayo *et al.*, 1998).

While the precocenes have been seen as fourth-generation insecticides, the drawback is that they have been shown to cause hepatotoxicity in rats (Hammond *et al.*, 1995). It is not certain if the precocenes are the only toxins responsible for the effects of ageratum plants, but due to the extensive exposure of humans and animals to this plant, it is important to identify the toxins involved in its adverse effects. The pollination season of the plants between November and January results in allergy in the exposed human beings. In a study, the pollens of ageratum caused naso-bronchial allergy in 5 out of 50 patients (Arbat and Patil, 1985). People working in ageratum infested fields suffer nausea, giddiness and fainting. Farmers have been reporting toxicity of ageratum to animals while grazing or when the plant is mixed in fodder, but data on morbidity and mortality are not available. However, poisoning in farm animals fed forage contaminated with *A. houstonianum* has been reported from Cuba (Alfonso *et al.*, 1989). It caused an acute haemorrhagic and photosensitization syndrome.

Eupatorium

The fast growth of plants of the *Eupatorium* genus is disturbing the overall ecology by encroaching upon pastures and replacing the forest biomass; it is a major concern for farmers, agriculture, and animal and forestry scientists (Sharma, 1994) (Fig. 1C). The overt impact on farmers' economy is in terms of loss of pastures. In addition, the huge *Eupatorium* biomass is not useful in agriculture and animal husbandry operations. The common species of the genus *Eupatorium* which have been investigated in different parts of the world are *E. adenophorum*, *E. glandulosum* common name: crofton weed, *E. odoratum* common name: siam weed, *E. riparium*, *E. rugosum* and *E. inulifolium*.

Eupatorium spp. are known to have a number of adverse interactions with livestock and humans. There is a lot of variation in the chemistry of the natural products of the different species of the *Eupatorium* genus. So, different toxicosis syndromes have been observed in different parts of the world. The clinical signs on ingestion of various *Eupatorium* spp. by grazing animals and experimental animals, and the present knowledge about the nature of the toxins, are summarized in Table 1.

Table 1. Toxicosis of different species of *Eupatorium*

Plant	Animal affected	Clinical signs/lesions	Toxin(s)	Reference
E. adenophorum	Horses	Coughing, heaving respiration, exercise intolerance	Not identified	O'Sullivan (1985)
	Cattle	Anorexia, photosensitization	Not identified	Verma *et al.*, (1987)
	Mice	Jaundice, hepatotoxicity	9-oxo-10,11, dehydroagerohporone	Oelrichs *et al.*, (1995)
	Rats	Jaundice, cholestasis, hepatotoxicity	Not identified	Katoch *et al.*, (2000), Kaushal *et al.*, (2001)
	Rats	Hepatotoxicity, cholestasis	9-oxo-10,11, dehydroagerohporone	Bhardwaj *et al.*, (2001)
	Mice	Jaundice, cholestasis, hepatotoxicity	Not identified	Singh *et al.*, (2012)

Plant	Animal affected	Clinical signs/lesions	Toxin(s)	Reference
E. riparium	Horses	Same as for *E. adenophorum*	Not identified	Gibson and O'Sullivan (1984)
E. rugosum	Cattle	Trembles, acetone breath, constipation, difficult respiration, profuse nasal discharge	-	Beier and Norman (1990)
	Horse	Unsteady gait, difficulty in swallowing, acetone breath, cardiac arrhythmias, constipation, trembling of muscles	-	White *et al.*, (1985)
	Sheep	Trembles, anorexia, laboured respiration stiffness of limbs, ataxia	Tremetol	Beier and Norman (1990)
	Goats	Depression, anorexia, photosensitization, no trembles	-	Beier and Norman (1990)
	Chicken	Trembles, cyanosis, acetone breath severe acidosis	Tremetol	Beier and Norman (1990)
E. inulifolium	Cattle	Liver cirrhosis	Not identified	Bahri *et al.*, (1988)
	Rats	Hepatotoxicity	Not identified	Bahri *et al.*, (1988)
E. odoratum	Mammal	-	High levels of nitrate, Antinutritional factors	Nwokolo (1987)

Oak

Oak (*Quercus* spp.) tree leaves and twigs, available throughout the year, are often browsed by animals or lopped to be used as livestock fodder during lean periods (Fig. 1D). The common species include *Quercus leucotricophora*, *Q. semicarpifolia* and *Q. dilata*. The toxic effects of oak leaves have been attributed to the presence of tannins which interact with various macromolecules, mainly proteins. The young oak leaves have higher levels of tannins. Oak poisoning has been observed during the months of March-April when young leaves are fed to the animals. Oak toxicity has been reported from Himachal Pradesh and Uttar Pradesh where the leaves form an integral part of livestock feed (Makkar *et al.*, 1986, Sharma *et al.*, 2001). The symptoms of oak toxicity are anorexia, watery nasal discharge, depression, abdominal pain, excessive thirst, rumen stasis, constipation, presence of mucus and sometimes white flakes in the urine, and blood in faeces. The principal lesions of oak toxicity are nephritis and gastritis.

In our laboratories, the pathological effects of experimental chronic toxicity of sole feeding of fresh *Q. leucotricophora* leaves in native Gaddi breed of goats were studied.

The duration of the trial was six weeks. The animals developed signs of toxicity characterized by depression, inappetence, emaciation, ruminal atony, weakness, anaemia, prostration and death. Out of six, two goats died within five weeks of the trial. The necropsy examination revealed severely emaciated carcasses with marked loss of subcutaneous and abdominal fat, and presence of straw-coloured fluid within the peritoneal cavity. The lungs showed diffuse large areas of haemorrhages and patchy consolidation and emphysema. The heart showed pale myocardium and gelatinization of pericardial fat. The kidneys appeared swollen, severely congested with presence of diffuse haemorrhages in the cortex. The liver appeared shrunken, hardened and showed patches of pale areas. The abomasum mucosa was swollen, edematous and showed multiple petechial hemorrhagic spots. The intestines revealed congestion and swollen mucosa. Mesenteric lymph nodes appeared congested, swollen and edematous. On histopathological examination, the renal cortex revealed severe hydropic degeneration in the lining epithelial cells of proximal convoluted tubules. The medulla showed severely congested interstitial blood vessels and presence of protein droplets in the tubules at multiple places. Liver revealed focal degeneration and swelling of hepatocytes. The heart showed severe atrophy of myocardiocytes and edema between the myofiber bundles (Bhar *et al.*, 2013).

Ferns

In India, fern-associated enzootic bovine haematuria (EBH) has been reported from Arunachal Pradesh, Himachal Pradesh, Jammu & Kashmir, Karnataka, Kerala, Nagaland, Sikkim, Tamil Nadu, Uttarakhand, Uttar Pradesh and West Bengal. This information is mainly based on the reports in Veterinary Hospitals. In a recent survey (Sharma, 2011, unpublished data), the following ferns were identified in the Chohar valley of Himachal Pradesh where EBH is endemic: *Pteris vittata* L., *Thelypteris erubescens* (Wall.ex Hook.) Ching, *Pseudocyclosorus canus* (Baker) Holttm & Grimes, *Hypolepis punctata* (Thunb.) Mett., *Pteris wallichiana Ag*, *Pseudophegopteris pyrrorhachis subsp. Laterepens, Dryopteris nigropaleacea (Fraser-Jenkins), Pteris pseudo-quadriaurita Khullar, Onchyium contiguum Wall., Polystium stimulans, Pteridium aquilinum* (bracken fern).

Besides causing EBH in cattle and associated environmental and human effects of ptaquiloside of the bracken fern (Sharma *et al.*, 2013), these ferns are also responsible for inducing toxicity in grazing animals (Fig. 1E). Toxicity has been reported in both ruminants and non-ruminants. Among the non-ruminants, horses, mules and pigs have been known to be affected in natural episodes of bracken poisoning. The effect of bracken poisoning is essentially those of vitamin B1 (thiamine) deficiency. The symptoms observed in horses and mules include in-coordination, staggering, muscular tremor, generalised congestion, pulmonary oedema, serosal & mucosal haemorrhages. The symptoms in pigs are characterized by loss of appetite, vomiting and constipation. Death occurs due to damage to the heart. The toxicity of bracken fern to non-ruminants has been ascribed to presence of thiaminase (EC 3.5, 99.2) in the fern which destroys vitamin B1 resulting in the deficiency of the vitamin and symptoms that respond to vitamin B1 therapy if started at an early stage.

The thiaminase activity in *Chelianthus sieberi* has been reported to be many times higher than that of *Pteridum aquilinum* (Chick *et al.*, 1985). Other ferns such as *Equisetum palustre* L and *Equisetum arvense* also cause toxicity in these species due to the presence of thiaminase. Biochemical changes are those of thiamine deficiency with hypoglycemia during the latent period and reduced tolerance to carbohydrates. There is an increase in plasma concentration of oxalic acid, phosphate and potassium and increased activity of alkaline phosphatase and elevated plasma cholinesterase. All biochemical changes respond to treatment with vitamin B1 (Wintzer, 1986). Pathological changes include atrophic degeneration of neurons in the cortex, caudate nucleus and corpora quadrigemina and loss of Purkinje cells in the cerebellum with proliferation of glial cells and haemorrhages. There is also hepatic and myocardial degeneration (Wintzer, 1986).

The toxicity symptoms in ruminants are characterized by an acute haemorrhage syndrome. The main symptom is progressive failure of blood forming bone marrow tissue. There is thrombocytopenia resulting in the increase in blood coagulation time (Evans, 1968). Unlike in non-ruminants, it is not vitamin B1 deficiency and it doesn't respond to thiamine treatment. The disease is noticed sporadically, mainly in young stock. They exhibit loss of appetite, watery discharge from eyes and nostrils, swelling of throat and difficult breathing, high temperature and death within 3 to 5 days. The symptoms in adult cattle include lack of appetite, watery discharge from eyes and nostrils, cessation of rumination, weak pulse and temperature, blood-tinged discharges, laboured respiration and constipation, blood in feces, dark urine sometimes containing blood.

Poisoning with the fern *Dryopteris filixmas* and *Dryopteris borreii* has been reported in cows reared in pastures containing these ferns. Affected animals showed anorexia and were found standing and later lying blind and comatose (MaCleod *et al.*, 1978). The lesions at necropsy included petechiation on the epicardium and major blood vessels; infarcts in the mouth, and ulcers in the oesophagus, omasum, caecum and colon; Zebra crossing (striped appearance) in small intestine and anterior colon; and focal retinal haemorrhages and scleral congestion (MaCleod *et al.*, 1978). Aplin *et al.*, (1983) have reported that *Chelianthus distans, C. sieberi, C. tenuifloia, Lindsaea linearis, Marsilea durmmondi, Pteridium aquilinum* and *Platysoma microphyllum* are toxic to animals. These ferns contain thiaminase and may contain other toxic constituents.

EBH is a disease of cattle that is characterized by the intermittent presence of blood in urine caused by malignant lesions in the urinary bladder. The disease causes anemia, progressive emaciation, and death. This neoplastic disease is primarily caused by chronic ingestion of ferns, and affliction with the papillomavirus is often associated with it. Two comprehensive reviews on the disease have been published (Dawra and Sharma, 2001; Sharma *et al.*, 2013). The erythrocyte membrane enzymes and chemical constituents were studied in animals presenting EBH and in normal animals. There were significant decreases in Mg^{2+}-ATPase, Na^{+}, K^{+} activity in erythrocyte membranes of the EBH-affected animals as compared to that of the control group.

The cholesterol: phospholipid and sialic acid: phospholipid ratios also decreased in animals suffering EBH (Dawra *et al*., 1988). A comparative study of areas where the disease is prevalent (enzootic), and where it is absent (non-enzootic), to determine the type of vegetation (including ferns), the grazing patterns, the animal husbandry practices and the agroclimatic conditions in animal-plant interaction was conducted (Dawra *et al*., 1989). Most of the ferns were common to both enzootic and non-enzootic areas. Bracken fern, a known source of carcinogens was present in both enzootic and non-enzootic areas. The authors concluded that different environmental conditions and animal husbandry practices may result in the cattle in the enzootic areas being exposed to carcinogenic brackens and other ferns at a time when there is a shortage of other alternative feedstuffs. For the first time, a fern other than bracken, *Onchyium contiguum*, was found capable of producing urinary bladder lesions and intestinal tumors in guinea pigs. *O. contiguum* may contribute significantly to the development of bovine urinary bladder tumors and haematuria under field conditions (Dawra *et al*., 2001). In one of the studies, the fern, *P. aquilinum* was collected from an area where cases of EBH had not been recorded. In these areas, animals were left for grazing during the rainy season. This fern when fed to guinea pigs for 30 months at the rate of 30% (w/w) produced toxicity and neoplastic changes in urinary bladders of the exposed animals. The incidence of tumours was 18.6%. The fern was found positive for the carcinogen ptaquiloside (3.74 ± 0.6 mg/kg). The low level of ptaquiloside as compared to the values reported from elsewhere (0 to 9,776 mg/kg; mean 1,257 mg/kg) and grazing during the period when grasses are abundant were perhaps the reasons for absence of the disease in such areas (Dawra *et al*., 2002).

In a recent study, the disease pattern was studied in Himachal Pradesh. Field surveys were conducted in Kangra, Mandi, Kullu, Chamba, Shimla and Lahaul & Spiti districts of Himachal Pradesh. Out of the total 103 plant samples collected, a total of 95 samples were identified as ferns. The major ferns identified included, *Onychium japonicum* (Thunb.) Kunze, *Polystichum piceopaleaceum*Tagawa, *Dryopteris juxtaposita*Christ, *Pseudocyclosorus canus (Baker)* Holttum & J.W. Grimes, *Onychium contiguum* C.Hope, *Dryopteris nigropaleacea* (Fraser-Jenk.), *Pteridium aquilinum* (L.) Kuhn, *Diplazium esculentum* (Retz.) Sw., *Allantodia maxima (D. Don) Ching*, *Woodwardia unigemmata* (Makino) Nakai, *Pteris cretica* L., *Pteris vittata* L., *Asplenium trichomanes* L., *Thelypteris phegopteris* (L.) Sloss. ex Rydb, *Adiantum venustum* D.Don and *Paraceterach vestita* (Hook.) R.M. Tryon. The concentration of ptaquiloside (PTA) and pterosin B (PtB) in some of the ferns collected from Kullu and Chamba regions ranged from 0 to 358.6±70.5 µg/g and 0 to 652.4±50.0µg/g, respectively. In addition, field cases of the disease in cattle were also studied in the EBH-endemic districts. A total of sixteen cattle urine samples and one urinary bladder of EBH affected cattle were collected. On physical, chemical (benzidine test) and microscopic examination of urine sediment, all the sixteen field samples were found to be positive for erythrocytes and the cases were diagnosed as macro haematuria. The clinico-pathological studies on the field cases and the presence of PTA and PtB in the ferns indicated that EBH is a prevalent disease and that there is an association between chronic fern ingestion and EBH in cattle. A case of transitional cell adenocarcinoma with chronic lymphocytic cystitis was diagnosed in cattle (Rai *et al.*, 2017).

Conclusions

Plant toxicity in animals is one of the major hindrances in the growth of the animal husbandry sector, particularly in North-Western India. The spread of lantana, eupatorium, ageratum and ferns is so extensive that eradication is very difficult. Under these circumstances, it is important to make use of the biomass of these plants and simultaneously develop strategies for combating toxicosis. No systemic database on plant toxicosis exists in India. These databases need to be prepared to get the exact figures of plant toxicosis so that effective strategies may be worked out to prevent it.

References

Alfonso HA, Rivera M, Aparicio JM, Ancisar J, Marrero E, Cabrera JM (1989) Natural and experimental poisoning by Ageratum houstonianum Mill. in cattle. Revista Cubana de Ciencias Veterias 20: 113-120.

Aplin TEH, Steele P, Nottle MC (1983) Toxic ferns of Western Australia, South Perth 6151, Western Australia, Dept. Agril. Jurral Road. 15 pages Technical Bulletin 63.

Arbat A, Patil GV (1985) Common allergenic pollens and spores causing respiratory allergy from Central India, Nagpur. Journal of Society of Pure Applied Natural Science 1: 5-7.

Bahri S, Stoltz DR, Paramardini D (1988) Hepatotoxic effect of Eupatorium *inulifolium* in the rat. Penyakit Hewan 20: 88-90.

Beier RC, Norman JO (1990) The toxic factor in white snakeroot: identity, analysis and prevention. Veterinary and Human Toxicology 32:81-88.

Bhar R, Ajith MK, Sharma R, Kannan A, Singh B, Bhat TK (2013) Chronic toxicity in Gaddi goats fed on Quercus *leucotricophora* leaves as sole feed. Proceedings of the 100thIndian Science Congress, Section of Animal, Veterinary and Fishery Sciences, Kolkata 3-7th January, 2013 pg. 329-330.

Bhardwaj R, Singh A, Sharma OP, Dawra RK, Kurade NP, Mahato SB (2001). Hepatotoxicity and cholestasis in rats Induced by the sesquiterpene, 9-oxo-1 0,11-dehydroageraphorone, isolated from E. *adenophorum*. Journal of Biochemical and Molecular Toxicology 15: 279-286.

Chick BF, Quinn C, McCleary BV (1985) Pteridophyte intoxication of livestock in Australia. In: Plant Toxicology, Proceedings of the Australia-USA Poisonous Plants Symposium, Brisbane, 1984 [edited by Seawright, A.A.; Heagarty, M.P.; James, L.F.; Keeler, R.F.] Queensland Poisonous Plants Committee Queensland, Department of primary Industries Animal research institute, Yeerogpilly, Queensland, pp. 453-464.

Day MD, Wiley CJ, Playford J, Zalucki MP (2003). Lantana: Current management status and future prospects. Australian Center for International Agricultural Research, Canberra.

Dayson R (1989). A guide to noxious north coast weeds. BGF-Bulletin 53: 13–16.

Ekundayo O, Sharma A, Rao EV (1988) Essential oil of A. conyzoides. Planta Medica 54: 55-57.

Evans IA (1968) The radiomimetic nature of bracken toxin. Cancer Research 28: 2252-2261.

Ghisalberti EL (2000) Lantana *camara* L. (Verbenaceae). Fitoterapia 71: 467–486.

Gibson JA, O'Sullivan BM (1984) Lung lesions in horses fed mist flower (Eupatorium riparium). Australian Veterinary Journal 61: 271.

Gopinath C, Ford EJH (1969) The effect of Lantana *camara* on liver of sheep. Pathology 99: 75–85.

Hammond AH, Garle MJ, Fry JR (1995) Journal of Biochemical Toxicology 10:265.

James LF (1984) Solving poisonous plant problems by a team approach. In: Plant associated toxins, Agricultural, Phytochemical and ecological aspects, S.M. Colgate, and P.R. Dorling, eds., pp. 1-6. CAB International Wallingford, U.K.

Katoch R, Sharma OP, Dawra RK, Kurade NP (2000) Hepatotoxicity of E. *adenophorum* to rats. Toxicon 38: 309-314.

Kaushal V, Dawra RK, Sharma OP, Kurade NP (2001) Biochemical Alterations in the Blood Plasma of Rats Associated with Hepatotoxicity Induced by Eupatorium *adenophorum*. Veterinary Research Communications 25: 601-608.

Kharwal M (2017) Evaluation of berberine in lantadene -induced toxicity in guinea pigs. M.V.Sc. thesis submitted to Deemed University, ICAR-Indian Veterinary Research Institute, Izatnagar, UP, India.

Kumar R (2015) Toxicopathological effects of sub-chronic exposure to lantadenes of Lantana *camara* in guinea pigs. M.V.Sc. thesis submitted to Deemed University, ICAR-Indian Veterinary Research Institute, Izatnagar, UP, India.

Lal M, Kalra DB (1960) Lantana poisoning in domesticated animals Lantana poisonining domesticated animals. Indian Veterinary Journal 37: 263–269.

MaCleod NSM, Greig A, Bonn JM and Angus KW (1978) Poisoning of cattle associated with Dryopteris flix-max. Veterinary Record 102: 239-240.

Makker HPS, Singh B, Dawra RK (1986) Can oak leaves be fed to animals? Farmers and Parliament 24: 17-18.

McSweeney CS, Pass MA (1983) The mechanism of ruminal stasis in lantana poisoned sheep. Q J. Exper. Physiol. Cogn. Med. Sci. 68: 301– 313.

Negi GC (1988). Problems of Lantana and Ageratum in Himachal Pradesh - an overview. In: Singh, C. M. and Angiras, N.N. (eds), Proceedings of the Seminar on Control of Lantana and Ageratum, HPKV, Palampur, pp. 1-5.

Nwokolo E (1987). Leaf meals of cassava (Manihot *esculenta* Crantz) and siam weed (E. odoratum L.) as nutrient sources in poultry diets. Nutrition Report International 36: 819-825.

Oelrichs PB, Calanasan CA, MacLeod JK, Seawright AA, Ng JC (1995) The isolation of a compound from Eupatorium *adenophorum* (Spreng.) (Ageratina *adenophora* (Spreng.) causing hepatotoxicity in mice. Natural Toxins 3: 350-354.

O'Sullivan BM (1985) Investigations into Crofton weed (Eupatorium *adenophorum*) toxicity in horses. Australian Veterinary Journal 62: 30-32.

Parimoo HA, Sharma R (2014) Orally induced sub-acute toxicity of lantadenes of Lantana *camara* in guinea pigs: a haematological study. J Pathol Toxicol 1: 12-15. Parimoo HA, Sharma R, Patil RD, Patial V (2015) Sub-acute toxicity of lantadenes isolated from Lantana *camara* leaves in guinea pig animal model. Comp Clin Pathol 24(6): 1541-1552.

Pass MA (1991) Poisoning of livestock by lantana plants. In: Handbook of Natural Toxins, Toxicology of Plant and Fungal Compounds R. Keeler, and T. Anthony, eds., Marcel Dekker, Inc., New York 6: 297–311.

Pass MA, McSweeney CS, Reynoldson JA (1981) Absorption of the toxins of Lantana camara L. from the digestive system of sheep. Journal of Applied Toxicology 1: 38–42.

Rai SK, Sharma R, Kumari A, Rasmussen LH, Patil RD, Bhar R (2017) Survey of ferns and clinico-pathological studies on the field cases of Enzootic Bovine Haematuria in Himachal Pradesh, a North-Western Himalayan State of India. Toxicon DOI 10.1016/j. toxicon.2017.08.010

Seawright AA, Allen JG (1972) Pathology of the liver and kidney in lantana poisoning of cattle. Australian Veterinary Journal 48: 323–331.

Sharma OP (1994) Plant toxicosis in north-western India. In: Plant associated toxins, Agricultural, Phytochemical and ecological aspects, S.M. Colgate, and P.R. Dorling, eds., pp. 19–24. CAB International Wallingford, U.K.

Sharma OP, Makkar HPS (1981) Lantana-the foremost livestock killer in Kangra district of Himachal Pradesh. Livestock Advisor 6: 29–31.

Sharma OP, Sharma S, Pattabhi V, Mahato SB, Sharma PD (2007) A Review of the Hepatotoxic Plant Lantana camara. Critical Reviews in Toxicology 37: 313-352.

Sharma OP, Vaid J, Pattabhi V, Bhutani KK (1992) Biological action of lantadene C, a new hepatotoxicant from Lantana *camara* var. aculeala. Journal of Biochemical and Molecular Toxicology 7: 73–79.

Sharma R, Bhat TK, Sharma OP (2013). The environmental and human effects of ptaquiloside-induced enzootic bovine haematuria: a tumorous disease of cattle. Reviews of Environmental Contamination and Toxicology 224: 53-95.

Sharma, R, Mandial RK, Gupta VK (2001) Oak poisoning in a cow- a case report. Indian Veterinary Journal 78:1054-1055.

Singh YD, Mukhopadhyay SK, Shah MAA, Ali MA, Tolenkhomba TC (2012) Pathology of E. adenophorum (Sticky snakeroot) toxicity in mice. International Multidisciplinary Research Journal 2:16-21.

Stirton CH (1977) Some thoughts on the polyploidy complex Lantana *camara* L. (verbenecae). Proc. 2nd National Weeds Conference., Balkenia, pp. 321-340.

Verma A, Yadava BPS, Sampath KT (1987). Possible use of Eupatorium *adenophorum* Spreng. in animal feeding. Indian Journal of Animal Nutrition 4: 189-192.

White JL, Shivaprasad HL, Thompson U, Buck WB (1985) White snakeroot (Eupatorium *rugosum*) poisoning. Clinical effects associated with cardiac and skeletal muscle lesions in experimental equine toxicosis. In: Seawright AA Hegarty MP, James LF, Keeler RF, eds. Plant Toxicology. Melbourne: Dominion Press, Hedges & Bell, 411-422.

Wintzer HJ (1986) Equine Diseases, Verlag Paul Parley, Berlin. pp. 415-416.

22

Agro-industrial Wastes as Animal Feed for Economic Livestock Production

Gauri Jairath, Devi Gopinath, Sudesh Radotra
Gorakh Mal and Birbal Singh
ICAR-IVRI, Regional Station, Palampur-176061, Himachal Pradesh

Introduction

Though, India is bestowed with large livestock population (512.05 million) to which cattle buffaloes, goats and sheep contribute 190.90, 108.70, 135.2 and 65.07 numbers in millions, respectively (DADF, 2018), but at the same time, facing with a great shortage of crop residues, greens and concentrates for animal sustainability (NIANP, 2013). The shortage of these conventional feeds and fodders tropical and sub-tropical regions has already been documented and well recognized (Maneerat *et al*., 2015). The feed and fodder resources are gradually decreasing throughout India owing to many factors like shrinkage of common property resources and shift towards the cultivation of commercial crops etc. (Biradar and Kumar, 2013). Based on feed production and feed requirement calculated as above, India falls short by 219.2 Mt of green fodder and 226.73 MT of dry fodder (Earagariyanna *et al*., 2017). India faces a green fodder shortage of 63.5 percent and a dry fodder shortage of 23.5 percent and if the current situation continues then India's green fodder shortage will reach 66 percent and dry fodder will reach 25 percent by 2030 (Jitendra, 2017). This scenario demands the utilization of alternate non-conventional feed resources to sustain and economize livestock farming. The issues can be addressed by those unconventional resources like agricultural wastes which are widely available at low or zero cost and too with minimal treatment may serve as potential nutritional feeding material for animals.

Agriculture wastes are the residues or the byproducts which are left behind after growing, harvesting, or processing of raw agriculture products like fruits, vegetables, meat, poultry, dairy products and crops. Thus, can be classified into different categories, such as crop waste and residues, byproducts from fruit and vegetable-processing industry, sugar, starch and confectionary industry byproducts, byproducts from grain and legume-milling industry and oil industry and byproducts from distilleries and breweries. The handling and technologies used for the processing of agro-wastes are mainly based on their type (Ajila *et al*., 2012). The composition of these wastes is quite variable and depends upon the type and extent of processing (Obi *et al*., 2016). Generally, these wastes are discarded on landfills if not fed to ruminants, which result in environmental load (Mirzaei-Aghsaghali and

Maheri-Sis, 2008). Agricultural-based industries like fruit juice industries, cereal industries, coffee industries produce a huge lot of residues every year, which mostly remain underutilized or untreated and thus create a disposal problem resulting in a great environmental load which is very difficult to estimate (Obi *et al.*, 2016; Rodríguez Couto, 2008; Sadh *et al.*, 2018).

For example, world-wide total apple production in 2017 was 83.1 million metric tons and generally, 20-25% is processed, where juice factories share 65% of the total processed apples and generate apple pomace in several million metric tons every year (Kammerer *et al.*, 2014; Lyu *et al.*, 2020). The recovery rate of later in the form of animal feed or dry product is quite low (1%) (Shalini and Gupta, 2010) and mostly disposed directly to the soil in a landfill or burned road side (Bajar *et al.*, 2020). This land disposal directly increases the environmental load due to high biodegradable organic load (chemical and biochemical oxygen demand) of apple pomace (Bhushan *et al.*, 2008; Perussello *et al.*, 2017; Shalini and Gupta, 2010; Singha and Muthukumarappan, 2018). The high moisture content and total soluble carbohydrates of apple pomace make it very perishable and fermentable (Bhushan *et al.*, 2008). Similarly, spent mushroom compost, the residue of mushroom growing industry which use mushroom substrate composed of sawdust, corn cob, and rice bran, etc. is either dumped on road side or used as manure (Chauhan and Sharma, 2015). Likewise, many agro-industrial wastes are dumped which are directly contributing towards environmental load and public health hazards too (Bhushan *et al.*, 2008). Thus, effective utilization of these waste in the form of animal feed may give returns to farmers as feed alone comprises 60-70% of total cost of animal production (Sagar *et al.*, 2009; Sindhu *et al.*, 2002). Formulation of least-cost rations, by exploring the use of more economical alternative sources is need based research area in current scenario.

The above-mentioned issues like fodder shortfall, agro-industrial associated environmental pollution and higher feeding cost can be well addressed in an integrated way by using these wastes as livestock feed. Many researchers have worked over the feeding of agriculture wastes to livestock e.g., olive cake to ewes, cucumber and tomato wastes in dairy goats, pomegranate seed pulp in goat kids, pomegranate byproduct silage in growing lambs, olive cake in lambs (Emami *et al.*, 2015; Kotsampasi *et al.*, 2014; Luciano *et al.*, 2013; Modaresi *et al.*, 2011; Romero-Huelva *et al.*, 2012; Vargas-Bello-Pérez *et al.*, 2013).

Therefore, recovering byproducts to use as animal feed can help the agro-industry to save money by reducing waste discharges, cutting waste-management costs and also preventing environmental pollution. Most of the agro-residues offer an inexpensive source of nutrients as compared to traditional feeds and also support acceptable animal performance (Ajila *et al.*, 2012). Thus, these wastes can be used as an economic nutritional feed resource to the animals and would definitely aid in enhancing the livelihood of farmers. Further, both environmental and economic issues can be resolved by utilizing food industrial by-products as animal feed (Tufarelli *et al.*, 2013). This chapter will focus over on the various agro-industrial wastes, their composition and limiting factors that hinder their use as livestock feed.

Agro-industrial wastes as non-conventional feed sources

About 1.3 billion tonnes that account for one third of the total food produced for human consumption is either lost or wasted annually out of which 40-50% i.e., 520–650 million tonnes of wastage is contributed by fruits and vegetables, plus roots and tubers. The European Union contributes 89 million tonnes of food wastage every year, 39% of which is due to manufacturing processes and 367 million tonnes of total agricultural residue production per year which are either crop residues, or parts of cropped plants that are not consumed as food (Ravindran *et al*., 2018).

In India, approximately, 20% of the total fruit and vegetables production have been reported to be wasted every year which mainly includes apple, cotton, soy bean, and wheat being the larger producer of the same (Rudra *et al*., 2015). The increase in wastage is directly linked up with the increase in production rate (Sadh *et al*., 2018). Thus, thousands of tonnes of these agricultural byproducts viz. sugarcane bagasse, citrus bagasse, fruit peel, corn straw, and corncobs are generated from agro-industrial activities which consequently increase the BOD, COD, and other suspended solids (Sadh *et al*., 2018) in the environment. The percentage of wastes that comes from fruits and vegetable processing have been detailed in table 1 and may be utilized as a non-conventional feed source for the livestock. Further, table 2 briefs the characteristics and utilization of some non-conventional feed resources.

Table 1: Percentage of wastes generated from different fruits and vegetable processing (Ajila et al., 2012).

S. No.	Fruits/vegetables	Residues	Percentage of wastes
1.	Apple	Peel, pomace, seed	25
2.	Mango	Peel, stones	45
3.	Citrus	Peel, rag, seed	50
4.	Tomato	Skin, core, seed	20
5.	Pineapple	Skin, core	33
6.	Grape	Stem, skin, seed	20
7.	Guava	Peel, core, seed	10
8.	Potato	Peel	15
9.	Onion	Outer leaves	10
10.	Banana	Peel	35
11.	Pea	shell	40

Table 2: Characteristics and utilization of some non-conventional feed resources (Devendra, 1987)

Agro-industrial residues	Characteristics	Targeted animal as feed
Rice Bran, coconut cake, soyabean meal, poultry litter	High energy and high protein	Poutry, pigs, ducks, cattle
Cassava peels, cereal grain waste, animal waste	High energy and high protein	Pigs, ducks, cattle

Nonconventional food sources are those which have neither been used before in animal feeding nor in commercially prepared rations for animals and mainly consist of a variety of feed from perennial crops like palm press fiber (oil palm byproducts), single-cell proteins, feed materials derived from agro-industrial byproducts of plant origin, poor-quality cellulosic roughages from farm residues, such as slaughterhouse byproducts and byproducts from processing of sugar, cereal grains, citrus fruits and vegetables from the processing of food for human consumption (Devendra, 1987). The below mentioned characteristics are those which are mainly applicable to non-conventional food sources (Ajila *et al.*, 2012)

1. They are mainly organic and can be in a solid, slurry, or liquid form.
2. Their economic value is often less than the cost of their collection and transformation for use, and consequently, they are discharged as wastes.
3. Nonconventional food sources are generally excellent sources of fermentable carbohydrates e.g., cassava and sweet potato.
4. Fruit byproducts like apple pomace have sugars which are energetically very beneficial.
5. Most of the nonconventional food sources are bulky, poor-quality cellulosic roughage with a high crude fiber (CF) and low nitrogen contents, suitable for feeding to ruminants.
6. Some of these feeds have deleterious and toxic effects on animals and there is not enough information about the nature of the active principles and ways to detoxify these effects.
7. They have considerable potential as feed materials by the modern technological applications.
8. Further information is needed on chemical composition, nutritive value, toxic factors, and value in feeding systems.

These waste residues can either be fed as such to the livestock or after value addition through processing like fermentation. On similar lines, agro-industrial waste residues like sunflower seed hull (SSH), brewer's spent grain (BSG) and sugar beet pulp (SBP) were bioprocessed in to value-added ruminant feed and found that the fermented SBP, SSH and BSG together with immobilized pro-biotic biomass have great potential for use as a probiotic enriched source of nutrients in compounded ruminant feeds due to favorable probiotic characteristics of *Lactobacillus paracasei* (Mladenović *et al.*, 2019).

Types of agro-industrial wastes

There are different types of agro-industrial wastes and can mainly be categorized into agricultural residues and Industrial residues which have been discussed below:

Agricultural residues

Agriculture residues are of two types. First type is field residues which are present in the field after the process of crop harvesting and include stems, stalks, leaves and seed pods. Gram husk, arhar, urad, moong and masoor chunies are the most commonly available by-products used for feeding the animals (Verma, 1997) and second type is process residues that are produced after crop processing and include husks, seeds, roots, bagasse and molasses. Both can be well utilized as livestock feed (Sadh *et al.*, 2018). For example, ground straw can be safely fed with wheat bran and can sufficiently meet the nutritional requirements of a lactating cow producing up to 5L of milk/day (Ranjhan, 1993).

However, its high content of phosphorous and crude fiber (38%) inhibit feed intake during summer season, but may be overcome by sprinkling a mixture of molasses and diammonium phosphate or preferably a balanced liquid supplement on chopped groundnut straw (Maglad *et al.*, 1986). Maize husk can be incorporated up to 50% of the dry roughage portion in the rations of adult non-producing cattle (Ranjhan, 1993). Similarly, wheat bran is a well-known protein rich ingredient while formulating livestock feed and contains about 10% DCP, 65% TDN, 0.07% calcium and 0.35% phosphorus. It can be incorporated up to 50% of TMR for young calves and can also be fed to sick animals without any ill effects (Verma, 1997). Moreover, amino acid balance of wheat bran is much better than whole wheat. It is a rich repository of water-soluble vitamins, except niacin and phosphorous content, though low in calcium (Cheeke, 1999). Wheat middlings have digestible energy than bran as have lower fiber and higher flour contents and contain 10-14% crude protein and 9.5% crude (Cheeke, 1999). Rice husks which 8 to 11% water, 15.6 to 22.6% ash, 14.5 to 17.5% acid insoluble ash, 2.9 to 3.6% crude protein, 0.8 to 1.2% ether extract, 39 to 42% crude fiber and 25 to 29% nitrogen free extract not palatable (Ranjhan, 1993) and should be used as a part of ration (Deschard *et al.*, 1988) and always be mixed with concentrates. Rice bran, an excellent source of energy and a rich repository of vitamin B-complex has high oil content (13%) (Cheeke, 1999) and is a good feed for Livestock. Furthermore, maize gluten feed is a rich source of protein (45 to 48%) and very useful for livestock feeding (Verma, 1997).

Industrial residues

Sugar and fruit and vegetable industries are the two main industries whose left overs are a quite nutritious and potential source of feed. Both have been discussed below in detail:

Sugar Industry

Cane and sugar beet are the main raw materials for sugar industry and harvesting of later results in beets and beet roots. which accounts for 2.5-5% of beets. These residues which are generated while harvesting is either sold directly to the farmer for animal feeding or mixed with cleaned beat or beat pulp. The yield of pulp is 5% and is a nutritive livestock feedstuff which can be either fed as such with dry matter content of 10-12% or pressed to dry matter content of 20-25% or in dried form with 88-90% dry matter content. Further juice processing to finished purified and crystalized product i.e., sugar result in scums and molasses generation as residues. Molasses are further used in animal nutrition which is well documented (Bodas *et al.*, 2007; Mirzaei-Aghsaghali and Maheri-Sis, 2008).

Fruit and vegetable industry

Fruit pomace is the main left over of fruit industry containing pulp and seed and can be fed to the animals to a certain extent. For example, pineapple waste has also been found suitable for feeding of draught animals as a source of energy together with maize grain, wheat bran, and molasses (Verma, 1997). Similarly, citrus pulp can replace one-third of animal feed mixture without ill effects on the health and utilization of nutrients in buffaloes and contains a high level of soluble sugars with a digestibility of 85%, contains about 6.0% CP (NRC, 2001; Wadhwa and Bakshi, 2013).

A study in Philippines on 5000 feedlot beef cattle which were raised on fresh as well as ensiled pineapple wastes containing peel, pomace, and leaves, revealed that 90% waste material and 10% concentrate mixture when fed to animals, a growth rate of 600–700 gm /day was achieved in growing and finishing steers (Ranjhan, 1993). Mango byproducts, such as mango-seed kernels contain 6% DCP and 70% TDN, and 5–7% tannin and can also be used as an ingredient in livestock rations (Sanon and Kanwe, 2010). The dried apple pomace contains 7.7 % protein (CP) and 5.0 % ether extract (EE) and has 1.86 Mcal metabolizable energy (ME)/kg DM and 1.06−1.12 Mcal net energy (NE)/kg DM for lactating dairy cows (NRC, 2001). It can be best incorporated at 15% incorporation in diet and can be incorporated up to 30%. The ensiled apple pomace, incorporated up to 30 percent in the diet of lactating multiparous Holstein cows, did not show any adverse effects on milk yield or its composition. However, the best feed conversion ratio was observed at 15 percent incorporation in the diet (Ghoreishi *et al.*, 2007).

The vegetable-based industries like baby corn, pea, tomato wastes, etc. produce a huge amount of wastes. Baby corn cob has a 15% of edible portion and 85% of inedible i.e., outer peels with a silky thread like structure called baby corn husk which is a waste material and a pollutant. The other leftover includes tassels and green plant material such as baby corn fodder. Fresh baby corn husk (BCH) contained 11.7% CP and 1.8% EE and can be fed either fresh or ensiled BCH as both all highly acceptable and palatable. Moreover, both are comparable with conventional maize fodder (Bakshi and Wadhwa, 2012; Wadhwa and Bakshi, 2013). Similarly, baby corn fodder's daily DM intake, nutrient utilization, purine nitrogen index and N-retention all comparable to conventional maize fodder when fed ad libitum alone or with other feedstuffs as a total mixed ration to adults. However, same study showed that digestibility of nutrients, total volatile fatty acid (TVFAs) production and ME availability are significantly higher for baby corn (Bakshi *et al.*, 2017; Wadhwa *et al.*, 2018). Pea vine is the left-over plant after harvesting the vegetable and can be fed as fresh or ensiled. The digestion kinetic parameters for DM of fresh pea vines revealed that it had 60.8% degradable fraction, with effective and true degradability of 52.3 and 75.1%. The *in-vitro* gas production study revealed the presence of 41.7% NDF digestibility, 64.1% OM digestibility and 7.1Mcal ME/kg DM in pea vines (Wadhwa and Bakshi, 2005). However, the ensiled pea vines have been reported to contain 13 percent CP and 3.3 percent EE with 2.09 Mcal ME/kg DM and 1.28 Mcal NE/kg DM for lactating dairy cows (NRC, 1989). Further, pea pods, the left-over material after extracting pea are quite palatable and nutritious containing 19.8% crude protein and high total soluble sugars, total phenolics and macro and microelements (Wadhwa *et al.*, 2006). Furthermore, pea straw that is dried leftover after harvesting sweet peas contains 5–10% CP, 53–63% NDF and 7–12% minerals, notably calcium. Thus, owing to higher protein content and less fibre, it has higher nutritive value than cereal straws (Wadhwa and Bakshi, 2013). Tomato waste combined of culled tomatoes and tomato pomace. a waste of tomato can also be used as a part of animal feed up to 35% level and contains 14.3% DCP and 65% TDN (Ranjhan, 1993; Verma, 1997).

Other agro-industrial wastes

Byproducts of guar gum, starch, lemongrass oil industry are also the potential sources of livestock feed. Guar gum industry byproduct contains 42.52% DCP and 83.49% TDN and is being used as a cattle feed (Verma, 1997). Starch industry byproducts are quite proteinaceous source of cattle feeding (Ranjhan, 1993). Lemongrass oil industry byproducts are more nutritious than straw and contain 0.64% DCP and 49.76% TDN and can be fed to livestock (Cheeke, 1999). Similarly, tapioca wastes containing 2.0% DCP and 64% TDN on dry matter basis have been successfully used in growing and lactating animals (Ranjhan, 1993).

Nutritional aspects of agro-industrial wastes

Fibrous residues and brans are two types of agro-industrial residues in terms of nutritional aspects. Fibrous residues can be of high digestibility or low. The examples of high digestible fibrous residues include citrus pulp, corn gluten bran, soy husk, and brewing residues (barley), and those with low digestibility include sugarcane bagasse, cereal, corn, soy and cotton straw, cotton husk, soy husk, peanut husk, and harvest remnants of forage grass seeds.

Broadly, nonconventional and agro-industrial byproducts can be divided into three categories (Ajila *et al.*, 2012):

1. Energy-rich feeds which include bananas, citrus fruits, pineapple, sugarcane, and root crop wastes
2. Protein supplements which include oilseed cakes and meals,
3. Byproducts from milling and refining processes which include cereal milling and palm-oil refining

The composition of different agro-industrial wastes has been tabulated in table 3. In addition to the agro-industrial wastes mentioned in table 3, oil industry residues play an important role as livestock feed. The oil industries produce a huge amount of processed residues after oil extraction from the seeds; these residues are known as oil cakes.

Table 3: The composition of various agro-industrial wastes

Agro-industrial waste	Chemical composition (% w/w)				
	Moisture	Ash	Lignin	Cellulose	Hemicellulose
Sugarcane bagasse (El-Tayeb *et al.*, 2012; Singh nee' Nigam *et al.*, 2009)	4.8	1.9	13.4	30.2	56.7
Rice straw (El-Tayeb *et al.*, 2012)	6.58	12.4	36.1	39.2	23.5
Corn stalk (El-Tayeb *et al.*, 2012)	6.40	10.8	6.9	61.2	19.3
Sawdust (El-Tayeb *et al.*, 2012; Martin *et al.*, 2012)	1.12	12	24.2	45.1	28.1
Sugar beet waste (El-Tayeb *et al.*, 2012)	12.4	4.8	25	26.3	18.5
Barley straw (Singh nee' Nigam *et al.*, 2009)	-	11	13.8	33.8	21.9
Cotton stalks (Singh nee' Nigam *et al.*, 2009)	7.45	9.98	21.5	58.5	14.4
Oat straw (Martin *et al.*, 2012)	-	8	17.5	39.4	27.1
Soya stalks (Motte *et al.*, 2013)	11.84	10.39	19.8	34.5	24.8
Sunflower stalk (Motte *et al.*, 2013)	-	11.17	13.4	42.1	29.7
Wheat straw (Martin *et al.*, 2012; Singh nee' Nigam *et al.*, 2009)	7	6.7	8.9	32.9	24.0
Potato peel waste (Al-Weshahy and Rao, 2012)	9.89	7.7	-	2.2	-
Orange peel (Rivas *et al.*, 2008)	11.86	3.5	0.84	9.21	10.5
Coffee skin (Ballesteros *et al.*, 2014)	-	5.36	28.58	23.77	16.68
Pineapple peel (Prabhudessai *et al.*, 2013)	91	-	1.37	18.11	-
Apple pomace (Masood *et al.*, 2018)	77.30	4.73	-	21.23	27.63
Bagasse (Maneerat *et al.*, 2015)	91.64	11.31	14.30	44.19	20.59

(Contd.)

Agro-industrial waste	Chemical composition (% w/w)				
	Moisture	Ash	Lignin	Cellulose	Hemicellulose
Vinasse (Maneerat *et al.*, 2015)	32.85	17.58	-	-	-
Baby corn fodder (Wadhwa and Bakshi, 2013)	7.8	-	-	37.1	28.8

Different cakes which are produced are: canola oil cake, sunflower oil cake, coconut oil cake, sesame oil cake, mustard oil cake, palm kernel cake, soy bean cake, groundnut oil cake, cotton seed cake, olive oil cake, rape seed cake (Ramachandran *et al.*, 2007). These discussed agro-industrial residues are relatively economic rich repositories of proteins and energy (Sadh *et al.*, 2018). Their proximate composition has been detailed in table 4.

Table 4: The proximate composition of various agro-industrial wastes (%w/w) (Sadh *et al.*, 2018)

Oil cakes	Dry matter	Crude protein	Crude fiber	Ash	Calcium	Phosphorous
Canola oil cake	90	33.9	9.7	6.3	0.79	1.06
Coconut oil cake	88.8	25.2	10.8	6.0	0.08	0.67
Cotton seed cake	94.3	40.3	15.7	6.8	0.31	0.11
Groundnut oil cake	92.6	49.5	5.3	4.5	0.11	0.74
Mustard oil cake	89.8	38.5	3.5	9.9	0.05	1.11
Olive oil cake	85.2	6.3	40.0	4.2	-	-
Palm kernel cake	90.8	18.6	37	4.5	0.31	0.85
Sunflower oil cake	91	34.1	13.2	6.6	0.30	1.30

Challenges associated with the use of agro-industrial waste as feed

Nutritional and technological aspects are the two main challenges that come across while using agro-industrial wastes as animal feed (Ravindran and Blair, 1992). Variability in nutritional level and quantity, presence of naturally occurring antinutritional and toxic factors, presence of pathogenic microorganisms and need for nutrient supplementation are the nutritional aspects which need to be tackled. Whereas, technological aspects include seasonal and unbelievable supply, bulkiness, wetness, and /or powdery structure, requirement of further processing and lack of proper research and development efforts. These limiting factors associated with agro-industrial residues are needed to be addressed. Many antinutritional factors have been reported in various agro-industrial wastes that lead to toxicity in animals. Such toxic effects can be avoided by specific treatments of these residues as mentioned in table 5.

Table 5: Antinational factors and ways to neutralize or detoxify these factors (Benerjee, 1993).

Feedstuff	Inhibitor(s) toxins/ antinutritional factors	Deactivation process
Cottonseed meal	Gossypol, cyclopropane fatty acids	Adding iron salts; rupturing pigment gland
Soyabean meal	Trypsin inhibitors an unidentified factor	Heating; autoclaving
Linseed meal	Crystalline water-soluble substance	Water treatment
Raw fish	Thiaminase	Heating
Lucerne meal	Saponins: pectin methyl esterase	Limit amount feed
Groundnut meal	Aflatoxin	Treatment with ammonia or ammonium hydroxide

Conclusions

Efficient utilization of agro-industrial byproducts would not only strengthen the farmers economically but also reduce the environmental load. These byproducts are quite nutritious, but underutilized. Thus, they may be fed directly or in dried form or processed form like after ensiling.

References

Ajila CM, Brar SK, Verma M., Tyagi RD, Godbout S and Valéro JR (2012) Bio-processing of agro-byproducts to animal feed. Critical Reviews in Biotechnology 32(4): 382–400. https://doi.org/10.3109/07388551.2012.659172

Al-Weshahy A and Rao VA (2012) Potato Peel as a Source of Important Phytochemical Antioxidant Nutraceuticals and Their Role in Human Health—A Review. Phytochemicals as Nutraceuticals - Global Approaches to Their Role in Nutrition and Health. https://doi.org/10.5772/30459

Bajar S, Singh A, and Bishnoi NR (2020) Exploration of low-cost agro-industrial waste substrate for cellulase and xylanase production using Aspergillus *heteromorphus*. Applied Water Science, 10(6), 153. https://doi.org/10.1007/s13201-020-01236-w

Bakshi MPS and Wadhwa M (2012) Nutritional evaluation of baby corn husk—A new feed resource for livestock. Indian Journal of Animal Sciences, 82(12), 1548–1550.

Bakshi MPS, Wadhwa M and Kumar B (2017) Nutritional evaluation of baby corn fodder and conventional maize fodder in buffaloes. Livestock Research for Rural Development, 29(7). https://www.cabdirect.org/cabdirect/abstract/20173292908

Ballesteros LF, Teixeira JA, Mussatto SI (2014) Chemical, Functional, and Structural Properties of Spent Coffee Grounds and Coffee Silverskin. Food and Bioprocess Technology, 7(12), 3493–3503. https://doi.org/10.1007/s11947-014-1349-z

Benerjee GC (1993) Animal Husbandry. Oxford and IBH Publishing Co. Pvt. Ltd.

Bhushan S, Kalia K, Sharma M, Singh B, Ahuja PS (2008). Processing of Apple Pomace for Bioactive Molecules. Critical Reviews in Biotechnology, 28(4), 285–296. https://doi.org/10.1080/07388550802368895

Biradar N, and Kumar V (2013) Analysis of fodder status in Karnataka. The Indian journal of animal sciences 83(10): 1078-1083.

Bodas R, Giráldez FJ, López S, Rodríguez AB, Mantecón AR (2007) Inclusion of sugar beet pulp in cereal-based diets for fattening lambs. Small Ruminant Research 71(1): 250–254. https://doi.org/10.1016/j.smallrumres.2006.07.006

Chauhan SK, Sharma KD (2015) A study on production potential economic viability and marketing system of varied size mushroom units in Himachal Pradesh. Dep Agric Econ Ext Educ Rural Sociol Coll Agric CSKHPKV Palampur ICSSR. Research Project File No. 02/196/2012-RPR, dated 24.04.2013.: 157.

Cheeke PR (1999) Applied Animal nutrition: feed and feeding 2nd ed. Prince Hall. Inc., New Jersey. 525.

DADF. Annual report 2017-18. Published online 2018. Accessed November 5, 2020. https://dahd.nic.in/sites/default/filess/Livestock%20%205_0.pdf

Deschard G, Mason VC, Tetlow RM (1988) Treatment of whole-crop cereals with alkali. 4. Voluntary intake and growth in steers given wheat ensiled with sodium hydroxide, urea or ammonia. Anim Feed Sci Technol 19(1): 55-66. doi:10.1016/0377-8401(88)90054-5

Devendra C (1987) Expanding the utilisation of agro-industrial by-products and non-conventional feed resources in Asia. Tokyo Jpn Asian Product Organ. Published online 51.

Earagariyanna M, Venkayala J, Kammardi S, Sriramaiah M (2017) Fodder Resource Management in India- A Critical Analysis. Int J Livest Res. Published online 1. doi:10.5455/ijlr.20170513095912

El-Tayeb TS, Abdelhafez AA, Ali SH, Ramadan EM (2012) Effect of acid hydrolysis and fungal biotreatment on agro-industrial wastes for obtainment of free sugars for bioethanol production. Braz J Microbiol 43(4): 1523-1535. doi:10.1590/S1517- 83822012000400037

Emami A, Ganjkhanlou M, Fathi Nasri MH, Zali A, Rashidi L (2015) Pomegranate seed pulp as a novel replacement of dietary cereal grains for kids. Small Rumin Res 123(2-3):238- 245. doi:10.1016/j.smallrumres.2014.12.001

Ghoreishi S, Rasoul P, Teimouri A (2007) Effects of Ensiled Apple Pomace on Milk Yield, Milk Composition and DM Intake of Holstein Dairy Cows. J Anim Vet Adv 6. Bakshi MPS, Wadhwa M (2012) Nutritional evaluation of baby corn husk - a new feed resource for livestock. Indian J Anim Sci 82(12): 1548-1550.

Jitendra (2017). How is fodder crisis rendering livestock vulnerable? Down to earth. https://www.downtoearth.org.in/coverage/agriculture/drought-of-fodder-52671.Published March 24, 2017. Accessed November 5, 2020.

Kammerer DR, Kammerer J, Valet R, Carle R (2014) Recovery of polyphenols from the by-products of plant food processing and application as valuable food ingredients. Food Res Int 65: 2-12. doi:10.1016/j.foodres.2014.06.012

Kotsampasi B, Christodoulou V, Zotos A, Liakopoulou-Kyriakides M, Goulas P, Petrotos K, Natas P, Bampidis VA (2014) Effects of dietary pomegranate byproduct silage supplementation on performance, carcass characteristics and meat quality of growing lambs. Animal Feed Science and Technology 197: 92-102.

Luciano G, Pauselli M, Servili M, Mourvaki E, Serra A, Monahan FJ, Lanza M, Priolo A, Zinnai A, Mele M (2013) Dietary olive cake reduces the oxidation of lipids, including cholesterol, in lamb meat enriched in polyunsaturated fatty acids. Meat Science. 93(3): 703-14.

Lyu F, Luiz SF, Azeredo DRP, Cruz AG, Ajlouni S, Ranadheera CS (2020) Apple Pomace as a Functional and Healthy Ingredient in Food Products: A Review. Processes 8(3): 319. doi:10.3390/pr8030319

Maglad MA, Lutfi AA, Gabir S (1986) The effect of grinding groundnut hulls either with or without alkali treatment on digestibility of diet and on ruminal and blood components. Anim Feed Sci Technol 15(1): 69-77.

Maneerat W, Prasanpanich S, Tumwasorn S, Laudadio V, Tufarelli V (2015) Evaluating agro-industrial by-products as dietary roughage source on growth performance of fattening steers. Saudi J Biol Sci. 22(5): 580-584. doi:10.1016/j.sjbs.2015.01.015

Martin JGP, Porto E, Corrêa CB, de Alencar M, de Aquino LM (2012) Antimicrobial potential and chemical composition of agro-industrial wastes. J Nat Prod 5:11.

Masood D, Ganai AM, Gull G, Farooq J, Beigh YA, Ishfaq A (2018) Effect of feeding graded levels of apple pomace on growth performance, haemato-biochemical parameters and rumen metabolites in crossbred calves. Indian J Anim Res 52. doi:10.18805/ijar.B-3229

Mirzaei-Aghsaghali A, Maheri-Sis N (2008) By-products from fruits and vegetable generation, characteristics and their nutritional value. In Proceeding of Third national congress of recycling and reuse of renewable organic resources in agriculture pp. 13-15.

Mirzaei-Aghsaghali and Maheri-Sis (2008) Nutritive Value of Some Agro-Industrial By product.pdf.

Mladenović D, Djukić-Vuković A, Stanković M, Milašinović-Šeremešić M, Radosavljević M, Pejin J, Mojović L (2019) Bioprocessing of agro-industrial residues into lactic acid and probiotic enriched livestock feed. Journal of the Science of Food and Agriculture 99(12): 5293-302.

Modaresi J, Fathi Nasri MH, Rashidi L, Dayani O, Kebreab E (2011) Short communication: effects of supplementation with pomegranate seed pulp on concentrations of conjugated linoleic acid and punicic acid in goat milk. J Dairy Sci 94(8): 4075-4080. doi:10.3168/ jds.2010- 4069

Motte JC, Trably E, Escudié R, Hamelin J, Steyer JP, Bernet N, Delgenes JP, Dumas C (2013) Total solids content: a key parameter of metabolic pathways in dry anaerobic digestion. Biotechnology for biofuels 6(1): 1-9.

NIANP (2013) . Vision 2050. Published online 2013. Accessed November 5, 2020. http://nianp. res.in/ static/docs/Nianp_vision_2050.pdf

NRC (1989) Nutrient Requirements of Dairy Cattle. In: 6th revised. National Research Council, National Academy of Sciences

Obi F, Ugwuishiwu B, Nwakaire J (2016) Agricultural waste concept, generation, utilization and management. Niger J Technol. 35(4): 957. doi:10.4314/ njt.v35i4.34

Perussello CA, Zhang Z, Marzocchella A, Tiwari BK (2017) Valorization of Apple Pomace by Extraction of Valuable Compounds: Valorization of apple pomace. Compr Rev Food Sci Food Saf 16(5): 776-796. doi:10.1111/1541-4337.12290

Prabhudessai V, Ganguly A, Mutnuri S (2013) Biochemical Methane Potential of Agro Wastes. J Energy:1-7. doi:10.1155/2013/350731

Ramachandran S, Singh SK, Larroche C, Soccol CR, Pandey A (2007) Oil cakes and their biotechnological applications–A review. Bioresour Technol 98(10): 2000-2009. doi:10.1016/j.biortech.2006.08.002

Ranjhan SK (1993) Agro-industrial by-products as component of livestock rations. In: In: Animal Nutrition in the Tropics. New Dehli, India: Vikas Publishing House PVT Ltd 222–258.

Ravindran R, Hassan S, Williams G, Jaiswal A (2018) A Review on Bioconversion of Agro-Industrial Wastes to Industrially Important Enzymes. Bioengineering 5(4):93. doi:10.3390/ bioengineering5040093

Ravindran V, Blair R (1992) Feed resources for poultry production in Asia and the Pacific.

II. Plant protein sources. Worlds Poult Sci J. 48(3): 205-231. doi:10.1079/WPS19920017 Benerjee GC (1993) Animal Husbandry. Oxford and IBH Publishing Co. Pvt. Ltd.

Rivas B, Torrado A, Torre P, Converti A, Domínguez JM (2008) Submerged Citric Acid Fermentation on Orange Peel Autohydrolysate. J Agric Food Chem 56(7): 2380-2387. doi:10.1021/ jf073388r

Rodríguez Couto S (2008) Exploitation of biological wastes for the production of value-added products under solid-state fermentation conditions. Biotechnol J 3(7): 859-870. doi:10.1002/ biot.200800031

Romero-Huelva M, Ramos-Morales E, Molina-Alcaide E (2012) Nutrient utilization, ruminal fermentation, microbial abundances, and milk yield and composition in dairy goats fed diets including tomato and cucumber waste fruits. J Dairy Sci 95(10): 6015-6026. doi:10.3168/jds.2012-5573

Rudra SG, Nishad J, Jakhar N, Kaur C (2015) Food industry waste: mine of nutraceuticals. Int. J. Sci. Environ. Technol 4(1): 205-29.

Sadh PK, Duhan S, Duhan JS (2018) Agro-industrial wastes and their utilization using solid state fermentation: a review. Bioresour Bioprocess. 5(1): 1. doi:10.1186/s40643-017- 0187-z

Sagar M, Ahlawat O, Raj D, Vijay B, Indurani C (2009) Indigenous technical knowledge about the use of spent mushroom substrate. Indian Journal of Traditional Knowledge 8(2): 242-248.

Sanon H, Kanwe A (2010) Valorisation of mango peels and seed kernels in animal feeding: Nutritive value and voluntary feed intake by sheep. Adv Anim Biosci 1(2): 445-446. doi:10.1017/S2040470010000695

Shalini R, Gupta DK (2010) Utilization of pomace from apple processing industries: a review. J Food Sci Technol 47(4): 365-371. doi:10.1007/s13197-010-0061-x

Sindhu AA, Khan MA, Sarwar M (2002) Agro-Industrial By-Products as a Potential Source of Livestock Feed. 4(2): 5.

Singha P, Muthukumarappan K (2018) Single screw extrusion of apple pomace-enriched blends: Extrudate characteristics and determination of optimum processing conditions. Food Sci Technol Int 24(5): 447-462. doi:10.1177/1082013218766981

Singh nee' Nigam P, Gupta N, Anthwal A (2009) Pre-treatment of Agro-Industrial Residues. In: Singh nee' Nigam P, Pandey A, eds. Biotechnology for Agro-Industrial Residues Utilisation: Utilisation of Agro-Residues. Springer Netherlands 13-33. doi:10.1007/978-1-4020- 9942-7_2

Tufarelli V, Introna M, Cazzato E, Mazzei D, Laudadio V (2013) Suitability of partly destoned exhausted olive cake as by-product feed ingredient for lamb production. J Anim Sci 91(2): 872-877.

Vargas-Bello-Pérez E, Vera RR, Aguilar C, Lira R, Peña I, Fernández J (2013) Feeding olive cake to ewes improves fatty acid profile of milk and cheese. Anim Feed Sci Technol 184(1):94-99. doi:10.1016/j.anifeedsci.2013.05.016

Verma DN (1997) A Text Book of Animal Nutrition. 1st edition. New Delhi, India: New Rajinder nagar publications

Wadhwa M, Bakshi M (2005) Vegetable wastes-a potential source of nutrients for ruminants. Indian J Anim Nutr 22: 70-76.

Wadhwa M, Bakshi MPS (2013) Utilization of fruit and vegetable wastes as livestock feed and as substrates for generation of other value-added products. Published online 2013. NRC (2001) Nutrient Requirements of Dairy Cattle: Seventh Revised Edition, 2001. National Academies Press 9825. doi:10.17226/9825

Wadhwa M, Kaushal S, Bakshi MPS (2006) Nutritive evaluation of vegetable wastes as complete feed for goat bucks. Small Rumin Res 64(3): 279-284. doi:10.1016/j.smallrumres.2005.05.017

Wadhwa M, Kumar B, Bakshi M (2018) Nutritional Evaluation of Ensiled Baby Corn Fodder as Livestock Feed. Anim Nutr Feed Technol 18: 267-272. doi:10.5958/0974-181X.2018.00025.2

23

Vectors and Vector Transmitted Diseases of Ruminants

Devi Gopinath, Gauri Jairath, Rinku Sharma, Ajayta Rialch Sudesh Radotra, Birbal Singh and Gorakh Mal
ICAR- IVRI Regional Station, Palampur-176061, Himachal Pradesh

Introduction

Incidence of ectoparasitism is on rise in the livestock population, impeding its production and performance. Those areas which were free of ectoparasites are now under great parasite load because of changing climatic conditions and global warming. Global warming has resulted in vectors shifting their habitats to temperate regions also. Ectoparasites are not only causing irritation to livestock by blood sucking and associated pruritus, they are serving as vectors for a variety of haemoprotozoan and rickettsiae leading to far-flung complications. Major ectoparasites infesting ruminants are ticks, lice, fleas and flies. Though ticks and flies are proclaimed as notorious for transmission of haemoprotozoans, now a days evidences are on rise reporting the role of fleas and lice as vectors for various haemoprotozoan and viral diseases. The need of the hour is to explore more and more ectoparasites to identify their vector potential and their effective control measures. While addressing the ectoparasitism in livestock, another major problem arises with their control. Most ectoparasitism is of seasonal nature at least in temperate areas, while it is a round the year phenomenon in tropics. Only very few compounds are available as ectoparasiticides and used by clinicians, and has resulted in onset of resistance among ectoparasites. New compounds need to be developed and marketed to counter this and at the same time it should be environment friendly also. Lest their rising use can lead to eradication of friendly fauna which can be more detrimental to the ecosystem. Now a days researches are focusing on the development of integrated tick/vector control measures which are making use of minimal chemical compounds and utilizing the synergistic application of farming techniques/practices and cultivating plants of acaricidal properties. In this era of pandemic, zoonotic nature of various haemoprotozoan/rickettsiae affecting livestock is also of concern to the mankind. So, they need to be addressed at the earliest considering their impact. The susceptibility to ectoparasitism varies from animal to animal. This is mostly of genetic peculiarities and this has led to resistance of certain breeds of livestock to various ectoparasites. Such breeds should be found out and their genetic potential needs to be tapped to develop new breeds of resistant livestock.

Major ectoparasites of concern

Arthropods are the major ectoparasites infesting ruminants. They include insects, ticks, lice, fleas, flies and mites. Almost 80% of the world's cattle population is exposed to tick infestation and they are causing an economic loss of 7.3 US dollar/head/year (FAO, 2004). Losses caused by ticks involve poor health associated with blood loss as well as tick borne diseases and their treatment costs and impact on production. Few of the tick borne diseases are zoonotic and they are listed as notifiable by the World Organisation for Animal health. Major dipterans parasitizing animals are blood sucking, causing nuisances, myiasis, and serve as biological as well as mechanical vectors for many pathogens (Pérez de León *et al.*, 2020). They include horn fly (*Haematobia irritans*), stable fly (*Stomoxys calcitrans*), face fly (*Musca autumnalis*), black fly (family *Simuliidae*), mosquitoes, etc. Tsetse flies are responsible for transmission of Trypanosomes responsible for African animal trypanosomiasis (nagana). Many flies are vectors for viral diseases as well eg: culicoides transmits blue tongue virus.

Myiasis is the name for maggot worm infestation caused by another group of flies, whose immature stage is responsible for the condition. They feed on the live/necrotic tissue of living animals and cause extensive damage and nuisance to the animals. Some flies causing myiasis are belonging to families *Sarcophagidae* and *Calliphoridae* (flesh flies and blow flies). The degree of damage caused by them varies from species to species. Heavy infestations are fatal (Cortinas and Jones, 2006). Bot flies are the dipterans belonging to Family *Oestridae*, their larvae called as grubs, penetrate the skin, eat up the dermis and connective tissue causing extensive hide damage to cattle.

Ticks are the most common ectoparasites of ruminants with world-wide distribution, and the most notorious vectors for haemoprotozoan and rickettsiae. Ticks are broadly divided into soft ticks and hard ticks based on their morphology. Ticks' life cycle varies according to the number of hosts they parasitize. Other than blood sucking and associated irritations, they are responsible for inflammatory reactions in some hosts (Brain and Bohrmann, 1992). They even cause tick paralysis like complications by the toxins released by some members of the species Ixodes and Argas even though they account for only 8% of the total tick species (Pienaar *et al.*, 2018). The economic impact of tick infestation is so high that countries like India are spending 498.7 million US dollars/annum for the control of ticks and tick borne diseases (Mondal *et al.*, 2013). Their impact is immense in case of small and marginal farmers who are the majority in our country.

Lice are the next group of ectoparasites mostly species specific, even though very few exceptions also exist. They are of two types according to their feeding pattern *i.e.,* sucking lice or anoplura and biting lice or mallophaga. Their predilection sites vary according to their species. Though their control is comparatively easy, they are responsible for skin irritations, alopecia and in extreme cases anaemia and abortions (Ruano *et al.*, 2016). Sucking lice are reported to act as vectors for anaplasma, theileria and dermatophytes (Cortinas and Jones, 2006).

Mites are microscopic obligate ectoparasites that penetrate deep into the skin. Infestation with mites is called as mange which varies in severity from species to species. Mites cause severe dermatitis in response to host immune reactions and secondary infections. They localize in hair follicles and sebaceous glands (Pérez de León *et al.*, 2020). Mites can also mechanically transmit viruses (Maggi, 2014). Major mites infesting ruminants are *Sarcoptes*, *Psoroptes*, *Chorioptes* and *Demodex* (Pérez de León *et al.*, 2020). *Psoroptes are located* peripherally and are less damaging in comparison with *Sarcoptes*, which is deep burrowing.

Impact of climate change on ectoparasites

Global warming is a phenomenon putting the vulnerable population at risk. Global temperature is rising and it is expected to rise by 0.4°Celcius in next 2 decades (IPCC, 2007). It is going to have a great impact on biodiversity as well. Climate change is affecting vector biology and dynamics. A metadata analysis of 1700 species has shown that as an adaptive measure the range of distribution of these species has shifted an average of 6.1 km towards poles per decade (Wall *et al.*, 2011). The change in temperature is leading to far flung complications and irreversible changes to the whole living beings on earth. However, climate change is something which is a hard truth, every living thing is to cope up with, though measures of mitigating global warming are progressing worldwide.

The impact of climate change on husbandry is immense, because it will lead to alteration in breeding times of livestock, availability of nutritive forage, disease susceptibility and last but not the least stress and immunity. Change in vector population size and their distribution is also having its impacts on livestock. Elongated blow fly season and fly strikes in sheep is a sign of impact of rising temperature on insect parasites in England (Taylor, 2012). Lice infestation will increase in confined environments, and tick infestation will also see a rise because of longer grazing seasons in warm and wet forages and exposures (Wall *et al.*, 2011). Vectors like ticks spending most of their time in the environment is greatly influenced by changing climatic conditions. Their abundance and distribution are few important factors responsible for the prevalence of diseases they transmit. As a result, a boom in the number of zoonotic diseases transmitted by Ixodes species is observed in Europe (Gray *et al.*, 2009). The Arctic region, where the rate of climate change is faster, has enough population of bot flies and winter ticks allowing opportunities for studies (Dobson *et al.*, 2015). Tick dispersal is also impacted by the host movement as well (Moghaddam *et al.*, 2014). Host abundance by various policy decisions is responsible for rise in vector population (Gray *et al.*, 2009).

Response of vectors to climate change varies according to their degree of dependence on the environment. However new species of vectors are identified from various locations, which were once free of them. Another problem expected to crop up in most populated third world countries will be competing for limited resources. It will lead to conflicts among different groups of livestock rearers especially headers. Nigeria has witnessed one such incidence in recent past and it is likely to repeat in other areas also unless we are shifting our husbandry practices more towards less methane producing and temperature tolerant livestock (Alaanuloluwa Ikhuoso *et al.*, 2020).

Hemoprotozoa and rickettsiae of ruminants

Major hemoprotozoa and rickettsiae of ruminants are Theileria, Anaplasma, Babesia and Borrelia. Most of them are zoonotic and notifiable diseases by WHO. It reveals their importance under the One Health approach. The most important fact is that they all are insect vector transmitted diseases. As we have already discussed, their spread is altered by vector dynamics and distribution. However, host susceptibility cannot be ignored. Altered climatic conditions too have an impact on the epidemiology of vector transmitted diseases. One such example is the number of vector borne zoonotic diseases rising in Europe due to warmer winters causing prolonged vector periods of *Ixodes ricinus* (Gray *et al.*, 2009). As the vectors started spreading their range away from tropics, the diseases they transmit have also followed the same course. Host immunity got impacted by non-availability of nutritious forage, and untimely onset of these diseases.

Order Rickettsiales are host cell-dependent obligate intra-cellular prokaryotic organisms. They grow inside the gut epithelium of ticks and host endothelial cells. They are pathogenic to animals as well as humans (Storz, 1990). They are gram negative cocco-bacilli or bacilli (Crossley *et al.*, 2008). They are maintained in rodents and transmitted to humans through arthropod vectors. The order Rickettsiales contain two families; Rickettsiaceae and Anaplasmataceae. Some examples of important Rickettsiae are *Rickettsia rickettsii* causing Rocky mountain spotted fever and *Ehrlichia ruminantium* causing heart water. Heart water is an acute disease of both domestic and wild ruminants, transmitted by *Amblyomma* species. Rickettsiosis are the oldest vector-borne diseases and their importance is growing because many of them are having zoonotic potential (Parola *et al.*, 2013). Ticks are second to mosquitoes in disease transmission. Tick borne rickettsiae are belonging to Spotted Fever Group of rickettsiae, one among the 4 major classifications of genus *Rickettsia.* Family Anaplasmataceae contain genera Anaplasma, Ehrlichia and Candidatus neoehrlichia (Abdelkadir *et al.*, 2019).

Regarding haemoprotozoan diseases, small ruminants are least studied groups. But sheep and goats are the major source of income to the resource poor communities in developing third world countries. These diseases are highly economically important because of their long time implications and herd mortality (Taha *et al.*, 2015). Theileriosis and babesiosis are the most economically important tick-borne haemoparasitic diseases of ruminants caused by *Theileria* spp. and *Babesia* spp. respectively (Aouadi *et al.*, 2017). In small ruminants, babesiosis is caused by *Babesia ovis* and *B. motasi*. *Theileria lestoquardi* is most pathogenic in sheep (Zobba *et al.*, 2020).

Cattle is more susceptible to anaplasmosis than buffaloes. Anaplasmosis caused by *Anaplasma marginale* previously called gallsickness is having world-wide distribution (Ashuma *et al.*, 2013). *Anaplasma*, intra cellular bacteria, having no conventional LPS cell wall is found inside RBC. The affected animals are showing anaemia, icterus and cachexia and sometimes become fatal. Their wide distribution is attributed to their large and variety of vector population and managemental lacunae. It is even reported to transmit to susceptible hosts through using the same used needle.

Haemoprotozoa and rickettsiae can be diagnosed microscopically by Giemsa stained blood smear examination. But only acute phases of infection could be diagnosed by this method. To be more precise and to identify the disease at all phases, recently we are using molecular techniques like Polymerase Chain Reaction (PCR). It has the advantage that it facilitates identification of the organism till species level by the sequencing of the specific amplicons.

Babesia and Theileria are major piroplasms affecting ruminants and turn fatal in severe infections. Their infection is commonly called piroplasmosis and it has a worldwide distribution. Some of them are responsible for emerging zoonosis eg: *Babesia divergens*. (Remesar *et al.*, 2019). Till date, no zoonotic Theileria have been identified. *Babesia bigemina, B. divergens, B. bovis* cause severe disease conditions in cattle (Zobba *et al.*, 2020). *Theileria annulata* and *T. parva* are highly pathogenic while *T. buffeli/orientalis/sergenti* group causes subclinical conditions in large ruminants (Aktas *et al.*, 2006). Though several Theileria and Babesia species have been identified in many wild ungulates, they never expressed any clinical symptoms, therefore wild life is considered as reservoirs of these piroplasms.

Vector control measures: old vs new concepts

Ectoparasiticides are used commonly in the control of parasitic arthropods. For efficient control various methods should be combined like drugs, mechanical, biological, environmental and genetic (Pérez de León *et al.*, 2020). Owing to availability of only few compounds as ectoparasiticides, and their lower price, livestock farmers often use them indiscriminately. This has led to another major problem of development of drug resistance among the parasites in the same way as microbes developing anti microbial resistance. In north western Uganda, it is reported that indiscriminate use of chemical acaricides, poor rotation of acaricides and lacunae in proper spraying has resulted in heavy ectoparasitism and development of acaricide resistance. There was a heavy rate of ectoparasitism among exotic cattle breeds, pointing towards breed variation in susceptibility/immunity to ectoparasites (Vudriko *et al.*, 2018). Tick control measures include use of topical acaricides, arsenic trioxide previously and organochlorines, organophosphates, carbamates, pyrethroids and ivermectin recently (Mondal *et al.*, 2013). The topical application involves dipping, spraying, dusting, jetting, back line application etc. These methods become effective only when properly applied and concentration of insecticides are maintained (Plant and Lewis, 2011). Many alternative methods of tick control eg: spraying engine oil, manual removal of ticks, pecking with chicken, ethno-veterinary practice of using medicinal plants are used by resource poor farmers and are found effective to some extent (Moyo and Masika, 2009). The adoption of such unconventional methods needs to be checked to identify their toxic impacts on animal and human health. Ethno veterinary practices are to be validated with proper scientific evidence.

Future of tick control is integrated pest management (IPM) where environment friendly and cost-effective technologies are combined (Ghosh *et al.*, 2006). Some specialists are of the opinion that vaccination and natural resistance are the most effective. Few native breeds of livestock are highly resistant to ectoparasites. Genetic control measures involve the utilization of genetic potential of resistant breeds in ectoparasite control. This is widely accepted as a new option of vector control. Veterinary scientists are fast progressing in the field of vaccine development in spite of the many odds they face. Tick vaccines are the need of the hour because the environmental impact of chemical acaricides is on rise. The risk of emergence of acaricide resistant ticks cannot be ignored.

Migratory pastoralism and ectoparasitism

Transhumance is migratory nomadism practiced by different communites like *Gaddis*, *Gujjars* and *Bakharwals*. They are traditional shepherds depending solely on the environment and nature in their minimum input livestock rearing system. Spending most of the time in migration, with flocks of sheep and goats they are typical examples of co-inhabitations and greatly influenced by climate change and the first people who can give evidence of changing weather patterns and global warming.

Ectoparasitism is one of the major health implications of migratory sheep and goats. Since they are mostly staying outdoors, their contact time during grazing is relatively longer than their intensively reared counterparts. No much study is conducted on the migratory small ruminants, because they spend most of the time in migration. Gaddi sheep and goats, the native breeds of Himachal Pradesh are highly adapted to the harsh climate and terrain of the area. The breed is famous for its sturdiness and is reported to be immune to many disease conditions. Gaddi breed deserves to be explored extensively especially their immune status and disease resistance potential. If the breed could be genetically utilized with ectoparasitism resistance, it will be a boon to the conservationists. It will in turn pave the way to the upgradation of the species.

Their migratory routes are away from human inhabitations and therefore timely veterinary help is not received. Traditional knowledge about medicinal plants is for their help during such situations. There is evidence of 9 plant species used by Gaddi shepherds as a therapy for ectoparasitism (Dutt *et al*., 2015). These Oral traditional Knowledge (OTK) are at the risk of extinction since they are not documented till date.

Conclusion

Ectoparasitism is one of the most common cause for reduced productivity in livestock of tropical and subtropical countries. Their ill effects not only involve blood loss and irritation, but also they are vectors for many life threatening and zoonotic haemoprotozoa and rickettsiae. The control of ectoparasitism is the need of the hour because their number is increasing due to climate change and they are shifting their habitat to previously naïve areas. Moreover the problems caused by acaricide resistant parasites also need to be addressed. Newer compounds with fewer side effects are to be developed along with herbal formulations to achieve this. Integrated Pest Control, the newer and cheaper technique is gaining acceptance among the resource poor farmers of developing countries. Tick vaccine research is also progressing at a great pace in spite of the many odds. Genetic improvement of the susceptible livestock is the most advanced technique offering great scope for native ectoparasite resistant breeds of livestock. Ultimately, this will be the future of combating livestock ectoparasitism.

References

Abdelkadir K, Palomar AM, Portillo A, Oteo JA, Ait-Oudhia K, Khelef D (2019) Presence of Rickettsia aeschlimannii, 'Candidatus Rickettsia barbariae' and Coxiella burnetii in ticks from livestock in Northwestern Algeria. Ticks and Tickborne Diseases 10: 924– 928. https://doi.org/10.1016/j.ttbdis.2019.04.018

Aktas M, Altay K, Dumanli N (2006) A molecular survey of bovine Theileria parasites among apparently healthy cattle and with a note on the distribution of ticks in eastern Turkey. Veterinary Parasitology 138: 179–185. https://doi.org/10.1016/j.vetpar.2006.01.052

Alaanuloluwa Ikhuoso O, Adegbeye MJ, Elghandour MMY, Mellado M, Al-Dobaib SN, Salem AZM (2020) Climate change and agriculture: The competition for limited resources amidst crop farmers-livestock herding conflict in Nigeria - A review. J Clean Prod 272 123104. https://doi.org/10.1016/j.jclepro.2020.123104

Aouadi A, Leulmi H, Boucheikhchoukh M, Benakhla A, Raoult D, Parola P (2017) Molecular evidence of tick-borne hemoprotozoan-parasites (Theileria ovis and Babesia ovis) and bacteria in ticks and blood from small ruminants in Northern Algeria. Comp. Immunol. Microbiol. Infect. Dis. 50: 34–39. https://doi.org/10.1016/j.cimid.2016.11.008

Ashuma Sharma A, Singla L, Das Kaur, P, Bal MS, Batth BK, Juyal PD (2013) Prevalence and haemato-biochemical profile of Anaplasma marginale infection in dairy animals of Punjab (India). Asian Pacific Journal of Tropical Medicine 6: 139–144. https://doi.org/10.1016/S1995-7645(13)60010-3

Brain C, Bohrmann R (1992) Tick infestation of baboons (Papio ursinus) in the Namib Desert. Journal of Wildlife Diseases 28: 188–191. https://doi.org/10.7589/0090-3558-28.2.188 Cortinas R, Jones CJ (2006) Ectoparasites of Cattle and Small Ruminants. Veterinary Clinicians of North America - Food Animal Practice 22: 673–693. https://doi.org/10.1016/j.cvfa.2006.06.003

Crossley EC, Jordan JM, Walker DH, Medical T (2008) Rickettsiae and Orientia 582– 590.

Dobson A, Molnár PK, Kutz S (2015) Climate change and Arctic parasites. Trends in Parasitology 31: 181–188. https://doi.org/10.1016/j.pt.2015.03.006

Dutt HC, Bhagat N, Pandita S (2015) Oral traditional knowledge on medicinal plants in jeopardy among Gaddi shepherds in hills of northwestern Himalaya, J&K, India. Journal of Ethnopharmacology 168: 337–348. https://doi.org/10.1016/j.jep.2015.03.076

FAO (2004) Resistance Management and Integrated Parasite Control in Ruminants: Guidelines. Animal Production and Health Division., Food and Agriculture Organization of the United Nations, Rome, pp. 25-77

Ghosh S, Azhahianambi P, De La Fuente J (2006) Control of ticks of ruminants, with special emphasis on livestock farming systems in India: Present and future possibilities for integrated control - A review. Experimental and Applied Acarology 40: 49–66. https://doi.org/10.1007/ s10493-006-9022-5

Gray JS, Dautel H, Estrada-Peña A, Kahl O, Lindgren E (2009) Effects of Climate Change on Ticks and Tick-Borne Diseases in Europe. Interdisciplinary Perspectives on Infectious Dis eases 1–12. https://doi.org/10.1155/2009/593232

Maggi RG (2014) Animal Health: Ectoparasites. Encyclopedia on Agric Food Syst 1:315–326. https:// doi.org/10.1016/B978-0-444-52512-3.00192-3

Moghaddam AG, Seyed MR, Rasouli M, Hosseinzade S, Darvishi MM, Rakhshanpour A, Rahimi MT (2014) Survey on cattle ticks in Nur, north of Iran. Asian Pacific. Journal of Tropical Biomedicine 4: 209–212. https://doi.org/10.1016/S2221-1691(14)60233-1

Mondal DB, Sarma K, Saravanan M (2013) Upcoming of the integrated tick control program of ruminants with special emphasis on livestock farming system in India. Ticks and Tick. Borne Diseases 4: 1–10. https://doi.org/10.1016/j.ttbdis.2012.05.006

Moyo B, Masika PJ (2009) Tick control methods used by resource-limited farmers and the effect of ticks on cattle in rural areas of the Eastern Cape Province, South Africa. Tropical Animal Health and Production 41: 517–523. https://doi.org/10.1007/s11250-008-9216-4

Parola P, Paddock CD, Socolovschi C, Labruna MB, Mediannikov O, Kernif T, Abdad MY, Stenos J, Bitam I, Fournier PE, Raoult D (2013) Update on tick-borne rickettsioses around the world: A geographic approach. Clinical Microbiology Reviews 26: 657–702. https://doi.org/10.1128/CMR.00032-13

Peres de León AA, Mitchell RD, Watson DW (2020) Ectoparasites of cattle. Veterinary Clinics: Food Animal Practice 36(1): 173-85.

Plant JW, Lewis CJ (2011) Treatment and Control of Ectoparasites in Sheep. Veterinary Clinicians North America - Food Animal Practice 27: 203–212. https://doi.org/10.1016/j.cvfa.2010.10.01

Remesar S, Díaz P, Prieto A, Markina F, Díaz Cao JM, López-Lorenzo G, Fernández G, López CM, Panadero R, Díez-Baños P, Morrondo P (2019) Prevalence and distribution of Babesia and Theileria species in roe deer from Spain. International Journal of Parasitology Parasites Wildl. 9: 195–201. https://doi.org/10.1016/j.ijppaw.2019.05.005

Ruano P, Delgado LL, Picco S, Villegas L, Tonelli F, Merlo M, Rigau J, Diaz D, Masuelli M (2016) We are IntechOpen, the world ' s leading publisher of Open Access books Built by scientists, for scientists TOP 1 %. Intech 13.

Storz J (1990) Rickettsiae and Chlamydiae, Fifth Edit. ed, Diagnostic Procedure in Veterinary Bacteriology and Mycology. Academic Press, Inc. https://doi.org/10.1016/b978-0-12-161775-2.50029-3

Taha HA, Shoman SA, Alhadlag NM (2015) Molecular and serological survey of some haemoprotozoan, rickettsial and viral diseases of small ruminants from Al- Madinah Al Munawarah, KSA. Tropical Biomedicine 32: 511–523.

Taylor MA (2012) Emerging parasitic diseases of sheep. Veterinary Parasitology 189: 2–7. https://doi. org/10.1016/j.vetpar.2012.03.027

Vudriko P, Okwee-Acai J, Byaruhanga J, Tayebwa DS, Okech SG, Tweyongyere R, Wampande EM, Okurut ARA, Mugabi K, Muhindo JB, Nakavuma JL, Umemiya Shirafuji R, Xuan X, Suzuki H (2018) Chemical tick control practices in southwestern and northwestern Uganda. Ticks and Tick Borne Diseases 9: 945–955. https://doi.org/10.1016/j. ttbdis.2018.03.009

Wall R, Rose H, Ellse L, Morgan E (2011) Livestock ectoparasites: Integrated management in a changing climate. Veterinary Parasitology 180: 82–89. https://doi.org/10.1016/j.vetpar.2011.05.030

Zobba R, Chisu V, Pinna Parpaglia ML, Spezzigu A, Masala G, Schianchi E, Alberti A (2020) Molecular characterization and phylogenetic analysis of Babesia and Theileria spp. in Sardinian ruminants. Veterinary Parasitology Regional Studies and Reports 22: 100453. https://doi. org/10.1016/j.vprsr.2020.100453

24

Sustainable Control Measure for Gastro-Intestinal Nematodes of Small Ruminants

Ajayta Rialch, Gauri Jairath, Devi Gopinath, Rinku Sharma Gorakh Mal, Birbal Singh and Sudesh Radotra

ICAR-Indian Veterinary Research Institute, Regional Station, Palampur-176061 Himachal Pradesh

Introduction

Gastro-intestinal parasites are considered as the 'silent killers' and remain hidden or undiagnosed by the livestock owners or veterinarians as the infected animals manifest meagre clinical signs. These parasites often have detrimental effects on the growth and development of animals where they can potentiate mortality especially among young, weak or nutritionally compromised animals. They negatively impact animal health in terms of reduced weight gain, anorexia, digestive disturbance, impaired reproductive performance, condemnation of affected organs, mortality in infected animals and ultimately affect animal production, contributing to huge economic losses to the livestock owners. At present, chemotherapy is the most practical and widely practiced approach to curb these infestations. But frequent and indiscriminate use of anthelmintics imposes a threat on the sustainability of current control measures. Thus, there is an urgent need for incorporation of alternate control approaches while designing our worm control programs, so that we can reduce the usage of anthelmintics and prolong their effectiveness. The effectiveness or success of any worm control strategy is evaluated based on integrated parameters like the ultimate goal of increasing production, minimizing risks regarding drug resistance and considering consumer's concerns about health and environment-associated problems. In general, gastro-intestinal nematode control strategies can target either the parasite population inside the host or the free-living stages of parasites in the environment. Here, we are discussing some of the components of sustainable control measures for these parasites in detail.

Strategic chemotherapeutic measures

Anthelmintics (also commonly called dewormers) are the drugs which are used for the prevention and control of gastrointestinal nematodes (GIN). They are widely used by field veterinarians as they are cheap, simple and cost-effective. But, over a period of time, prescription of these drugs without proper diagnosis of these parasitic infestations or their frequent administration by livestock owners without even proper consultation of vets, has led to the country-wide emergence of anthelmintic drug resistance. This scenario imposes a question on their efficacy and sustainability to control GIN infestations in the future. To maintain the effectiveness of these drugs, they should be used wisely and judiciously which include selective or target selective treatment of animals. The concept of selective treatment depends on the "overdispersion phenomenon" which says that 80% of the worm burden lies in the 20% of the animals in the flock (Gowane *et al.,* 2019). So, if we identify this 20% of the animals and selectively treat these animals only, we will successfully decrease the worm burden to an acceptable level and will be able to maintain the susceptible worm population. Simultaneously, the cost of treatment will be lowered and the efficacy of anthelmintic will be maintained or prolonged. Another basis of implementing selective treatment is by using the FAMACHA chart (Prashanth *et al.,* 2020). This is a laminated eye color chart and is specifically used to identify and treat only those animals with high haemonchosis levels by predicting the levels of anemia using their eye color. Farmers can compare the color of their sheep's conjunctivae using a scientifically developed FAMACHA chart and treat accordingly.

Table 1. List of commonly used anthelmintics against gastro-intestinal nematodes in small ruminants

Chemical group	Anthelmintic	Prescribed dose (in mg/kg body weight of animals)
Benzimidazole	Albendazole Fenbendazole Oxfendazole	5 mg/kg 5-10 mg/kg 5 mg/kg
Imidazothiazole	Levamisole	7.5 mg/kg
Macrocyclic lactones	Ivermectin Moxidectin	0.2 mg/kg 0.2 mg/kg
Salicylanilides	Closantel	10 mg/kg

Potential use of vaccines against gastrointestinal nematodes (GINs)

The most pathogenic gastro-intestinal nematode is barber's pole worm, *Haemonchus contortus*, a blood-feeding parasite that attaches to the abomasum of ruminants (sheep, goats and cattle) causing production losses due to malaise and mortality of susceptible young animals. This is the most prevalent parasite in most parts of India followed invariably by *Oesophagostomum, Trichostrongylus, Trichuris, Strongyloides, Bunostomum, Ostertagia/ Teladorsagia, Cooperia* etc. To date, "Barbervax" (WormVax, Australia Pvt Ltd) that contains purified native H-gal-GP and H11 from the guts of adult *H. contortus* is commercially available (Bassetto *et al.*, 2014) in Australia. This is a native gut antigen-based vaccine, recently launched for the control of haemonchosis in sheep in Australia and a similar vaccine under the name of "Wirevax" (Afrivet Business Management Pvt Ltd) is launched in South Africa (Claerebout and Geldhof, 2020).

Although, the vaccine is only registered in Australia and South Africa, it can be used in the United Kingdom under Special Treatment Certificate and veterinary prescription. In India, it is neither registered nor commercialized. As it is a native antigen-based vaccine and we know that recombinant antigen-based vaccines have advantages over them in terms of reproducibility of product batches, biosafety, and global distribution. Thus, many attempts have been made to identify and express a range of antigens from *H. contortus*, but most recombinant proteins were unsuccessful in eliciting protective immunity. Recently, an adult somatic recombinant protein, rHc23 is showing promise achieving an overall reduction of more than 80% in fecal egg counts and parasite burdens in vaccinated lambs (Fawzi *et al.*, 2015). These latter antigens are currently being developed further for a next-generation subunit vaccine against *H. contortus*.

Table 2. Overview of commercially available vaccine 'Barbervax' against *Haemonchus contortus*

Commercial Name	Barbervax® (in Australia), Wirevax® (in South Africa)
Used against	*Haemonchus contortus* in sheep
Dose	1ml subcutaneous, 3 priming doses 3-4 weeks apart + 2 boosters 6 weeks apart
Components	5 µg native protein purified from integral membrane glycoprotein (containing H-11 and H-gal-GP) adjuvanted with 1 mg saponin
Level of Protection	93%–95% (decrease in egg counts) and 72%–94% (decrease in worm burden)
Miscellaneous	Barbervax was commercialized first in 2014 in Australia, developed by Moredun Research Institute, Scotland (U.K.) and marketed by Albany Lab, Deptt of Agriculture and Food, Western Australia

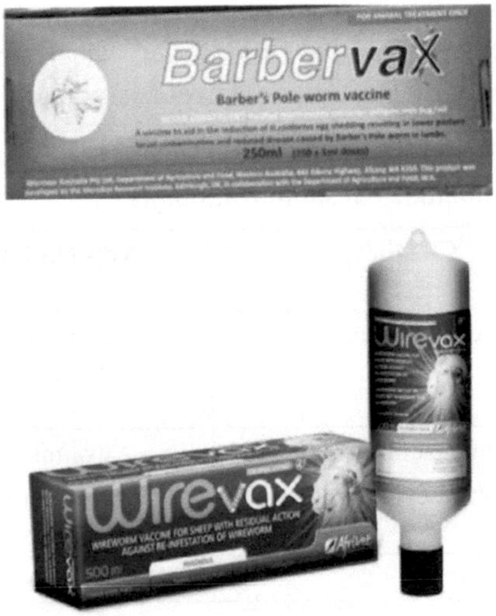

Among other important GINs, against *O. ostertagi*, *Teladorsagia circumcincta* several native or subunit vaccine preparations based on excretory/secretory or membrane targets have been shown to reduce worm fecundity by ±50% (Halliday and Smith, 2010, Nisbet *et al.*, 2016) and still, we have not come up with something very promising.

Nutritional management

Managing the nutritional plan of the animals is also a very important aspect with respect to parasitic disease management. Voluntary feed intake (VFI) depression with reductions of intake between 10 and 30% is generally recognized as a major feature of the pathogenesis of GIN infections (van Houtert and Sykes, 1996). Modifications in feed components including nutrient enrichment can offset the negative impacts of infection even at low levels of feed intake. Studies have shown that extra protein supplementation could overcome some degree of anorexia and pathogenicity in the experiments with *H. contortus* (Datta *et al.,* 1998). Minerals like phosphorus, copper, cobalt, selenium and vitamin supplementation containing Vitamin A, D, B etc. also helps animals to sustain the parasitic infestation. Copper oxide wires when given orally to small ruminants they have shown a decrease in the *Haemonchus contortus* infestation (Chartier *et al.*, 2000).

Selection of Resistant breeds or propagation of superior germplasm

There are certain animals in the population which is less susceptible to the harmful effects of parasitic infestation, this ability of the host to maintain a relatively undepressed production level under parasite challenge is called "resilience". Combining the concept of resilience and overdispersion phenomenon we can identify the superior germplasm and breed them to get a better host population. Apart from this, there is a concept of "breed resistance" where there are certain breeds of animals that are resistant to GIN infestations. Breeding and selecting these animals which are less reliant on anthelmintics for maintaining health and productivity is a good component to be incorporated in GIN control (Saddiqi *et al.,* 2011). For eg. for gastro-intestinal parasitic infestation Red masai, Garole, Hissardale are some sheep breeds and West African dwarf, Small east African goat, Jamnapari are few goat breeds that are resistant to GIN infestations.

Grazing management

This is another useful component of GIN management and can be very useful when common grazing areas are exploited. There are several components of grazing management which includes (Maqbool *et al.,* 2017)

a. **Pasture rotation system**: Here subdivision of pasture into paddocks is done and each paddock is grazed for short time after that it is given rest for a relatively much longer period.

b. **Safe pasture system**: The number of larvae in pasture are reduced to a very less number so that if they are ingested they will not cause pathogenic conditions. This is done by either resting for long or growing crop of hay or silage.

c. **Alternate grazing system**: Here the young ones are grazed first and then adults are grazed later on that pasture land.

d. **Mixed grazing system**: Different species are grazed together in the same pasture as among these species the parasitic species are different. For example, the free living stages of parasites of cattle are if ingested by horses, they will not develop inside horse and thus will simultaneously decrease the pasture larval burden of cattle parasites.

e. Pasture resting for 2 months in semi-arid places and 6 months in cool, moist environment will be useful to kill the larvae on the pastures.
f. Less stock rate should be maintained.
g. Herbage height should be more as 80% of parasitic stages are present in first 5 cm of herbage towards the ground.
h. Grazing should be avoided in the early morning and late evening due to vertical migration of infective stages on parasites.

Biological control

The biological control of gastro-intestinal nematodes utilizes their natural enemies to reduce the infection level in the environment or pastures and animals grazing on these areas will ultimately avoid both clinical and subclinical effects due to these parasites. A lot of work has been carried out on the use of nematophagous fungi in GIN control throughout the world including India (Sanyal, 2000) and this area is speedily becoming an area of applied research with the possibility of becoming an important integrated element in developing new sustainable control strategies. Thus, this control program is directed against the free-living stages and will lower the pasture larval burden. So, the grazing animals will constantly receive a small number of parasitic larvae and thereby should be able to develop a natural immune response. Fungal species like *Duddingtonia flagrans, Arthrobotrys oligospora* displayed the ability of ruminant gut survival with the genus *Duddingtonia* performing significantly better. After passing through the gastrointestinal tract, spores germinate and looped hyphae trap the developing larval stages in the faecal environment (Sahoo and Khan, 2016). *Bacillus thuringiensis*, dung beetles, chicken, ants, birds can also be used.

Ethno-veterinary practices

Condensed tannin-rich plants can be fed to host e.g., *Sesbania* for prevention of gastro-intestinal nematodes. Cysteine proteinase, Saponin-rich plants or other herbal can also be fed for the same. A variety of Indian medicinal plants like garlic, tulsi leaves, Eucalyptus, Oak leaves, Ananas etc, (Ahmed *et al.*, 2013; Kanojiya *et al.*, 2015) have been tested and the results are promising to show a potential herbal anthelmintic formulation can be the outcome.

Conclusion

The concerns like ever-increasing anthelmintic resistance, awareness of consumers regarding environmental contamination and their pressure to reduce drug residues in meat and meat products demand alternate non-chemical parasite control strategies. Here, only integrated control strategies will withstand time and we need to implement these approaches at ground level. As far as helminth vaccines are concerned, though there are few commercial successes, still they encourage the researchers to explore this area with a multidisciplinary approach. *D. flagrans* is considered the most promising species for biological control against GIN infestation of livestock. Other components include, high plan of nutrition, strategic deworming and adoption of good grazing practices. Herbal anthelmintics can also be explored in a streamlined way.

References

Ahmed M, Laing MD, Nsahlai IV (2013) *In vitro* anthelmintic activity of crude extracts of selected medicinal plants against *Haemonchus contortus* from sheep. J Helminthol 87(2):174-9.

Bassetto CC, Picharillo ME, Newlands GF, Smith WD, Fernandes S, Siqueira ER, Amarante AF (2014) Attempts to vaccinate ewes and their lambs against natural infection with *Haemonchus contortus* in a tropical environment. Int J Parasitol 44(14):1049-54.

Chartier C, Etter E, Hoste H, Pors I, Koch C, Dellac B (2000) Efficacy of copper oxide needles for the control of nematode parasites in dairy goats. Vet Res Comm 24(6):389-99.

Claerebout E, Geldhof P (2020) Helminth vaccines in ruminants: from development to application. Veterinary Clinics: Food Animal Practice 36(1):159-71.

Datta FU, Nolan JV, Rowe JB, Gray GD (1998) Protein supplementation improves the performance of parasitised sheep fed a straw-based diet. Int J Parasitol 28(8):1269-78.

Fawzi EM, González-Sánchez ME, Corral MJ, Alunda JM, Cuquerella M (2015) Vaccination of lambs with the recombinant protein rHc23 elicits significant protection against *Haemonchus contortus* challenge Vet Para 211(1-2):54-9.

Gowane GR, Swarnkar CP, Misra SS, Kumar R, Kumar A, Prince LLL (2019) Genetic parameter estimates for fecal egg counts and their relationship with growth in Avikalin and Malpura sheep. Animal 13(9):1788-1796.

Halliday AM, Smith WD (2010) Protective immunization of calves against *Ostertagia ostertagi* using fourth stage larval extracts Parasit Immunol 32(9-10):656-63.

Kanojiya D, Shanker D, Sudan V, Jaiswal AK, Parashar R (2015) Anthelmintic activity of Ocimum sanctum leaf extract against ovine gastrointestinal nematodes in India. Res Vet Sci 99:165-70.

Maqbool I, Wani ZA, Shahardar RA, Allaie IM, Shah MM (2017) Integrated parasite management with special reference to gastro-intestinal nematodes. J Parasitic Dis 41(1):1-8.

Prashanth V, Kiran H, Rupner RK, Patil S, Prakash V (2020) The "FAMACHA" Chart-An Alternate to Manage Haemonchosis in Small Ruminants–A Review Article. Int J Current Microbiol and Appl Sci 9:1908-13.

Nisbet AJ, McNeilly TN, Greer AW, Bartley Y, Oliver EM, Smith S, Palarea-Albaladejo J, Matthews JB (2016) Protection of ewes against *Teladorsagia circumcincta* infection in the periparturient period by vaccination with recombinant antigens Vet Para 228:130-6.

Saddiqi HA, Jabbar A, Sarwar M, Iqbal Z, Muhammad G, Nisa M, Shahzad A (2011) Small ruminant resistance against gastrointestinal nematodes: a case of *Haemonchus contortus*. Parasitol Res 109(6):1483-500.

Sahoo A, Khan F (2016) Nutritional and biological control synergism against gastrointestinal nematodes in small ruminants. J Vet Sci Anim Husb 4(1):104.

Sanyal PK (2000) Screening for Indian isolates of predacious fungi for use in biological control against nematode parasites of ruminants. Vet Res Commun 24(1):55-62.

van Houtert MF, Sykes AR (1996) Implications of nutrition for the ability of ruminants to withstand gastrointestinal nematode infections. Int J Parasitol 26(11):1151-67.

Appendix

Some native breeds and their characteristics

Breed	Habitat	Important feature
Aseel	Andhra Pradesh is home, but now in the whole country	Game bird, known for its pugnacity, high stamina, majestic gait and dogged fighting qualities, large body size
Ankaleshwar	Ankaleshwar	Small body, single comb, hardy, poor layer
Bursa	Gujarat and Maharastra	Small to medium sized bird having non-significant characters
Brown Desi	Uttar Pradesh	A light to deep brown layer type single combed bird
Chittagong or Malay	North-eastern states	A large, heavy bird, strong and hardy, quarrelsome temperament
Daothigir	Assam	A fairly heavy breed with good juvenile growth mostly reared by the Bodo community
Denki	Andhra Pradesh	Fairly heavy breed, glossy and lustrous plumage, single comb, long necks and legs
Kalasthi	Andhra Pradesh	Birds closely resembles Denki, but are smaller
Frizzle fowl	Hot and humid coastal regions and North Eastern regions	The feathers are curved due to curving of rachis of the feather. The birds have better heat dissipation, hence show good adaptability in tropical climate especially for arid zones
Ghagus	Andhra and Karnataka	Small sized-bird, small comb and wattles, thick neck, feathered shank
Haringhata	Black West Bengal	Small bodied black bird, good layer
Kadakanath	Madhya Pradesh	Known as *Kalamasi* and characterized by presence of black pigments on external and internal surfaces
Faverolla	Kashmir	Small sized birds, small comb and wattles. Feathered Comb is the peculiarity of this breed
Miri	Assam	A small sized black bird, mostly reared by Miri tribes of Assam
Naked Neck	Hot and humid coastal regions and North Eastern states	Birds are characterized by having no feather or small tuft of feather on the neck. The birds are well adapted to high temperature due to better heat dissipation mechanism
Punjab Brown	Punjab and Haryana	Heavy breed, brown plumage, yellow beak, legs and feet
Tellichery	Kerela	Small bird, black skin, plumage range from black to grey in colour or various combination of colour
Titri	-	Small bird, speckled black and white feathers, yellow beak and legs

Breed	Habitat	Important feature
Teni	All parts of country	It is a small bird, active forager and excellent sitter. It tolerates high temperature
Nicobari	Nicobar group of isolands	Small size birds, short legs, compact and round body, stout back, brown matte coloured plumage, good layer

Genetically superior poultry strains developed in public sector

Name of commercial stock	Type of stock	Name of the Institute
ILI 80 (White egger)	Commercial layer	Central Avian Research Institute, Izatnagar
ILM 90 (White egger)	Commercial layer	Kerala Agricultural University, Mannuthy
ILR 90 (White egger)	Commercial layer	Andhra Pradesh Agricultural University, Hyderabad
HH 260 (White egger)	Commercial layer	Central Poultry Breeding Farm, Bangalore
BH 78 (White egger)	Commercial layer	Central Poultry Breeding Farm, Bombay
Kalinga Brown (Brown egger)	Commercial layer	Central Poultry Breeding Farm, Bhubaneswar
CARI Gold 92 (Brown egger)	Commercial layer	Central Avian Research Institute, Izatnagar
CARI-RAINBRO (B-77) (Coloured Plumage)	Commercial Broiler	Central Avian Research Institute, Izatnagar
IBL 80 (Coloured plumage)	Commercial Broiler	Punjab Agricultural University, Ludhiana
IBB 83 (Coloured plumage)	Commercial Broiler	University of Agricultural Sciences, Bangalore
CARIBRO-VISHAL (91) (White plumage)	Commercial Broiler	Central Avian Research Institute, Izatnagar
CARIBRORANGEELA (Multicoloured Plumage)	Commercial Broiler	Central Avian Research Institute, Izatnagar
CARIBRO MRITUNJAI (CARI Naked Neck)	Commercial Broiler	Central Avian Research Institute, Izatnagar

Poultry germplasm for the rural-based poultry production

Name	Type	Characteristics			Developed at
		56-day body wt. (kg)	Feather colour	Purpose	
Vanraja	Breed cross	1.40	Graded brown	Dual/meat	PDP, Hyderabad
Giriraja	Breed cross	1.53	Graded brown	Dual/meat	Bangalore
AVM coloured	Breed cross	1.05	Mixed	Meat	Coimbatore
Croiler	Synthetic	1.20	Graded brown	Meat	Keggs, Delhi

Maines T	Synthetic	0.70	Mixed	Tandori	Hyderabad
Krishipriya	Breed cross	0.90	Graded brown	Dual	Kerala
Grampriya	Breed cross	1.00	Wheatish brown	Dual	PDP, Hyderabad
Krishna J	Synthetic	0.60	Mixed	Egg	Jabalpur
CARI-Gold	Breed cross	1.00	Brown	Dual	Izatnagar

High yielding Germplasm (other than broiler and layer chicken) developed at CARI, Izatnagar

Germplasm Developed	Plumage	Utility	Performance Status
Desi type (cross)			
CARI-Nirbhik (Aseel Cross)	Coloured	Backyard	190 eggs/year and plentiful meat
CARI-Shyama (Kadaknath Cross)	Coloured	Backyard	210 eggs
UPCARI (Frizzle Cross)	Coloured	Backyard	220 eggs, Adopted to hot climate
HITCARI (Naked neck Cross)	Coloured	Backyard	220 eggs, Adopted to hot climate
Quail (Japanese)			
CARI-Shweta	White	Meat type	165g at 5 wk, 245 eggs/year
CARI-Uttam	Wild	Meat type	182g at% wk, 285 eggs/year
CARI-Ujjwal	White breasted	Meat type	167g at 5 wk, 270 eggs/year
CARI-Pearl	Wild	Egg type	113g at 5 wk, 280 eggs/year
Guinea Fowl			
Guncari-Swetambri	White	Meat	Body weight of 964.1g at 12 weeks.
Guncari-Kadambri	Pearl	Meat	Body weight of 1084.2g at 12 weeks.
Guncari-Chitambri	Lavender	Meat	Body weight of 1068.6g at 12 weeks.
Turkey			
CARI-Virat	White	Meat	Body weight at -8th wk, M- 1860g; F- 1750g. -16th wk M- 4640g; F- 3123g. -24th wk M- 6123g; F- 3957g.

Source: Saran *et al.*, 2005

Colour Plates

Chapter 12: Freshwater Fish Transgenics Implications and Issues

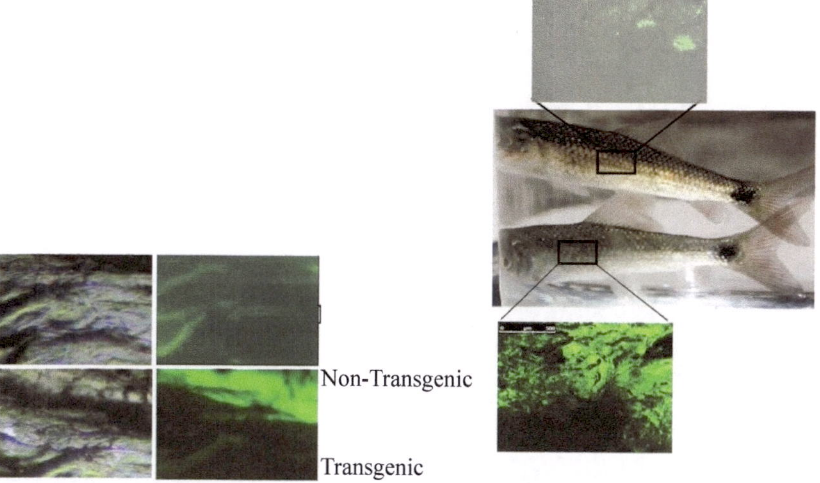

Fig. 1: GFP expressions driven by the mylz 2 promoter in the skeletal muscle of rohu (*L. rohita*): **(a)** Histological slides of skeletal muscle following direct muscular injection of DNA construct; **(b)** Massive GFP expressions in transgenic rohu fishes. *(See black & white version on page 133)*

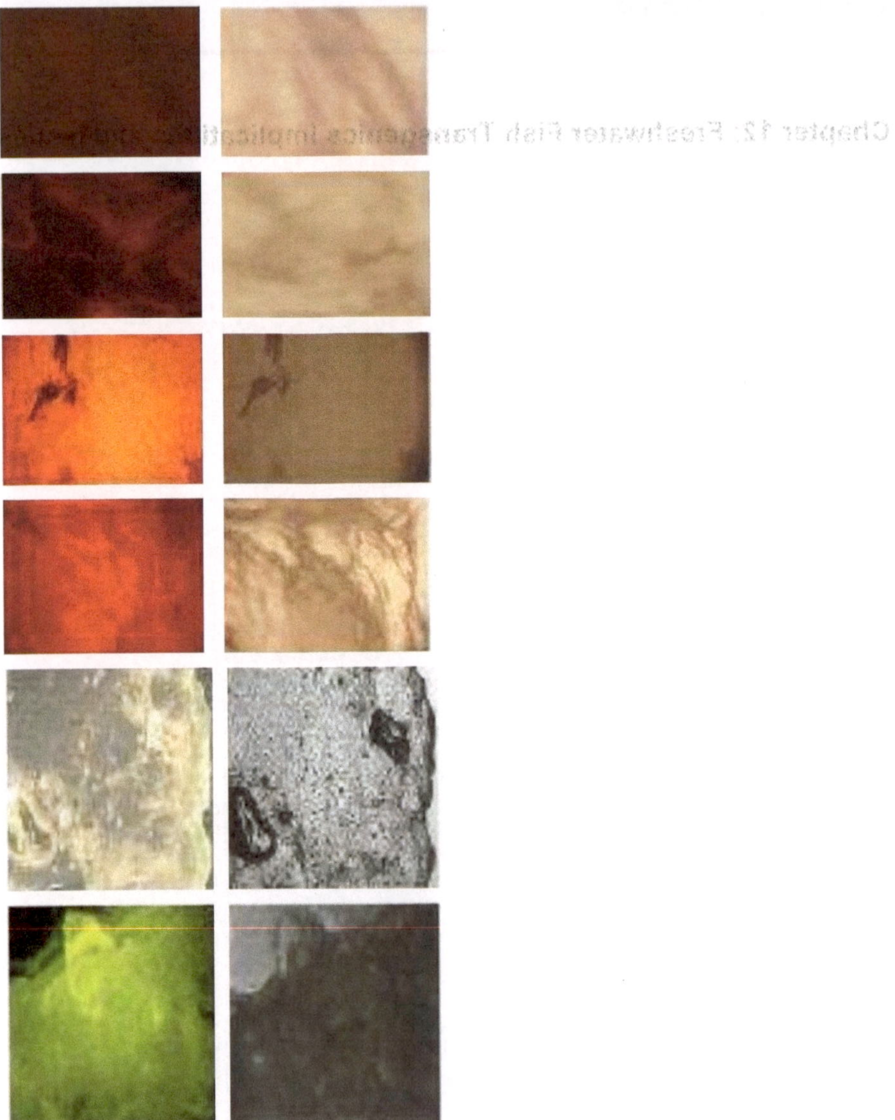

Fig. 2. Fluorescence protein expressions driven by the full-length promoter at the site of injection of the skeletal muscle. Images are taken under fluorescence- (left panel) and bright-field (right panel). RFP expressions driven by the full-length *mylz2* promoter at 15, 30 and 60 days in *L. laubuca* (upper panel). Control is the muscle of non-injected fish. GFP was expressed in the skeletal muscle of *L. rohita* at 15 days of examination (lower panel). *(See black & white version on page 134)*

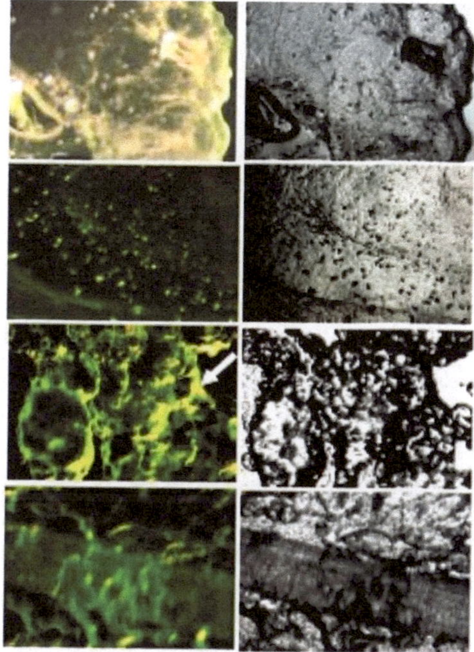

Fig. 3. Green fluorescence protein expression in muscle at the site of injection at 15, 30 and 55 days. Control is the muscle of non-injected fish. Images are taken under fluorescence (left) and bright-field (right). Arrow indicates autofluorescence. (Reproduced from our publication, *Current Science*, 99: 1030-1032) *(See black & white version on page 135)*

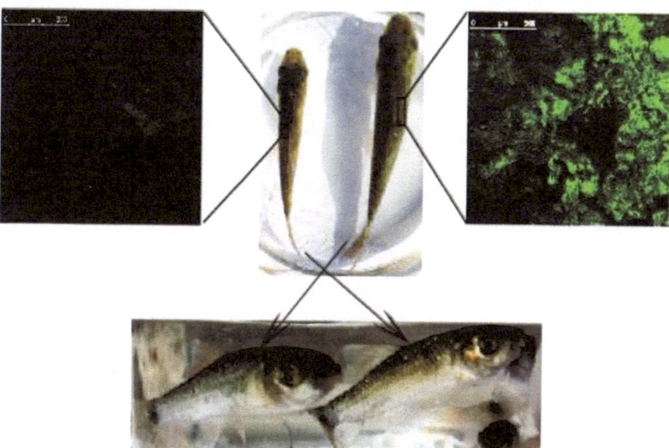

Fig. 4. Documented GFP expressions driven by the β-*actin* promoter in transgenic rohu (Reproduced from our publication, *Cellular & Molecular Biology Letters*, 20, DOI: 10.1515/cmble-2015-0010). *(See black & white version on page 135)*

Chapter 21: Toxicopathology of Important Plants of North-Western Himalayan Region of India

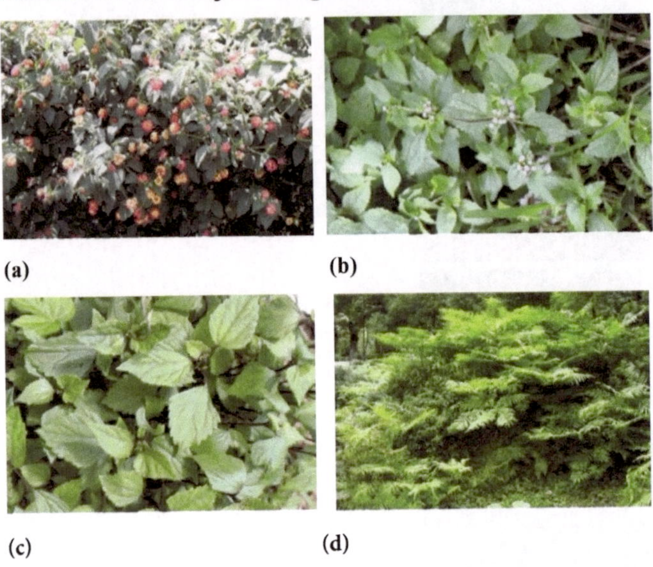

Fig. 1. (a) Lantana camara **(b)** Ageratum conyzoides **(c)** Eupatorium **(d)** Fern
(See black & white version on page 212)

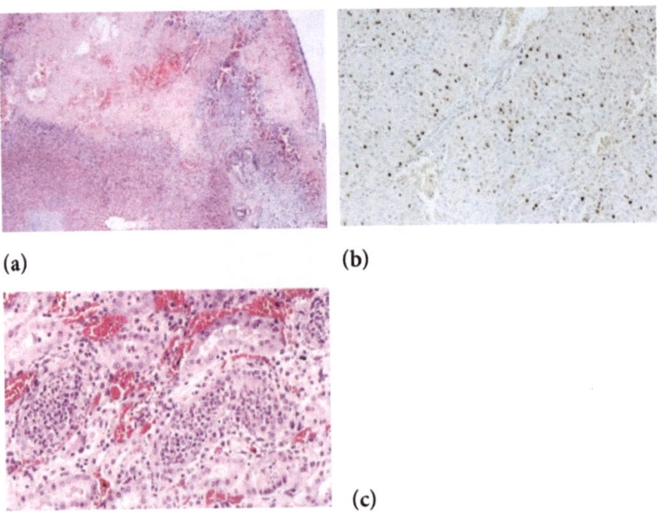

Fig. 2. Lantana intoxicated guinea pig: **(A)** Liver showing large area of coagulative necrosis, haemorrhages, infiltration of heterophils and proliferation of bile ducts. HE ×40. **(B)** Liver showing TUNEL positive apoptotic hepatocytes. Substrate, DAB; Counter stain, Mayer's Haematoxylin; TUNEL assay ×10. **(C)** Kidneys showing necrosis of the lining tubular epithelium and occlusion of the tubular lumen with inflammatory cells mainly heterophils. Degenerative changes in kidney tubules leading to formation casts in the lumen are also visible. HE x20
(See black & white version on page 212)